MEDICAL
INTELLIGENCE
UNIT 19

Coronary Sinus Interventions in Cardiac Surgery
Second Edition

Werner Mohl, M.D., Ph.D.

University of Vienna
Vienna, Austria

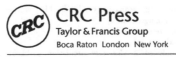

CRC Press
Taylor & Francis Group
Boca Raton London New York

CRC Press is an imprint of the
Taylor & Francis Group, an **informa** business

CORONARY SINUS INTERVENTIONS IN CARDIAC SURGERY
SECOND EDITION
Medical Intelligence Unit

First published 2000 by Landes Bioscience

Published 2018 by CRC Press
Taylor & Francis Group
6000 Broken Sound Parkway NW, Suite 300
Boca Raton, FL 33487-2742

© 2000 by Taylor & Francis Group, LLC
CRC Press is an imprint of Taylor & Francis Group, an Informa business

First issued in paperback 2019

No claim to original U.S. Government works

ISBN 13: 978-0-367-44734-2 (pbk)
ISBN 13: 978-1-58706-006-9 (hbk)

Visit the Taylor & Francis Web site at
http://www.taylorandfrancis.com

and the CRC Press Web site at
http://www.crcpress.com

Library of Congress Cataloging-in-Publication Data

Coronary sinus interventions in cardiac surgery / [edited by] Werner Mohl. -- 2nd ed.
       p. ; cm. -- (Medical intelligence unit)
Includes bibliographical references and index.
ISBN 1-58706-006-X (alk. paper)
       1. Cardiac arrest, Induced. 2. Coronary circulation. 3. Heart--Surgery. I. Mohl, W. (Werner) II. Series.
       [DNLM: 1. Heart Arrest, Induced. 2. Coronary Circulation--physiology. 3. Coronary Vessels--physiology. WG 169 C8228 2000]
RD598.35.I53 C67 2000
617.4'12--dc21

                                                                                    99-059771

CONTENTS

EDITORS

Werner Mohl, M.D., Ph.D.
University of Vienna
Vienna, Austria
Chapter 1

CONTRIBUTORS

Gabriel S. Aldea
Boston Medical Center
Boston, Massachusetts, U.S.A.
Chapter 8

Friedhelm Beyersdorf
Albert-Ludwigs-Universitat Freiburg
Abteilung Herz- und Gefasschirurgie
Freiburg, Germany
Chapter 11

Peter Boekstegers
Med. Klinik I
Klinikum Grobhadern
Universitat Munchen
Munchen, Germany
Chapter 14

Gerald D. Buckberg
UCLA Medical Center
Division of Surgery
Los Angeles, California, U.S.A.
Foreword

Shoji Chiba
Second Department of Anatomy
Hirosaki University
School of Medicine
Hirosaki, Aomori, Japan
Chapter 2

Steven R. Gundry
Loma Linda University Medical Center
Loma Linda, California, U.S.A.
Chapter 10

Rudolf Karch
University of Vienna
Department of Medical Computer
   Sciences
Vienna, Austria
Chapter 6

Sanjiv Kaul
Division of Cardiology
University of Virginia
Chalottesville, Virginia, U.S.A.
Chapter 8

Werner Heimisch
Deutsches Herzzentrum Munchen
Department of Cardiovascular Surgery
Munich, Germany
Chapter 14

Yukihoro Kaneko
University of Vienna
Vienna, Austria
Addendum and Chapter 1

Harold L. Lazar
Boston University School of Medicine
Department of Cardiothoracic Surgery
Boston, Massachusetts, U.S.A.
Chapter 13

Michael von Ludinghausen
Anatomisches Institut
University of Wurzburg
Wurzburg, Germany
Chapters 2 and 3

Samuel Meerbaum
Woodland Hills, California, U.S.A.
Chapter 12

Masahiro Miura
Institute of Anatomy
University of Wurzburg
Wurzburg, Germany
Chapter 3

Friederike Neumann
University of Vienna
Department of Medical Computer
 Sciences
Vienna, Austria
Chapter 6

Martin Neumann
University of Vienna
Institute of Experimental Physics
Vienna, Austria
Chapter 6

Nobuko Ohmachi
Department of Anatomy
Saitama Medical School
Saitama, Japan
Chapter 2

Katharina Palisek
Clinic of Cardiology
 and Clinic of Surgery
University of Vienna
Vienna, Austria
Chapter 7

Hubert Schad
Deutsches Herzzentrum Munchen
Department of Cardiovascular Surgery
Munchen, Germany
Chapter 4

Wolfgang Schreiner
University of Vienna
Department of Medical Computer
 Sciences
Vienna, Austria
Chapter 6

Richard S. Shemin
Department of Cardiothoracic Surgery
The University Hospital
Boston, Massachusetts, U.S.A.
Chapters 8 and 13

William D. Spotnitz
University of Virginia
Charlottesville, Virginia, U.S.A.
Chapter 9

Gunter Steurer
Clinic of Cardiology
 and Clinic of Surgery
University of Vienna
Vienna, Austria
Chapter 7

Flordeliza S. Villanueva
University of Pittsburgh Medical Center
Pittsburgh, Pennsylvania, U.S.A.
Chapter 9

FOREWORD

Development of Blood Cardioplegia and Retrograde Techniques, The Experimenter/Observer Complex

Gerald D. Buckberg

A surgical colleague, Dr. Mohl, asked me to describe the course of development in myocardial protection coming from our studies during the past 28 years, as all seems to flow logically. Such logic may be perceived since events do not normally progress in a coordinated way. It is uncommon that inadequate technical repair is the cause of perioperative low output syndrome after repair of adult and congenital defects. The usual cause is inadequate myocardial protection. This Foreword relates how studies in the UCLA cardiothoracic laboratory addressed this problem during the past 28 years and some clinical changes that developed from these studies. My interest started during my residency training. I quickly realized that one could do a perfect anatomic procedure in adult and pediatric cardiac disease, and wait anxiously to determine how the corrected heart will perform when cardiopulmonary bypass is discontinued. Failure to function normally made me realize that, at that moment, we had hurt the heart with our methods of myocardial protection more than we improved it anatomically. I decided that I must try to understand how this happened and try to define ways we can do better.

At that time, important observations by Najafi and Taber on subendocardial necrosis after ventricular fibrillation with valve disease made it clear that continuous perfusion via the coronary arteries was not the answer. We needed to understand the concept of supply (i.e., flow and its oxygen distribution) and demand (how much energy is required) during extracorporeal circulation. This would allow surgeons to develop a knowledge of physiologic balance of protective methods they could bring to the Operating Room, to allow them to make logical decisions. I participated in microspheres studies at the University of California at San Francisco, before returning to UCLA in 1971. This regional flow method led us to determine in 1973, with Christof Hottenrott from Heidelberg, Germany, that subendocardial blood supply was inadequate during ventricular fibrillation in hypertrophied ventricles. This information led us to abandon ventricular fibrillation during valve surgery. It seemed clear, at that time and now, that two elements are very important. These are technical perfection surgically and avoidance of cardiac damage during the mechanical process of correcting the cardiac lesion.

In 1865, Claude Bernard, a famous French physiologist, wrote a book entitled, *An Introduction to the Study of Experimental Medicine*. In that volume, he described the individual as either an experimenter or an observer. The observer, like an astronomer, watches the natural course of phenomena and reports them—he does not change them. Conversely, the experimenter perturbs the natural order of things (i.e., cardiopulmonary bypass or clamping the aorta), and Mother Nature provides a response. This response may be very different from the logic that led to the experiment and the expected outcome, but it is there. To use this new information, the experimenter must immediately become an observer and appreciate what has been revealed. One simply cannot persist in looking *only* for the expected, for such efforts will lead nowhere, as only Mother Nature speaks the truth and we must listen! Science and life are not different.

Acceptance of our role as an experimenter will allow us to make new decisions and ask new questions that must again pass the same test. During the course of these endless efforts at inquiry, we always meet other observers who sometimes surprisingly feel they know *all* that is true. This unfortunately occurs without generation of new knowledge by them or others. These obstructionists do not last, because growth and continued deeper understanding provide a clearer view, and each of these barriers to full comprehension will be removed.

To all, I recommend this wonderful Bernard book. I will relate to you how approaches to these changes from experimenter to observer and return to experimenter have allowed us to contribute new knowledge in myocardial protection. These data, of course, will be stepping stones for those in the future who will devise new studies. We must stimulate others to use our knowledge so that they can see further in a way that we cannot imagine.

Surgeon, Physiologist, Surgeon-Physiologist

The surgeon pays attention to the detail described in his findings. This information must be listened to by the physiologist. The physiologist does not believe the surgeon can think, while the surgeon thinks the physiologist cannot be practical. The surgeon-physiologist team is needed and this may occur in the same person. If so, the surgeon must possess basic physiologic knowledge and bring this to the practical area—the Operating Room. Solid surgical physiology must be converted to practical findings that are easily used clinically.

The all-too-frequent admonition that a major change in operation is needed to implement new knowledge reflects a clinical barrier placed by those who would rather deal with the problem than prevent it. This Foreword will describe two clinical phenomena; these are A) the retrograde cannula to deliver cardioplegic solution and B) the evolution of blood cardioplegia. It will become very clear that many new ideas come retrospectively or from the back door of an observation.

It is understood that myocardial failure due to inadequate protection may occur despite surgical success. This introduces the favorite surgical issue of prolonged aortic clamping versus cardiac damage. I will provide data to show this paradigm should be changed from "the longer the aorta is clamped, the more damage the heart undergoes," to "postoperative damage is determined more by how the heart is protected, than how long the aorta is clamped." Evidence comes from our studies showing that heart failure follows normal blood reperfusion after

45 minutes of ischemic arrest, versus near normal recovery after four hours of clamping when blood cardioplegia is used in normal hearts. These studies differed in the method of cardiac protection, whereby five times longer ischemia was tolerated well if myocardial protection was adequate.

Retrograde Cardioplegia

The back door approach exists because basic concepts remain basic concepts, even though the ideas underlying formation of a concept come from apparently unrelated sources. My studies of retrograde cardioplegia developed from lung experiments where I looked for a cause of pulmonary edema after massive transfusion. I was in the Air Force in 1968, and lung problems occurred in wounded Vietnam soldiers who were quickly removed from the battlefield and treated by massive fluid infusion; a "traumatic wet-lung syndrome" occurred.

Pulmonary venous spasm was thought to be a responsible mechanism by some surgeons. To look at this, we needed to cannulate the pulmonary vein, and used primates to simulate the clinical conditions in humans. In baboons, we did this by developing a cannula to enter the pulmonary veins from the left atrial appendage to avoid direct venous damage by dissection. This was easy and resulted in no atrial or pulmonary venous trauma. The firm stylet contained a handle to aid placement and had an internal hole for cannulation. I brought this to UCLA when I left the Air Force (Fig. 1A). We used this device to study myocardial metabolism in order to obtain effluent from the coronary sinus. It was facile to introduce the stylet into the right atrium and advance it into the coronary sinus by palpating the inferior vena cava/right atrial junction. In that approach we passed the cannula through the lumen of the stylet and taught this to all of our

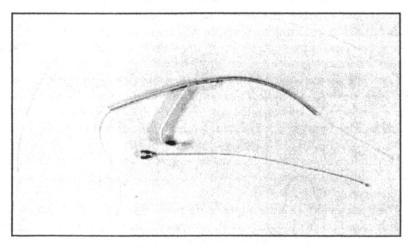

Fig. 1A.

residents. *In a sense, the right atrium became the left atrium, and the coronary sinus became the pulmonary vein—a back door approach that worked.*

The cannula we used to sample blood during measurements of myocardial metabolism allowed us to determine oxygen requirements in the beating, fibrillating, and arrested states. This was reported in 1977 and led us to make clinical decisions subsequently about control of cardiac activity during extracorporeal circulation. For example, it has become clear that the internal mammary grafts are the preferred left anterior descending conduit due to excellent late patency rates. We found, clinically, that this conduit was most useful when retrograde cardioplegia delivery provided satisfactory blood flow beyond an obstruction to avoid intraoperative myocardial damage. This mechanical method of delivery was unrelated to the solution composition or its temperature.

We introduced this concept by studying jeopardized muscle to evaluate antegrade and retrograde protection with Marshall Partington, M.D. The LAD was closed for 15 minutes before starting bypass to produce a dyskinetic anterior and apical region. We released the LAD ligature after 30 minutes on cardiopulmonary bypass to mimic performing coronary artery grafting into a myocardial segment with poor contractility. Cardioplegia was delivered either antegrade, retrograde (via the coronary sinus), or sequentially, first antegrade and then retrograde. With only antegrade cardioplegia, global performance was depressed because poor contractility developed in the anterior segment. Contractile recovery improved after retrograde or sequential antegrade and retrograde delivery, and we confirmed better flow distribution with radioactive microspheres. We then recommended using both antegrade and retrograde cardioplegia, and these benefits of laboratory studies are confirmed clinically.

Normally, the volume of cardioplegic delivery exceeds myocardial oxygen needs. Consequently, differences in antegrade and retrograde distribution can be seen every day by looking at the coronary venous effluent. We know that oxygen needs of the arrested cold heart are very low and further reduced to 98% of the beating working heart at 20°C. Sampling coronary sinus effluent blood during antegrade cardioplegic delivery shows it to be at first dark and then red in 15-30 seconds. The cardioplegic delivery provides more flow than needed, and there is little oxygen extraction. Following completion of antegrade delivery, transition to retrograde perfusion results in the aortic venous drainage (via the vent) becoming dark blue. This deoxygenated effluent from the coronary sinus perfusion develops *immediately after* bright red coronary sinus blood was seen during antegrade delivery. These changing effluent colors signify changes in distribution and suggest that different regions of the myocardium are supplied by the antegrade and retrograde route of delivery.

These changes in effluent are more marked in damaged hearts, where it is unlikely cardioplegic flow adequately supplies all areas when given in one direction. In contrast, with a normal heart with open coronary arteries, antegrade perfusion should supply the entire myocardium so that retrograde delivery may not be needed. Confirmation of this aforementioned concept by daily operative observations will allow all surgeons to see effluent oxygen color changes and determine if antegrade and retrograde delivery would be useful.

Our only clinical change in the coronary sinus catheter was alteration of the stylet containing a hole (into which a coronary sinus catheter could be introduced), *into* a cannula with a solid stylet to allow the coronary sinus catheter to be placed over it). This cannula is shown in Figure 1B, and includes a way to measure pressure and the self-inflating balloon. This balloon concept utilized the McGoon method of coronary artery perfusion during aortic valve replacement. He used a thinner cannula and placed smaller holes at the tip and larger holes in the balloon for self-inflation during perfusion. More than 200,000 of this type of cannula are used clinically today for retrograde perfusion and even more self-inflating balloons from other sources follow this Mayo Clinic approach to antegrade flow. Clearly, this clinical worldwide application has developed from experimental studies of the pulmonary vein, which were then changed to the coronary sinus. In one sense, basic pulmonary, then coronary sinus metabolism in animal investigation preceded the current patient related surgical/physiologic approach to retrograde perfusion.

Blood Cardioplegia

A similar back door approach led to our development of blood cardioplegia for myocardial protection. Not surprisingly, this concept emanated from carefully listening to the clear thinking and thoughtful questions of a master surgeon/physiologist named John Kirklin, M.D.

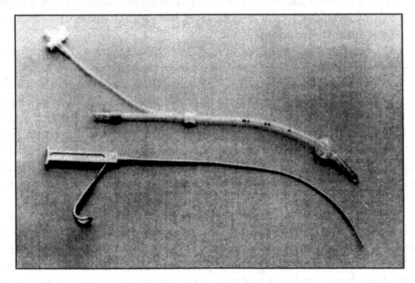

Fig. 1B.

In 1974, our studies using microspheres to measure perfusion showed sub-endocardial ischemia during ventricular fibrillation. This finding led to avoidance of ventricular fibrillation during valve replacement in hypertrophied hearts. At that time, we changed to intermittent ischemia (i.e., 15 minutes) to enhance direct vision during cardiac repair. This was followed by reperfusion flow to restore oxygen to the beating empty heart. My intent was to intermittently reoxygenate to facilitate metabolic repair after ischemia. Now we suspect that we also added some form of preconditioning. This ischemia technique was applied in patients with coronary disease, aortic and mitral valve replacement, and was associated with low morbidity and mortality. We reported these combined results in 1975 at the AATS meeting. Our intent was to limit ischemia and reduce the low output syndrome.

Some remember that I was in my "hippie" phase in 1975. I wore a suede coat jacket and had very long hair. I was concerned that my presentation at the AATS to avoid depressed myocardial performance was serious, and that I should wear a different outfit to avoid any suggestion that my unconventional appearance could modify the importance of delivering this information. I took a haircut and wore a three-piece suit (which was my wedding attire). Someone, knowing my standard dress previously, asked "Gerry, are you going to some type of formal, happy affair?" To this I answered, "No, I am here to bury the low output syndrome." The burial lasted only 15 minutes, as Dr. George Rodewald from Hamburg, Germany, made his comments about cardioplegia. That was all I could think about as I flew back to Los Angeles. Upon my return, I began studies on crystalloid cardioplegia with Myron Goldstein, M.D. These cardioplegic comments galvanized a series of studies over the next 20 years in our laboratory. These were done with a superb group of investigators who spent two years with me from several institutions, including UCLA.

My introduction into research started when I helped develop the early micro lin was Professor of Surgery at the University of Alabama.

Knowing of my work at the CVRI and UCLA, Dr. Kirklin was the first to invite me to give a lecture outside of Los Angeles in 1973. It is good to be a surgeon, as you can imagine my chagrin to give a physiologic/surgical lecture to the Master, sitting patiently in a shirt, pad in hands, and carefully scrutinizing this member of the New Age. Surgeons learn to deal with this focus problem as a way of life. My intent, going to Alabama, was to teach about what we had learned using intermittent ischemia, myocardial flow distribution, venting, maintaining pressure, and reducing hemodilution to limit damage.

Progress is always made by the teacher becoming the student. One must travel to learn, not only to teach. I vividly recall our first visit. As we left the Intensive Care Unit, we passed a patient having an internal mammary artery graft to the left anterior descending artery. John Kirklin told me two very important things. First, how wonderful it was to use an arterial graft in a coronary patient.

That is done routinely today, especially with retrograde cardioplegic protection of the ischemic distal ventricle. Second was his observation that while the myocardial muscle was soft during ischemia, it became rigid immediately after reperfusion. He asked me why this occurred. I did not know but suggested it may be related to changes in myocardial calcium accumulation—a now logical guess.

I reflected on this reperfusion issue during the plane trip home. I immediately discussed this with Dr. Glenn Langer at UCLA, who is a superb cardiologist and physiologist—he is "Mr. Calcium" today. Glenn advised me that calcium accumulated during ischemia and even more during reperfusion and referred me to studies by Reimer and Jennings.

We looked at this surgically, by developing a globally ischemic model where normal blood supply was restored by aortic unclamping. Protection from ischemic damage was with hypothermia only, an important modification that slowed myocardial metabolism as suggested by Dr. Norman Shumway of Stanford. We understood that hypothermia was only one method of protection. Consequently, functional recovery after cold ischemia occurred, but was only 40% after aortic unclamping. This seemed a clinically useful method to become our control studies to assess reperfusion damage. In that experiment we did not immediately unclamp the aorta and give normal blood following one hour of cold ischemia. Instead, we collected 500 ml of blood from the extracorporeal circuit, and reduced calcium citrate-phosphate dextrose (C.P.D.), a blood storage constituent was used to limit calcium influx. This low calcium reperfusate was given over five minutes before removing the clamp.

Drs. David Follette and James Livesay, surgical residents in 1976, who are now colleagues, did these studies. At that time we could not measure calcium directly to learn why adding 50 ml of C.P.D. to 500 ml of blood produced 85% recovery. We can measure calcium now and know that C.P.D. produced 500-600 μmol of calcium (1200 umol is normal), and this hypocalcemic concentration is still used in many centers that apply our technique. In another experiment, which included James Livesay, M.D., we changed only the pH to counteract the anaerobic metabolism during ischemia. Tham, an extracellular/intracellular buffer changed pH from 7.3-7.7 and allowed 80% recovery (versus 40%) with hypothermic ischemia alone.

Since low calcium and increased pH are independently effective, it seemed logical that combining them would be more helpful. Surprisingly, after delivering a hypocalcemic, alkalotic blood solution, functional recovery was 40% (versus 80-85% with either low calcium or high pH). Of course, my natural reaction was to be certain that Drs. Follette and Livesay were incorrect. Accordingly, I asked them to repeat these studies to deal with my bias. The truth, of course, is in the results, and they were precisely the same—decreased recovery.

With understandable confusion, we scheduled another seminar with Dr. Langer to help us solve our problem. It is important to realize the value of interchange is to listen to each other, rather than learn from only one participant. Glenn Langer could not immediately understand the in vivo changes we had found, despite reaching into his vast store of knowledge of in vitro systems. During that seminar, I asked David Follette to describe the condition of the ventricle during reperfusion.

In usual fashion, the surgeon did not look immediately into the mechanisms but rather initially used his observatory powers, as they are used intraoperatively daily. Dave Follette indicated that fibrillation was very vigorous during these initial five minutes of low calcium, high pH blood reperfusion. That seemed illogical, since hypocalcemic perfusion should limit calcium availability and reduce, rather than increase, the strength of ventricular fibrillation.

This observation suggested to me that the myocardium was healthier and could fibrillate better, perhaps because alkalosis optimized metabolism during reperfusion. We have subsequently learned that the pH/sodium exchange during alkalosis increases sodium influx and subsequent hypercalemic influx follows this. I now realize the reason for the increased vigor of initial fibrillation remains unclear 22 years after we observed its presence.

Unperturbed by mechanisms, the increased fibrillation had to be dealt with and avoided. This was because we understood from previous studies that fibrillation impeded subendocardial flow, especially during hypertrophy. We suspected that ischemia occurred when fibrillating fibers compressed the subendocardial vessels, and thereby decided to avoid ventricular fibrillation and induce global arrest during initial reperfusion.

The extracorporeal circuit during cardiopulmonary bypass perfused the systemic circulation so that we could independently allow the heart to beat, fibrillate, or arrest during reperfusion. Knowledge that oxygen requirements were low during arrest made asystole preferable. The normothermic environment was selected to optimize metabolic repair. We avoided the Q_{10} effect of hypothermia in an effort to enhance O_2 utilization during reperfusion.

These reperfusion studies were performed *before* we considered using cardioplegia during aortic clamping to prevent injury. They also occurred before Rodewald's concept of cardioplegia from Hamburg. The contributions of German physiologists are enormous, as Bretschneider's efforts on cardioplegic techniques have influenced our surgical knowledge profoundly. The Bretschneider crystalloid solution continues to be used in patients in Europe and Asia.

We began to study crystalloid solution immediately after the 1975 AATS meeting. Our crystalloid solution contained low calcium, alkalosis, and potassium. Recognizing that a blood cardioplegic reperfusate solution can resuscitate the heart made us realize that we should substitute blood for the crystalloid portion of the cardioplegic vehicle. This allowed us to "nourish" the heart while we were stopping it. Additionally, we had shown previously with Roy Nelson, M.D. the value of multidose crystalloid administration to replenish cardioplegia after noncoronary collateral flow washed out the cardioplegic solution. Blood would, of course, provide renourishment during dose replenishment. The method of delivering blood cardioplegia is shown in Figure 2, whereby blood is mixed with crystalloid, here in a ratio of four parts blood, one part crystalloid. This blood cardioplegic solution is pumped through a heat exchanger to alter its temperature and then delivered to the heart.

We had documented noncoronary collateral blood flow during aortic clamping several years ago with Dr. John Brazier. These studies were done because we had microspheres, and this allowed us to solve a paradox in laboratory observations that occurred before I returned to UCLA. Dr. Collin Bayliss, in 1968, showed that cardioplegic solutions were effective in the transplanted heart after 24 hours of storage. There is no noncoronary collateral flow in explanted hearts. These same solutions were associated with high mortality after only three hours of aortic clamping of in situ hearts on extracorporeal circulation. There are noncoronary collateral flow vessels in the intact animal. These studies were done two years *before* we ever contemplated using a cardioplegic solution.

The back door concept was clear, as this sequence shows that warm blood cardioplegic reperfusate preceded the introduction of cold blood cardioplegia. Acceptance of the blood cardioplegia approach has increased since 1977, and sanguineous cardioplegic solutions are used in 1998 in more than 85% of operations in the United States and more than 60% of procedures in Asia, Europe, and worldwide. This reflects the correlation between scientific truth and environmental utilization described repeatedly in Claude Bernard's volume. He states, "By the experimental method, we simply make a judgment on the facts around us. Taken

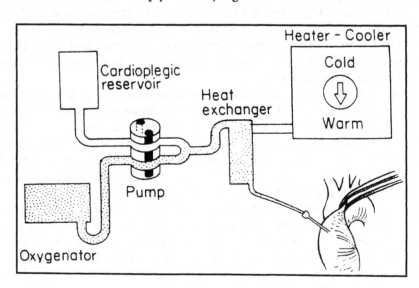

Fig. 2.

in this general sense, experience is the one source of human knowledge. The investigator, himself, must be analyzed into observer and experimenter; not according to whether he is active or passive in producing phenomena, but according to whether he acts on them or not, to make himself their master."

This new information about these blood cardioplegic studies made it clear that this was an advance over the ischemic arrest data that was very useful clinically. We had just completed evaluations of clinical intermittent ischemia with other members of our UCLA team; Drs. James Maloney and Donald Mulder, and our Chief Resident, Gordon Olinger, summarized our experience with normal blood reperfusion delivered after each 15 minutes of ischemic arrest. We reported our clinical data in coronary, mitral, and aortic procedures at many medical and surgical meetings in 1976. Our cardiology colleagues immediately understood the value of our "standard" approach, with intermittent ischemia and grew to expect improved mortality and morbidity without cardioplegia.

Of course the truth is always in the study rather than how we conceptualize the best way to proceed. The laboratory blood cardioplegic data showed improvement over intermittent ischemia so we began to clinically apply blood cardioplegia in 1977. I remember discussing this with Drs. Maloney and Mulder to inform them of our advances. To me it was not a question of "if they used blood cardioplegia," but rather "when they adopted this method."

It always seems easier for one surgeon to show other surgeons a completely new method. Understandably, the early surgical acceptance of a new method is slow and must await confirmation of findings by others. Change is, of course, facilitated through results after careful appreciation of the suggested approach from the clinical data. Change is not, however, easy when a surgeon addresses cardiologists. Our cardiology colleagues expect results to be immediately better in every possible way. They differ, however, in their expectations when they apply angioplasty for coronary artery disease. Here, they accept recurrence and recognize the need to repeat the procedure as normal.

A remarkable event occurred after we accumulated our early data with blood cardioplegia and compared clinical results with those of intermittent ischemia. Dave Follette presented this material in 1976 to the cardiologists in the library next to my office. The intent was to show how we continue to make progress, and that the 1976 technique of blood cardioplegia exceeded the excellent results of 1975 with intermittent ischemia. To my amazement, they questioned the data Dr. Follette presented, and blamed blood cardioplegia for some occasional late graft closures seen 4-6 months after the patient was discharged. For some reason, they believed that blood cardioplegia was responsible. There was frank concern about our "experiments" on their patients. They thought late graft closure could be interpreted in the cardiology/cardiac surgery local community to mean we used patients as guinea pigs; there was worry that this would be difficult for the University. Perhaps this is a universal view of how the world receives new information. This objection defines approaches when there is reluctance to receive and evaluate new ideas. None of these reactions retarded our ongoing commitment to achieve better myocardial protection and make further advancements. Blood cardioplegia is used in greater than 500,000 patients during 1998.

Time does not allow further recounting of other back door events, such as this description of warm blood cardioplegic reperfusate leading to cold blood cardioplegia during clamping. Similar events occur in the development of warm blood cardioplegic induction with Eliot Rosenkranz, M.D., adding glutamate and aspartate to the solution with Harold Lazar, M.D. and John Robertson, M.D., multidose cardioplegia, noncoronary collateral flow, changes in endothelial factors such as L-arginine with Asatoshi Mizuno, M.D. and Rufus Baretti, M.D., simultaneous antegrade/retrograde methods for enhancing delivery with Kai Ihnken and Kiyozo Morita, M.D., and treating acute ischemia with Bradley Allen, M.D., Fumiyuki Okamoto, M.D., and Jakob Vinten-Johansen, Ph.D. in a way that directs global reperfusion concepts to the region undergoing acute myocardial infarction. Each development had a similar tale of how concepts emerged.

My students who are now my colleagues believe I remain in my "hippie phase" in 1998 and that the experimenter/observer complex persists. We have a motto *that truth always wins, and that the data asks the questions even though it is generated to answer them.* I have said this frequently in the Operating Room and laboratory to my residents and research fellows. The experience of this surgeon/ physiologist makes plain the nature of our work. We are always changing, and this occurs because we must always perturb nature to learn something new. At that time, we must abandon the bias that led to altering natural phenomena and become an observer of the results (a surgeon) and record these. The final product is, hopefully, a step forward. It is wonderful to know that we can never resolve an issue, but only ask new questions. Clearly, this book directed toward pursuit of the method of coronary sinus perfusion will be helpful, and stimulate us to understand this approach more deeply.

References

1. Najafi H, Henson D, Dye WS. Left ventricular hemorrhagic necrosis. Ann Thorac Surg 1969; 7:550.
2. Taber RE, Norales AR, Fine G. Myocardial necrosis and the postoperative low cardiac output syndrome. Ann Thorac Surg 1967; 4:12.
3. Hottenrott CE, Towers B, Kurkji HJ et al. The hazard of ventricular fibrillation in hypertrophied ventricles during cardiopulmonary bypass. J Thorac Cardiovasc Surg 1973; 66:742-753.
4. Bernard C. An Introduction to the Study of Experimental Medicine. New York: Dover Publications, 1957.

5. Rosenkranz ER, Vinten-Johansen J, Buckberg GD et al. Benefits of normothermic induction of blood cardioplegia in energy-depleted hearts, with maintenance of arrest by multidose cold blood cardioplegic infusions. J Thorac Cardiovasc Surg 1982; 84:667-677.

6. Buckberg GD. Retrograde pulmonary venous pressure management—fact or artifact? J Thorac Cardiovasc Surg 1970; 59:393-400.

7. Buckberg GD, Brazier JR, Nelson RL et al. Studies of the effects of hypothermia on regional myocardial blood flow and metabolism during cardiopulmonary bypass. I. The adequately perfused beating, fibrillating and arrested heart. J Thorac Cardiovasc Surg 1977; 78:87-94.

8. Partington MT, Acar C, Buckberg GD et al. Studies of Retrograde Cardioplegia. I. Advantages of antegrade/retrograde cardioplegia in jeopardized myocardium. J Thorac Cardiovasc Surg 1989; 97:605-612.

9. Partington MT, Acar C, Buckberg GD et al. Studies of retrograde cardioplegia. II. Nutritive blood flow distribution in normal and jeopardized myocardium. J Thorac Cardiovasc Surg 1989; 97:613-622.

10. Loop F, Irarrazaval MJ, Bredee JJ et al. Internal mammary graft for ischemic heart disease: Effect of revascularization on clinical status and survival. Am J Cardiol 1977; 39:516-522.

11. Lazar HL, Foglia R, Manganaro AJ. Detrimental effects of premature use of inotropic drugs to discontinue cardiopulmonary bypass. Surg Forum 1978; 29:296-298.

12. Buckberg GD, Olinger GN, Mulder DG et al. Depressed postoperative cardiac performance. J Thorac Cardiovasc Surg 1975; 70:974-988.

13. Goldstein SJ, Nelson RL, McConnell DH et al. Cardiac arrest after aortic cross-clamping: Effects of conventional ischemic vs pharmacologic techniques on myocardial supply/demand balance. Surg Forum 1975; 26:271-273.

14. Reimer KA, Jennings RB. The "wavefront phenomenon" of myocardial ischemic cell death. Lab Invest 1979; 40:633-644.

15. Follette DM, Fey K, Buckberg GD et al. Reducing postischemic damage by temporary modification of reperfusate calcium, potassium, pH, and osmolarity. J Thorac Cardiovasc Surg 1981; 82:221-238.

16. Follette D, Livesay J, Maloney JV, Jr. et al. Citrate reperfusion of ischemic heart on cardiopulmonary bypass. Surg Forum 1976; 27:244-246.

17. Follette D, Fey K, Livesay J t al. Studies on myocardial reperfusion injury. I. Favorable modification by adjusting reperfusate pH. Surgery 1977; 82:149-155.

18. Bretschneider H J , Hubner G, Knoll D et al. Myocardial resistance and tolerance to ischemia: Physiological and biochemical basis. J Cardiovasc Su 1975; 16:241-260.

19. Nelson RL, Fey KH, Follette DM et al. Intermittent infusion of cardioplegic solution during aortic cross-clamping. Surg Forum 1976; 27:241-243.

20. Follette DM, Mulder DG, Maloney JVJr, Buckberg GD. Advantages of blood cardioplegia over continuous coronary perfusion or intermittent ischemia. J Thorac Cardiovasc Surg 1978; 76:604-619.

21. Brazier J, Hottenrott C, Buckberg GD. Noncoronary collateral myocardial blood flow. Ann Thorac Surg 1975; 19:425-435.

22. Foglia RP, Buckberg GD, Lazar HL. The effectiveness of mannitol after ischemic myocardial edema. Surg Forum 1980; 30:320-323.
23. Rosenkranz ER, Okamoto F, Buckberg GD et al. Safety of prolonged aortic clamping with blood cardioplegia. III. Aspartate enrichment of glutamate-blood cardioplegia in energy-depleted hearts after ischemic and reperfusion injury. J Thorac Cardiovasc Surg 1986; 91:428-435.
24. Ihnken K, Morita K, Buckberg GD et al. Prevention of reoxygenation injury in cyanotic immature hearts with coenzyme Q_{10}. J Heart Failure 1995; 2:691(Abstract)
25. Ihnken K, Morita K, Buckberg GD et al. The safety of simultaneous arterial and coronary sinus perfusion: Experimental background and initial clinical results. J Card Surg 1994; 9:15-25.
26. Allen BS, Okamoto F, Buckberg GD et al. Studies of controlled reperfusion after ischemia. XV. Immediate functional recovery after six hours of regional ischemia by careful control of conditions of reperfusion and composition of reperfusate. J Thorac Cardiovasc Surg 1986; 92:621-635.
27. Allen BS, Buckberg GD, Schwaiger M et al. Studies of controlled reperfusion after ischemia: XVI. Early recovery of regional wall motion in patients following surgical revascularization after eight hours of acute coronary occlusion. J Thorac Cardiovasc Surg 1986; 92:636-648.
28. Allen BS, Buckberg GD, Fontan F et al. Superiority of controlled surgical reperfusion vs. PTCA in acute coronary occlusion. J Thorac Cardiovasc Surg 1993; 105:864-884.

Chapter 1

Basic Considerations and Techniques in Coronary Sinus Interventions

Werner Mohl

Introduction

'Thank God for the ingenious device of coronary ventricular channels, which relieve the myocardium from the coronary blood and thus prevent accumulations of interstitial fluid' wrote Adam Christian Thebesius in 1703 in his thesis De circulo sanguine in corde.[17] The drainage pathway so described was later named the Thebesian system which is one part of the lesser coronary venous system draining about 5–10% of coronary venous blood.

It was only in the late 1800s that the significance of this system was rediscovered by Langer[8] stimulating further research in this area. In 1893 Pratt[16] provided the basis for today's concept of coronary sinus interventions, since he observed that isolated feline hearts could be kept alive by retroperfusing arterial blood through the coronary sinus thus reversing coronary flow and he concluded: The nutrition of mammalian hearts is not totally dependent on coronary arteries. Some 40 years ago, and preceeding many of the enormous advances associated with modern cardiovascular medicine, Beck,[2] Eckstein,[5] and Gregg[7] performed major experimental and clinical studies to relieve myocardial ischemia by permanent retroperfusion of the coronary sinus.

With today's understanding it was clear that this concept was the wrong goal and approach since it produced severe engorgement of the venous circulation. It is to the merit of a second generation (among them one of the contributors of the present book, S. Meerbaum[10]) to generate the modern concept of coronary sinus interventions for myocardial protection.

Today, coronary sinus interventions are generally understood to be methods of temporary protection of ischemic myocardium via the coronary sinus which include retroinfusion of cardioplegia during cardiac arrest in surgery, retroperfusion of arterial blood in settings of myocardial jeopardy (synchronized retroperfusion, SRP, and synchronized suction and retroinfusion, SSR), and manipulations of venous blood drainage by pressure-controlled intermittent coronary sinus occlusion, PICSO.[12]

There are two practical reasons why it makes logical sense to access the coronary circulation via the coronary sinus. First, the coronary venous vasculature remains unaffected by the atherosclerotic disease process. Second, the venous vasculature is a dense meshwork with numerous interconnections. By using this access, one has to keep in mind, however, that the coronary sinus drains only part of the venous blood (about 75%). Therefore, a considerable part of the myocardium (parts of the right ventricle, parts of the upper part of the septum) necessarily remain deprived of reversed coronary sinus blood flow (Fig. 1.1).

Coronary Sinus Interventions in Cardiac Surgery, Second Edition edited by Werner Mohl.
©2000 Eurekah.com.

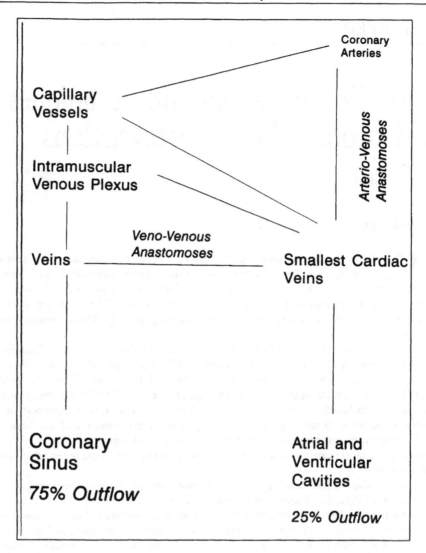

Fig.1.1. Schema of retroinfusion of cardioplegia.

Surgical Coronary Sinus Interventions for Myocardial Protection

Demographic changes in patients undergoing coronary artery bypass grafting, complex surgery for valve reconstructions, and an increasing number of reoperations warrant substantial myocardial protection. Retrograde delivery of cardioplegia is the best method to cool the myocardium extensively during prolonged aortic cross clamping times.

Practical Considerations

There are several coronary sinus catheters on the market with self-inflating ballons, or manual occlusion balloons, as well as special balloons that keep the catheter in place. The catheter is introduced through the right atrium and secured by a purse string suture. It is easiest to introduce the catheter just before going on bypass to avoid an air lock in the extra-corporeal circuit. Furthermore, it is more convenient to irrigate the coronary sinus during normal perfusion since venous drainage keeps the coronary sinus open. Otherwise, the orifice may collapse and remain inaccessible. The catheter has to be positioned so that the balloon does not occlude the posterior vein. The catheter position is very important to allow protection of the posterior septum as far as possible. Pressure monitoring is mandatory to document retroinfusion and to signal dislodgement of the catheter. Usually, the cannula can be inserted into the coronary sinus within 10-15 seconds after one to three efforts to probe the coronary sinus orifice. If the cannula is forced into place and becomes wedged into the distal coronary sinus or the posterior coronary vein, mechanical traumatization is possible. With three unsuccessful attempts to achieve cannulation, it is rather recommended to institute partial bypass (2-3 L/min) and free and elevate the heart in order to expose the surface of the coronary sinus. Now the cannula can be seen through the atrial wall and more easily advanced into the coronary sinus. Thus, hemodynamic changes can be kept at a minimum and aspiration of air can be avoided. Conventionally, coronary sinus pressure during retroinfusion should not exceed 50 mm Hg, although several sudies have shown that higher pressures can be tolerated without harm to the patient.[11]

Methods of Cardioplegic Delivery

There are several protocols of cardioplegic delivery in use. The most common methods aim to effectively use the coronary circulation to protect the heart during open heart surgery.

1. Combined method:
- Antegrade induction
- Retrograde continuation
- Rewarming of perfusate just prior to aortic declamping

Cardiac arrest is initiated with antegrade cardioplegia to effectively stop the heart and to access areas antegradely which are drained by the lesser cardiac veins. After cardiac arrest with initial 700 ml of cardioplegia, continuation with 300 ml of solution applied repeatedly through the coronary sinus will cool the heart effectively (Fig. 1.2). Shortly before reopening the coronary sinus, the perfusate is rewarmed to normal blood temperature to be applied as terminal cardioplegia.

2. Retrograde method:
- Retrograde induction
- Retrograde continuation

Cardioplegic delivery is started retrogradely until asystole and continued in the same way. This method should only be used in reoperations (to avoid embolization), aortic insufficiency, calcific aorta and aortic stenosis before opening the aorta. In all these cases aortic root pressure would not reach levels high enough to effectively perfuse the myocardium with cardioplegic solution.

3. Antegrade cardioplegia with coronary sinus occlusion.

Another possibility to perfuse the coronary circulatory system is to apply cardioplegia antegradely and occlude the coronary sinus at the same time. This method has experimentally[9] proven its potential to protect the myocardium by combining the potential benefits of both delivery pathways, i.e., the anatomical advantage of antegrade perfusion and the possibility of retrograde redistribution of the perfusate into deprived areas.

4. Reperfusion with additional coronary sinus interventions. There are basically two methods to enhance reperfusion recovery using coronary sinus techniques.

- Buckberg techniques. During rewarming of the cardioplegic substrate, retrograde flow is increased and then the perfusate is switched to normal blood. Proximal anastomoses are now done during aortic cross clamping.[4] Since at blood retroperfusion the rate of delivery has to be increased to 150-300 ml/min, it is one of the hazards that catheter dislodgements occur during this period, especially when the heart starts beating and the normal venous drainage

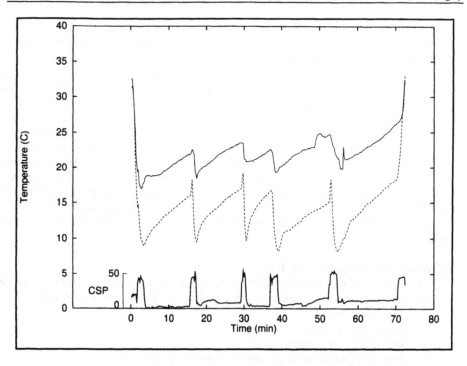

Fig. 1.2. Coronary sinus pressure (CSP) and myocardial temperature in the anterior (solid line) and posterior septum (dashed line) during surgery with retograde cardioplegia after antegrade induction. Note the pressure increase to approximately 50 mm Hg and concomitant temperature decrease during retrograde infusions.

competes with the retroperfusate. During this period pressure may reach peak levels of 60-80 mm Hg which are tolerated well. Normally, the aortic cross clamp is removed when the heart starts beating to allow normal unhindered perfusion, and then the coronary sinus catheter is removed. This method seems to have great potential but certainly needs further refinements.

• PICSO during reperfusion. This method has been clinically investigated by our own group in 30 patients undergoing coronary artery bypass grafting.[13] The PICSO mechanism is similar to the concept of antegrade cardioplegic delivery and coronary sinus occlusion. Coronary sinus pressure is elevated and thus effects a more homogeneous distribution of the perfusate, because the outflow impedance is increased. During reperfusion in the empty beating heart, coronary sinus pressure under sinus occlusion shows marked peaks during systole. After some seconds of coronary sinus occlusion, a curve connecting these peaks will show a plateau indicating that the filling capacity of the venous system has been reached. Then the coronary sinus blockade is released for a few seconds to allow unhindered blood flow (Fig. 1.3).

Evaluation of Coronary Sinus Interventions

Antegrade cardioplegic delivery with coronary sinus occlusion (A + CSO) has been investigated clinically by our own group. Twenty-four patients with three-vessel disease, undergoing coronary artery bypass grafting were divided into two groups according to the mode of cardioplegic delivery. Cardioplegic delivery in both groups essentially followed the Buckberg protocol,[4] using blood cardioplegia for cold induction (800 ml), multidose intermittent administration (400 ml after finishing each distal anastomosis), and warm reperfusion (500

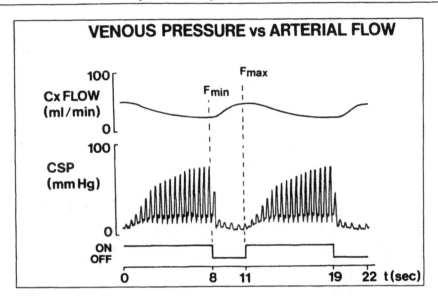

Fig. 1.3. Coronary sinus pressure during PICSO. Systolic pressure rises to reach a plateau during coronary sinus occlusion. Rise time of systolic peaks is used for occlusion time control.

ml) before removing the aortic clamp. In all patients cardioplegia was induced antegradely with the coronary sinus initially unobstructed, and topical cooling was used. After 30 seconds the coronary sinus was occluded continuously for the rest of the aortic cross-clamp time by inflation of the balloon of the retrograde cannula to achieve indirect delivery via venous redistribution of the antegradely infused cardioplegic solution. In group I (12 patients) initial cardioplegic delivery was subsequently continued and completed using the antegrade route. All subsequent applications in this group were performed similarly, i.e. by antegrade infusion only. In group II (12 patients) the coronary sinus was also continuously occluded, but antegrade delivery of the initial dose was discontinued after infusion of 50% of the volume. The rest was infused directly via the coronary sinus route. All subsequent applications in group II were performed in a similar way, i.e. by splitting the total volume equally into antegrade and retrograde delivery. In order to test the feasibility and safety of the A + CSO method, the first 10 patients were assigned to protocol II supporting A + CSO by additional direct retrograde cardioplegic delivery.

Two temperature probes were positioned into the anterior and posterior septum. Intra-operatively, septal temperatures and cardioplegic infusion pressures (ARP, CSP) were continuously monitored. There was a total of 73 individual applications of cardioplegia in group I and a total of 69 in group II. Temperatures of initial and terminal cardioplegia were analyzed separately from intermittent applications of cold cardioplegia.

To illustrate the typical temporal variation of infusion pressures during cardioplegic delivery (except initial and terminal cardioplegia), pressure readings from individual applications of cardioplegia were averaged point-wise for both groups. Adjustment was achieved by superimposing the points of onset of cardioplegic delivery (Fig. 1.4). Depending on whether protocol I or II was followed (antegrade supply of the total volume versus 1:1 splitting between antegrade and retrograde delivery), different pressure patterns could be observed. In group I the total 400 ml of blood cardioplegia was applied via the aortic root over 1.5-2 minutes and aortic root pressure increased from negative values (caused by ventricular venting) to an average level of approximately 50 mm Hg. In group II, it usually took less than 1 minute to infuse 200 ml of cardioplegic solution antegradely. Therefore, due to its negative initial values and relatively

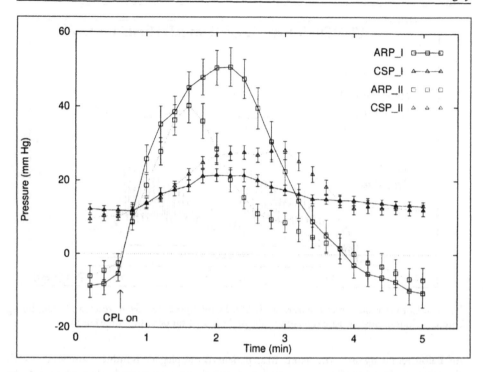

Fig. 1.4. Aortic root pressure (ARP) and coronary sinus pressure (CSP) during cardioplegic delivery in groups I and II. Data are means and standard errors of superimposed individual applications of cardioplegia. Note that due to ventricular venting ARP is negative before and after cardioplegic delivery. CPL: Cardioplegia.

slow rise time, aortic root pressure did not exceed values of approximately 40 mm Hg on average. Since the coronary sinus was continuously occluded, the increase of aortic root pressure was followed in both groups by an increase in coronary sinus pressure, usually no sooner than 20-30 seconds after the onset of cardioplegia. In group I coronary sinus occluded pressure levels were around 20 mm Hg when antegrade delivery was continued throughout. In group II switching from antegrade delivery to direct retrograde infusion resulted in a further increase of coronary sinus pressure to higher levels than in group I.

Although there were no statistically significant differences between temperature measurements of the two groups, there were some quantitative trends indicating a more effective distribution of cardioplegia in group I. During initial cardioplegia, the minimum temperature of the posterior septum was lower in group I than in group II (15.7 ± 3.09 vs. 16.95 ± 4.80). Therefore, initial cooling of the posterior septum seems to be slightly more effective when the total volume of cardioplegia is solely delivered via the aortic root. Similarly, during intermittent applications of cold cardioplegic solution the mean temperature was lower in group I than in group II (20.9 ± 2.07 vs. 21.83 ± 2.46 for the posterior septum). The same trend could be observed for the anterior septum. At terminal cardioplegic delivery, temperatures were similar in both groups.

As to the feasibility of the A + CSO method, we observed in 15% of 142 cardioplegic applications (22 infusion cycles in 12 patients) that aortic root pressure did not properly increase during antegrade infusion. In principle, this is a shortcoming of aortic root delivery which results from aortic valve opening due to loss of tissue tonus and drainage of perfusate into the left ventricle. In most cases we were able to restore adequate conditions by slightly squeezing the aortic valve and at the same time applying cardioplegic infusion flow rates of at least 250 ml/min.

The results presented above indicate an improvement of myocardial protection by antegrade cardioplegic delivery in combination with indirect venous redistribution. The effect seems to be particularly beneficial for the posterior region of the interventricular septum. For anatomical reasons any kind of retrograde infusion will penetrate the capillary network in a much more homogeneous fashion than when applied antegradely. At the same time, however, relatively large areas of the right ventricular free wall and of the interventricular septum necessarily remain un- or underperfused by retrograde cardioplegic infusion alone (cf. Fig. 1.1). These two considerations suggest the concept of combining antegrade cardioplegia with coronary sinus occlusion for retrograde redistribution. In this way, two complementary modes of cardioplegic delivery are expected to be mutually enhancing in their effectiveness in that each one can reach myocardial areas which are not or only partially accessible to cardioplegic solution applied via the other route.

Some practical comments on the method are necessary. Antegrade cardioplegic delivery is ruled out in the presence of aortic insufficiency of grade I or more, since substrate effusion into the ventricle is unavoidable in that case. Whenever antegrade delivery is feasible, however, the A + CSO method is simple in a technical sense. Even if retrograde catheterization is impossible for some reason, coronary sinus occlusion can be achieved by externally squeezing the coronary sinus and obstructing the outflow of cardioplegic solution during antegrade infusion. Antegrade administration of cardioplegia is in itself a simple and rapid procedure. Moreover, the coronary arteries are less sensitive to high infusion pressures than the venous system, thus rendering antegrade application a less demanding procedure in terms of accuracy of flow adjustment of the infusion pump. Nevertheless, aortic root pressure should be monitored and pump flow rates should be at least roughly adjusted to that pressure rather than to pump pressure alone, as is usually done. Also, aortic root pressure monitoring will be especially helpful in the case of cardioplegic malfunction due to aortic valve opening as described above.

In order to evaluate PICSO during reperfusion in our study, a randomized group of 15 patients had reperfusion in combination with PICSO after coronary artery bypass grafting and another 15 patients had reperfusion alone. PICSO was started immediately after aortic declamping and continued for 1 hour. Diastolic values under coronary sinus occlusion remained unaffected at about 5 mm Hg during the PICSO treatment, while the plateau values of coronary sinus occluded pressure rose from 36 ± 13 mm Hg to 49 ± 11 mm Hg. This effect shows the gradual recovery process of the myocardium. Reperfusion injury appeared to be less pronounced in the PICSO treated group. Intraoperative echocardiography of wall motion abnormalities demonstrated that originally hypokinetic segments were better preserved in PICSO treated patients than in controls ($p<0.04$). Since the values of systolic occluded pressure after the one-hour PICSO treatment were found to be directly related to washout of CK-MB from the venous system ($r=0.94$; $p<0.006$), we concluded from our results that the potential of PICSO in myocardial preservation during reperfusion is mainly due to the redirection of venous flow to otherwise low- or no-flow areas and to sebsequent washout of toxic metabilites. This washout is facilitated by periodic occlusion and release of the coronary sinus.

Coronary sinus techniques as described above can be used primarily in patients with severe atherosclerosis, difficult surgical techniques, and prolonged aortic cross clamping times as well as in patients with myocardial hypertrophy. The most beneficial method has to be chosen on the basis of the pathophysiological background of the patient, the surgical procedure and the available time.

Coronary Sinus Techniques in Interventional Cardiology

Coronary sinus interventions seem to be today's concept of myocardial protection in ischemic syndromes. Basically we discriminate between synchronized retroperfusion (SRP), PICSO, and synchronized suction and retroinfusion (SSR). There has been a long debate about the advantages of any of these methods which was misleading, manipulating and disasterous for all concepts. Coronary sinus interventions will come fully into effect when we clearly can define the patients' characteristics, inclusion/exclusion criteria and the proper indication for each of the methods.

SRP is applied by a catheter positioned into the coronary sinus to retroperfuse arterial blood into the venous system. The benefits of the method have been shown in several ischemic syndromes. However, it seems questionable whether blood can be forced upstream as far as to reach the ischemic area in the relatively large and interconnected venous meshwork.[1] Incomplete myocardial protection by synchronized coronary venous retroperfusion during ischemia might result from nonselective retroinfusion and solely passive drainage. Therefore, in a modified concept (SSR), the catheter is more selectively advanced into the venous circulation and an active suction system is added to the retroinfusion device. In this way, the obstacles of SRP seem to be mainly overcome, and better preservation of regional function could be proven experimentally.[3]

PICSO follows a different concept of using venous blood to maintain cell viability during ischemic syndromes. The rationale of PICSO holds that the beneficial effects are mainly due to forced redistribution of venous blood flow into the coronary beds. In contrast to retroperfusion and its primary effect of oxygen delivery, the effect of PICSO appears to result from redistribution and washout of toxic metabolites.[6] For a long time surgeons have been aware of the effect of oxygen toxicity and reperfusion injury and therefore it seems reasonable to start reperfusion with a modified reperfusate making use of the enormous metabolic and buffer potential of venous blood until ultimate reperfusion from the arterial side can be established, i.e., thombolysis in myocardial infarct. The concept of a substantial contribution of PICSO to myocardial metabolite washout resulting in improved tissue salvage and maintained function during acute ischemia is consistent with observations of Murry[14] and Neely.[15] These authors showed a relationship between cell integrity, viability, functional recovery, and catabolic accumulation during ischemia and reperfusion. Since numerous experimental studies showed that PICSO reduces infarct size, this method should be primarily used during myocardial infarction and unstable angina pectoris and to avoid reperfusion injury (cf. Table 1.1).

Bearing in mind the limitations of all these methods of coronary sinus interventions— i.e., the anatomy and pathophysiology of the venous vasculature and drainage pathways, feasibility, potential hazards, different concepts and indications—coronary sinus techniques can be applied beneficially during cardiac surgery as well as in the catheter lab and, even more important, during myocardial infarction (see Table 1.2).

References

1. Beatt KJ, Serruys PW, Feyter P et al. Hemodynamic observations during percutaneous transluminal coronary in the presence of synchronized diastolic coronpary sinus retroperfusion. Br Heart J 1988; 59:159-67.
2. Beck CS. Revascularization of the heart. Surgery 1949; 26:82-88.
3. Boekstegers P, Peter W, von Degenfeld G et al: Preservation of regional myocardial function and myocardial oxygen tension during acute ischemia in pigs: Comparison of selective synchronized suction and retroinfusion of coronary veins to synchronized coronary venous retroperfusion. JACC 1994; 23:459-469.
4. Buckberg GD. Antegrade/retrograde blood cardioplegia to ensure cardioplegic distribution: Operative techniques and objectives. J Cardiac Surg 1989; 4:216-238.

Table 1.1. Infarct size after (P)ICSO treatment in LAD occlusion and reperfusion experiments

Mohl et al. [JACC 1984, 53: 923-928]	56 ± 7	99 ± 3	< 0.001
Zalewski et al. [Circulation 1985, 71: 1215-1223]	84 ± 5	100 ± 5	n.s.
Ciuffo et al. [In: Mohl et al. (eds.): The coronary Sinus. Steinkopff, Darmstadt 1984]	15 ± 6	57 ± 8	< 0.001
Ciuffo et al. [In: Mohl et al. (eds.): The coronary Sinus. Steinkopff, Darmstadt 1984]	19 ± 7	49 ± 9	< 0.02
Jacobs et al. [Clin Res 1985, 33: 197A]	17 ± 4	33 ± 4	< 0.025
Jacobs et al. [In: Mohl et al. (eds.): The coronary Sinus. Steinkopff, Darmstadt 1984]	29 ± 6	45 ± 2	< 0.02
Diltz et al. [Circulation 1985, Suppl. III, 72: 120]	30 ± 8	33 ± 3	n.s.
Guerci et al. [JACC 1987, 9: 1075-1081]	30 ± 8	75 ± 4	< 0.01

Table 1.2. Summary of methods of coronary sinus interventions

CSI during surgery	Cardioplegia:	Retrograde cardioplegia Combined antegrade/ retrograde Antegrade + coronary sinus occlusion
	Modified reperfusion:	Blood retroperfusion under prolonged aortic cross clamping PICSO + normal reperfusion
Catheter lab	SRP, SSR	Protection during PTCA Perioperative support
Intensive care unit	PICSO	Myocardial infarction Instable angina Perioperative support

CSI: Coronary sinus interventions
PICSO: Pressure-controlled intermittent coronary sinus occlusion
SRP: Synchronized retroperfusion
SSR: Synchronized suction and retroinfusion

5. Eckstein RW, Smith G, Eleff M. The effect of arterialization of the coronary sinus in dogs on mortality following acute coronary occlusion. Circulation 1952; 6:16-20.
6. Gregg DE, Dewald D. The immediate effects of the occlusion of the coronary veins on the dynamics of the coronary circulation. Am J Physiol 1938; 124:444-456.
7. Kenner T, Moser M, Mohl W. Arteriovenous difference in the blood density in the coronary circulation. Proc Am Soc Mech Engin 1983:6770.
8. Langer L. Die Foramina Thebesii im Herzen des Menschen. Sitzungsberichte der mathematisch naturwissenschaftlichen Klasse der kaiserlichen Akademie der Wissenschaften 1881; 82:25.
9. Lazar HL, Khoury T, Rivers S. Improved distribution of cardioplegia with pressure-controlled intermittent coronary sinus occlusion. Ann Thorac Surg 1988; 46:202-207.

10. Meerbaum S, Lang TW, Osher JV et al. Diastolic retroperfusion of acutely ischemic myocardium. Am J Cardiol 1976; 37:588-598.
11. Mohl W, Simon P, Neumann F et al. PICSO workshop. In: Mohl W, Faxon DP, Wolner E (eds.): Clinics of CSI. Steinkopff Verlag, Darmstadt 1986:363-377.
12. Mohl W. The momentum of coronary sinus interventions clinically. Circulation 1988; 77:6-12.
13. Mohl W, Simon P, Neumann F et al. Clinical evaluation of pressure-controlled intermittent coronary sinus occlusion: Randomized trial during coronary artery surgery. Ann Thorac Surg 1988; 46:192-201.
14. Murry CE, Jennings RB, Reimer KA. Preconditioning with ischemia: A delay of lethal cell injury in ischemic myocardium. Circulation 1986; 74:1124-1136.
15. Neely JR, Grotyohann LW. Role of glycolytic products in damage to ischemic myocardium. Dissociation of adenosine triphosphate levels and recovery of function of reperfused ischemic hearts. Circ Res 1984; 55:816-824.
16. Pratt FH. The nutrition of the heart through the vessels of Thebesius and coronary veins. Am J Physiol 1898; 1:86-103.
17. Thebesius AC. De circulo sanguine in corde. Dissertatio medica, Leiden 1703.

Addendum

Update in Surgical Coronary Sinus Intervention

Yukihoro Kaneko and Werner Mohl

Introduction

Protection of the heart remains of crucial importance in cardiac surgery. Cardioprotection consists mainly of three actions 1) delivery of nutritive and protective substrates including oxygen, potassium, glucose, glutamate, aspartate, etc. to all parts of the myocardium; 2) wash-out of harmful metabolites including lactate, hypoxanthine, xanthine, oxygen-derived free radicals, etc. From the myocardium; and 3) hypothermia of the myocardium by cold cardioplegia. Cardioprotection must be feasible, and must not hinder or interrupt the conduct of surgical procedures. The clinical decision as to the method of cardioprotection to be used in cardiac surgery is a trade-off between cardioprotective actions and technical convenience.

Coronary sinus interventions including retrograde cardioplegia, antegrade cardioplegia with coronary sinus occlusion, and pressure-controlled intermittent coronary sinus occlusion (PICSO) became widely accepted as powerful tools in cardiac surgery. The combined antegrade/retrograde cardioplegia technique is used by more than 60% of surgeons in the United States.[1]

The clinical results of retrograde cardioplegia are excellent, whereas the experimental data are suboptimal in terms of inhomogeneous delivery and low perfusion efficacy. This discrepancy indicates that there may be a mechanism of retrograde cardioplegia that has scarcely been appreciated. We will discuss the importance of protection against deployment of cytokines in the venous vasculature which we believe is highly relevant to surgical cardioprotection. In this Chapter, we would like to elucidate the role of coronary sinus intervention in the paradigm of surgical cardioprotection at the beginning of the new millenium.

Clinical Effect of Coronary Sinus Interventions

The clinical results of retrograde cardioplegia are generally good. Talwalker and associates found that cardioplegia exclusively given retrogradely showed adequate cardiac protection in cardiac valve surgery.[2] Arom and associates compared the efficacy of retrograde cardioplegia and antegrade/retrograde cardioplegia in a non-randomized retrospective study in coronary surgery.[3] They found that retrograde cardioplegia alone provides as good myocardial protection as antegrade/retrograde cardioplegia. Jasinki and associates compared retrograde cardioplegia and antegrade cardioplegia in a prospective randomized study in coronary surgery.[4] Retrograde cardioplegia attenuated ischemic injury and permitted better early recovery of myocardial function than antegrade cardioplegia. Other techniques of coronary sinus intervention also turned out to be effective in cardiac surgery. Mohl and associates found that PICSO during the early reperfusion period in patients undergoing coronary surgery had beneficial effect on myocardial function.[5] the benefit of PICSO is attributable to re-direction of venous flow to hypoperfused myocardium. Antegrade cardioplegic delivery with coronary sinus occlusion was clinically found to be a feasible and effective technique for homogeneous cardioplegia delivery.[6]

Delivery of Nutritive Substrates and Wash-Out of Metabolites

Exchange of materials between the myocardium and perfusate occurs along capillary vessels. Therefore, delivery of substrates and wash-out of metabolites are believed to be accomplished by capillary perfusion. Several investigators reported inhomogeneous distribution and low capillary perfusion efficiency of retrograde cardioplegia.

The coronary sinus drains about 75% of coronary venous blood. The remaining coronary venous blood is drained through the Thebesian veins, the anterior right ventricular veins, and/ or the right marginal vein, which have egresses independent of the coronary sinus.[7] These veins are distributed throughout the right ventricle. Consequently, retrograde cardioplegia distributes less to the right ventricle that the left ventricle.[8] Densitometry of intraoperative contrast echocardiography demonstrated that capillary perfusion of retrograde cardioplegia in the right ventricular free wall was about half of the perfusion in the ventricular septum.[9] Higher infusion rates make distribution of cardioplegia more homogeneous.[10] Antegrade cardioplegia also distributes inhomogeneously unless coronary artery is free of stenosis. Antegrade and retrograde cardioplegia nourish different myocardial regions.[11] Coronary sinus occlusion causes the redistribution of antegradely delivered cardioplegia.[12] Therefore, the antegrade/retrograde cardioplegia and antegrade cardioplegia with coronary sinus occlusion are recommended to increase the homogeneity of cardioplegia delivery.[13]

Retrograde cardioplegia is delivered to the right ventricle through veno-venous networks. Cardioplegia reaching the right ventricle partly peruses the capillaries and thereby nutritive. However, it partly drains through the Thebesian veins without perfusing the capillaries (steal phenomenon). Perfusion efficacy (nutrient capillary flow/total flow) of antegrade cardioplegia reaches 90%, whereas perfusion efficacy of retrograde cardioplegia with the mouth of the coronary sinus occluded by a purse string suture is 0~70%.[11,14]

Myocardial Cooling

Cold cardioplegia need not perfuse capillary vessels to cool down the myocardium: cardioplegia shunted by steal the phenomenon also cools down the myocardium by thermal conduction. In experimental setting retrograde cardioplegia cools down the myocardium similar to, or more efficiently than, antegrade cardioplegia.[15]

With antegrade cardioplegia, retraction of the heart to expose coronary arteries or mitral valve causes aortic valve incompetence, resulting in insufficient cardioplegia perfusion and bloody surgical field. In aortic and aortic valve surgery, the surgeon must cannulate the coronary orifices to give antegrade cardioplegia. Consequently, each time antegrade cardioplegia is given, surgical manipulation is discontinued. Antegrade cardioplegia is frequently delayed for a few minutes until surgical manipulation reaches a good place to leave off, allowing warming of the heart.

With retrograde cardioplegia, the surgeon can usually continue the surgical procedure during cardioplegia unless extreme precision is required. Retrograde cardioplegia technically allows punctual and frequent cardioplegia delivery, keeping the heart adequately cool. In patients with coronary artery obstruction, retrograde cardioplegia cools down the myocardium more efficiently than antegrade cardioplegia.[16]

Position of the Coronary Sinus Cannula

The position of the balloon-tipped perfusion cannula in the coronary sinus has significant influence on perfusion efficacy. Rudis and associates compared perfusion efficacy of retrograde cardioplegia with the mouth of the coronary sinus closed and open. When purse-string suture around the coronary sinus was released, the efficacy fell from 60% to 30%.[11] Low efficacy is attributed to failure to perfuse all branches of coronary sinus. The posterior interventricular vein opens into the coronary sinus in 97% of human hearts.[7] The opening of the posterior interventricular vein is only 1.7 mm distal to the mouth of the coronary sinus on average.[8] Consequently, it is clinically impossible to place the balloon tipped cannula proximal to the opening of posterior interventricular vein.[17] Furthermore, the cannula is usually place 2-4 cm distal to the mouth of the coronary sinus for secure fixation of the cannula against retraction of the heart.[18] This makes additional veins open proximal to the cannula resulting in further decrease in perfusion efficiency. Low efficacy is a major theoretical drawback of retrograde cardioplegia.[19]

Transatrial coronary sinus cannulation made retrograde cardioplegia simple and rapid. Routine placement of a purse-string suture at the mouth of a coronary sinus is too cumbersome and impractical. Refinement in catheter design to perfuse or occlude proximal tributaries of the coronary sinus is desirable for improved perfusion efficacy. Bezon and associates clinically used a coronary sinus cannula with a 3 cm-long balloon to obliterate the opening of the posterior interventricular vein during cold retrograde cardioplegia delivery. They found better cooling of the left ventricular posterior wall with long balloon cannulae than with normal 8 mm-long balloon cannula.[20]

A question arises, therefore, why the clinical effect of retrograde cardioplegia is so good despite inhomogeneous delivery and low perfusion efficacy experimentally? We speculate that coronary sinus interventions including retrograde cardioplegia and PICSO reduce the inflammatory response of the heart.

Inflammatory Response in Cardiac Surgery

We will briefly review briefly the inflammatory response evoked by cardiac surgery. (Fig. 1.1A.) The interaction of blood with the cardiopulmonary circuit activates complement following commencement of cardiopulmonary bypass, leading to the formation of anaphylatoxins C3a and C5a mainly via the alternative pathway. P-selectin is expressed on endothelial surface as a result of endothelial cell exposure to C5a.[21] Endothelial cells, activated by C5a, adhere to neutrophils. Adherent neutrophils release cytotoxic proteases, and oxygen-derived free radicals that are responsible for tissue damage, resulting in capillary leak. Proinflammatory cytokines are released in response to cardiopulmonary bypass and tissue hypoxia. Levels of interleukin-1, interleukin-6, interleukin-8, and tumor necrosis factor rapidly increase following commencement of cardiopulmonary bypass. Cytokines are mainly deployed in the venous microcirculation and act as stimulants for neoangiogenesis. Another form of inflammatory activation is endotoxemia. Endotoxin is frequently detected in high concentrations after cardiopulmonary bypass.[22] Endotoxin stimulates both complement and endothelium, resulting in the surface up-regulation of adherence molecules and tissue factors.

As the aorta is cross-clamped, the cardiac tissue, especially the endocardium, becomes ischemic or hypoxic to some extent. Hypoxic insult causes local endothelial cells, monocytes, and tissue-fixed macrophages to release cytokines and oxygen-derived free radicals.[23] Activated endothelium promotes leukocyte adhesion molecules and tissue factor expression. The degree of cytokine response correlates with the length of cardiopulmonary bypass and aortic cross-clamp time.[24]

Reperfusion of myocardial and endothelial cells follows aortic clamp release. The influx of calcium causes reperfusion injury. Endothelial cells in the heart are activated further, causing neutrophils to plug the myocardial capillaries. Activated neutrophils release oxygen-derived free radicals and arachidonic acid metabolites, resulting in further endothelial injury and platelet activation.

As the early phase of complement-mediated neutrophil activation wears off, the second wave develops as new proteins, such as E-selectin, intercellular adhesion molecule, vascular cell adhesion molecule, and inducible nitric oxide synthetase are made and expressed by endothelial cells in response to exposure to cytokines, lipopolysaccharide and inflammatory mediators. The second wave comes 4 to 8 hours after cardiopulmonary bypass, because it requires de novo protein synthesis. The second wave lasts 24 to 48 hours, leading to prolonged endothelium-neutrophil adhesion.[25]

Inflammatory Response and Coronary Sinus Intervention

We speculate that coronary sinus interventions reduce inflammatory response in the heart through two possible mechanisms. Firstly, retrograde cardioplegia keeps the heart cool enough to suppress cytokine release. Secondly, PICSO enhances wash-out of toxic metabolites and thereby reduces the subsequent inflammatory response.

Concerning hypothermia, cardioplegia provides excellent homogeneous hypothermia of the myocardium as stated earlier.[26] Hypothermia not only reduces the oxygen demand of the myocardium but also suppresses activation of endothelial cells.[27] Suppression of endothelial cell activation by hypothermia results in decreased adhesion molecule and cytokine production followed by minimal deterioration in myocardial excitation-contraction coupling.[28] Menanché and associates found that body and cardiac temperatures profoundly affect neutrophil-endothelium interactions.[29] Patients submitted to normothermic cardiopulmonary bypass and continuous warm blood cardioplegia showed significantly higher levels of interleukin-1 receptor antagonist, soluble intercellular adhesion molecule 1, and elastase values than those submitted to hypothermic cardiopulmonary bypass (28-30°C) and cold crystalloid cardioplegia. Biagioli and associates explored the relationship between oxidative stress and myocardial function in patients undergoing coronary surgery by comparing warm continuous blood cardioplegia and cold intermittent blood cardioplegia.[30] They found that oxidative stress was significant in patients submitted to cold blood cardioplegia while continuous warm blood cardioplegia minimized the effects of ischemia. However, oxidative stress was not correlated with myocardial dysfunction. We assume that the deleterious effect of oxidative stress by cold intermittent cardioplegia was offset by the beneficial effect of reduced inflammatory responses in hypothermia.

Enhanced wash-out of toxic metabolites by PICSO has been reported previously by our group.[5,31-33] We measured blood density and calculated its gradient from arterial blood to coronary sinus blood in canine experiments.[31,32] Usually, coronary sinus blood has a higher density than arterial blood due to the loss of filtered fluid in the microcirculation, which is returned into the circulation again by the lymph flow. PICSO leads to a reduction or reversal of the density gradient, indicating that pressure-controlled coronary sinus occlusion enhanced wash-out of interstitial fluid from the myocardium. We also observed enhanced metabolite

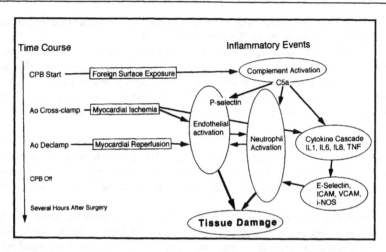

Fig. 1.1A. Schema of the inflammatory response in cardiac surgery. Ao=aorta, CPB=Cardiopulmonary bypass, ICAM=intercellular adhesion molecule, IL=interleukin, I-NOS=inducible nitric oxide synthetase, TNF=tumor necrosis factor, VCAM=vascular cell adhesion molecule.

wash-out by PICSO in clinical settings.[5,33] We evaluated the impact of PICSO during the early reperfusion period on wash-out of cardiac enzymes including CK-MB, alpha-HBDH, and myoglobin in patients undergoing coronary surgery. They found that clearance of enzymes during reperfusion was greater in PICSO-treated patients than in control patients.[33] Myoglobin value reached peak level during reperfusion in PICSO-treated patients, whereas further increase was observed in control patients. (Fig. 1.2A.) Increased blood level of myoglobin during PICSO, and its rapid decrease indicate that PICSO did not encourage myoglobin release, but accelerated wash-out from the myocardium into blood. In another similar clinical series, CK-MB value was inversely correlated with postoperative cardiac functional on echocardiogram in control patients. In PICSO treated patients, however, CK-MB value was correlated not with cardiac function but with peak coronary sinus pressure during coronary sinus occlusion.[5] These data show that PICSO enhances wash-out of enzymes released from the myocardium, and the efficacy of wash-out correlates with peak coronary sinus pressure. It is logical to assume that PICSO during reperfusion effectively washes out metabolites relevant to inflammatory response from the local environment of the cardiac tissue, and thereby attenuates subsequent inflammatory response.

Summary

The view on myocardial protection in cardiac surgery has changed dramatically since introduction of coronary sinus interventions. Off-pump and minimally invasive heart surgery are the pole opposite to surgical myocardial protection. Although these new methods are still considered the future of cardiac surgery, new developments and physiological insights are now available to improve our understanding of routine myocardial protection. The defects of retrograde cardioplegia including inhomogeneous delivery and low perfusion efficacy have been experimentally. Coronary sinus cannulae with improved access to the extensive area of the myocardium are now available or will soon be. The clinical application of retrograde cardioplegia turned out to be highly effective. Pressure-controlled intermittent coronary sinus occlusion during reperfusion is also clinically effective. New data on the inflammatory response in the myocardium during cardiac surgery in the presence of perioperative ischemia shed new light on the mechanism of action of coronary sinus intervention. We speculate that

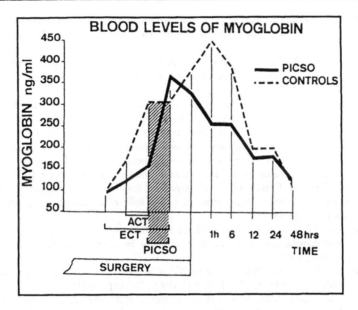

Fig. 1.2A. Time course of myoglobin levels in after coronary surgery. Note earlier peak level of myoglobin reached in PICSO-treated patients than in control patients. ACT=aortic cross-clamp time, ECT=extra corporeal circulation time. (With permission from Mohl W, Gloer D, Kenner T et al. Enhancement of washout induced by pressure controlled intermittent coronary sinus occlusion (PICSO) in the canine and human heart. In: Mohl W, Facon D, Wolner E editors. CSI—A new approach to inteventional cardiology. Darmstadt: SteinkopffVerlag; 1986, 537-48.

coronary sinus interventions including retrograde cardioplegia and pressure-controlled intermittent coronary sinus occlusion reduce the inflammatory response of the heart and thereby provide optimal myocardial protection.

References
1. Beyersdorf F, Allen BS, Buckberg GD. Myocardial protection with integrated blood cardioplegia. In: Franco KL, Verrier ED editors. Advanced therapy in cardiac surgery. Hamilton: BC Decker 1999; 159-65.
2. Talwalker NG, Lawrie GM, Earle N et al. Can retrograde cardioplegia alone provide adequate protection for cardiac valve surgery? Chest 1999; 115:135-9.
3. Arom KV, Emery RW, Petersen RJ et al. Evaluation of 7000+ patients with two different routes of cardioplegia. Ann Thorac Surg 1998; 63:1619-24.
4. Jasinski M, Kadziola R, Bachowski W et al. Comparison of retrograde versus antegrade cold blood cardioplegia: randomized trial in elective coronary artery bypass patients. Eur J cardiothorac Surg 1998; 12:620-6
5. Mohl W. Simon P, Neumann F et al. Clinical evaluation of pressure-controlled intermittent coronary sinus occlusion: randomized trial during coronary artery surgery. Ann Thorac Surg 1988; 46:12-201.
6. Mohl W. Basic considerations and techniques in coronary sinus interventions. In: Mohl W. edtior. Coronary sinus interventions in cardiac surgery. Austin: R.G. Landes Company 1994; 1-10.
7. Von Lüdinghausen M, Chiba S, Ohmachi N. The venous drainage of the myocardium in the human heart. In: Mohl W. editor. Austin: R.G. Landes Company: 1994; 11-16.

8. Farge A, Mousseaux E, Acar C et al. Angiograhic and electron-beam computed tomography studies of retrograde cardioplegia via the coronary sinus. J Thorac Cardiovasc Surg 1996; 112:1046-53.

9. Winkelmann J, Aronson S, Young CJ et al. Retrograde-delivered cardioplegia is not distributed equally to the right ventricular free wall and septum. J Cardiothorac Vasc Anethes 1995; 9:135-9.

10. Gundry SR, Wang N, Sciolaro CM et al. Uniformity of perfusion in all regions of the human heart by warm continuous retrograde cardioplegia. Ann Thorac Surg 1996; 61:33-5.

11. Rudis E, Gates RN, Laks H et al. Coronary sinus ostial occlusion during retrograde delivery of cardioplegic solition significantly improves cardioplegic distribution an efficacy.

12. Ihnken K, Morita K, Buckberg GD et al. Simultaneous arterial and coronary sinus cardioplegic perfusion: an experimental and clinical study. Thorac Cardiovasc Surg 1994; 42:141-7.

13. Sun SC, Diaco M, Couper GS et al. Improved distribution of antegrade cardioplegic solution with simultaneous coronary sinus occlusion following acute coronary artery occlusion. J Surg Res 1992; 53:98-102.

14. Partington MT, Acar C, Buckberg GD et al. Studies of retrograde cardioplegia. I. Capillary Blood flow distribution to myocardium supplied by open and occluded arteries. J Thorac Cardiovsc Surg 1989; 97:605-12.

15. Villanueva FS, Spotnitz WD, Glasheen WP et al. New insights into the physiology of retrograde cardioplegia delivery. Am J Physiol 1995; 268 (4pt 2):H1555-66.

16. Gundry SR, Kirsh MM, March R et al. Functional differences between retrograde and antegrade cardioplegia in heart with varying degrees of coronary artery obstructions. In: Mohl W, faxon D, Wolner E editors. CSI – A new approach to interventional cardiology. Darmstadt: Steinkopff Verlag; 1986; 189-94.

17. Gates RN, Laks H, Drinkwater DC. Angiographic and electron-beam computed tomography studies of retrograde cardioplegia via the coronary sinus. [Letter] J Thorac Cardiovasc Surg 1997; 114:518-9.

18. Tschabitscher M. The so-called "silent zone" of the coronary sinus. In: Mohl W, Faxon D, Wilner E, editors. CSI—A new approach to interventional cardiology. Darmstadt: Steinkopff Verlag; 1986; 11-14.

19. Tosson R, kuschkowitz F, Dasbach G et al. Relationship between position of the coronary sinus catheter and distribution of cardioplegia. J Heart Valve dis 1999; 8:120-3.

20. Bezon E, Barra JA, Mondine P et al. Retrograde cold blodd cardioplegia. Obliteration of the posterior interventricular vein in the coronary sinus improves cooling of the left ventricle posterior wall. Cardiovasc Surg 1997; 5:620-5

21. Chenoweth DE, Cooper SW, Hugli TE et al. Complement activation during cardiopulmonary bypass: evidence for generation of C3a and C5a anaphylatoxins. N Engl J Med 1981; 304:497-503.

22. Nilsson L, Kulander L, Nystrom SO et al. Endotoxins in cariopulmonary bypass. J Thorac Cardiovasc Surg 1990; 100:777-80.

23. Liebold A, Keyl C, Birnbaum DE. The heart produces but the lungs consume proinflammatory cytokines following cardiopulmonary bypass. Eur J Cardiothorac Surg 1999; 15:340-5.

24. Hennein HA, Ebba H, Rodriguez JL et al. Relationship of the proinflammatory cytokines to myocardial ischemia and dysfunction after uncomplicated coronary revascularization. J Thorac Cardiovas Surg 1994; 108:626-35.

25. Jegaden O, Eker A, Montagna P et al. Antegrade/retrograde cardioplegia in arterial bypass grafting: metabolic randomized clinical trial. Ann Thorac Surg 1995; 59:456-61.

26. Boyle EM Jr, Pohlman TH, Johnson MC et al. Endothelial cell injury in cardiovascular surgery: the systemic inflammatory response. Ann Thorac Surg 1997; 63:277-84.

27. Haque R, Kan H, Findle MS. Effect of cytokines and nitric oxide on myocardial E-C coupling. Basic Res Cardiol 1998; 93 (suppl 10):86-94.

28. Menanché P, Peynet J, Lariviére J et al. Does normothermia during cardiopulmonary bypass increase neutrophil-endothelim interactions? Circulation 1994; 90[part 2]: II-275-II-279.

29. Biagioli B, Borrelli E, Maccherini M et al. Reduction of oxidative stress does not affect recovery of myocardial function: warm continous versus cold intermittent blood cardioplegia. Heart 1997; 77:465-73.
30. Moser M, Mohl W, Kenner T. The arteriovenous density gradient as an index for myocardial function. In: Mohl W, Wolner E, Gloger D editors. The coronary sinus. Darmstadt: Steinkopff Verlag; 1984; 497-507.
31. Mohl W. Coronary sinus interventions: from concept to clinics. J Card Surg 1987; 2:467-93.
32. Mohl W, Gloger D, Kenner T et al. Enhancement of washout induced by pressure controlled intermittent coronary sinus occlusion (PICSO) in the canine and human heart. In: Mohl W, Wolner E, Gloger D, eds. The coronary sinus. Darmstadt: Steinkopff Verlag 1984; 537-48.

Chapter 2

The Venous Drainage of the Myocardium in the Human Heart

Michael von Lüdinghausen, Nobuko Ohmachi and Shoji Chiba

Introduction

The coronary sinus (cs) is the anatomically appropriate location for the placement of a balloon catheter for retrograde perfusion or revascularization, in particular of the vessels of the left ventricular myocardium, in a case of severe stenosing coronary heart disease and jeopardized myocardium. However, the results of invasive cardiological procedures via the cs are not satisfactory and are even inadequate in 1-5% of cases.[14,15] These cases reinforce the need not only for biochemical and physiological but also for anatomical reexamination. It was naturally impossible to carry out such examinations on patients who had undergone treatment; therefore we undertook a study of a large number of hearts from the dissection room.

The major venous drainage system of the human heart consists of four intercommunicating parts which generally open into the right atrium.[3] Very frequently the terminal veins of each drainage system are intramurally widened to form spaces, collectors, or sinuses, before emptying into the right atrium.[5] Among these collectors the cs, which is the main structure in the left posterior portion of the coronary sulcus, is of functional predominance. It collects the major cardiac veins: the great vein, the left marginal vein, the posterior vein of the left ventricle and the middle and small cardiac veins. In addition there are the oblique and the posterior veins of the left atrium, both of which empty into the cs.[2,9,21]

These major cardiac veins carry out, almost exclusively, the drainage of two-thirds of the left ventricular myocardium; they do not, however, drain the superior part of the interventricular septum, nor the myocardium of the right atrium and ventricle or the myocardium of the roof of the left atrium. In view of the fact that individual microanatomical conditions have to be taken into consideration when a catheter-tip is inserted into the coronary sinus,[14,15,17] it is the purpose of the present Chapter to clarify the anatomical situation of the cs and its tributaries so as to minimize the instances of failure of the technical procedure, damage, and hemorrhage of the endocardial-myocardial-endothelial complex.[3,5,12]

Material and Methods

This study was based on the examination of 240 human hearts, aged between 64 and 88 years, of which 132 were male and 108 female. After fixation the arteries and veins were injected with red and blue gelatin respectively.

Coronary Sinus Interventions in Cardiac Surgery, Second Edition edited by Werner Mohl.
©2000 Eurekah.com.

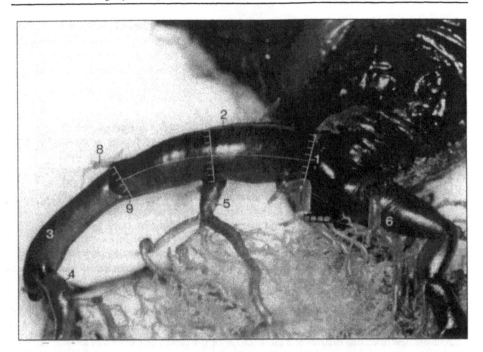

Fig. 2.1. Posterior surface of a corrosion cast of the cs of a human heart. The cs has a length of about 40 mm and a cylindrical shape. Its diameter at origin is about 6 mm, the midcoronary diameter is about 8 mm and the ostial diameter about 8 mm as well. (1) atrial ostium of the coronary sinus; location of the valve of Thebesius; (2) coronary sinus; (3) great cardiac vein (V. coronaria sinistra); (4) left marginal vein; (5) posterior left ventricular; (6) middle cardiac vein (V. interventricularis posterior); (7) small cardiac vein; (8) left atrial oblique vein of Marshall; (9) valve of Vieussens; (10) right atrium.

Microdissections were performed using a stereomicroscope (C. Zeiss, Oberkochen, F.R.G.). Photographs were taken with a Nikon AS camera fitted with a Medical Nikkor C Auto lens 1:5.6, f = 200, using Kodachrome 64 film.

All scales are given in millimetres.

The nomenclature is based on the Nomina anatomica, fifth edition, Mexico City, 1980 and sixth edition, Tokyo, 1989.

The Coronary Sinus

The Significance of the Coronary Sinus

The coronary sinus (cs) is the dominant structure in the left posterior portion of the coronary sulcus. It is the main collector of the cardiac venous blood. As wide and as long as one, two, or three phalanges of the little finger and either slightly or strongly curved, it accepts venous blood from the anterior half of the interventricular septum and anterior wall of the left ventricle via the great cardiac vein (V. interventricularis anterior and its continuation, the V. coronaria sinistra), from the lateral and posterior wall of the left ventricle via the left marginal and posterior veins, and from the posterior half of the interventricular septum via the middle cardiac vein (Fig. 2.1). In one third of the cases the left marginal and posterior veins replace each other.[5,23] When in existence (55% of the cases), the left marginal vein terminates in the v.

coronaria sinistra. When in existence (67% of the cases), the posterior vein of the left ventricle is represented in half of the cases by a very strong vein or a group of small vessels. These may empty either into the terminal great cardiac vein or the initial (left) or the terminal (right) half of the cs.[5,23] In addition the oblique vein and the posterior vein of the left atrium drain into the cs.[7,8]

Length, Shape and Position of the CS
The cs resembles a finger or part of a little finger in length and shape.

Length
The length was measured between the entrance of the oblique vein of Marshall[11] and the base of the Thebesian valve.[22] There were numerous variations in both length and shape. The average length was between 15-70 (37.0) mm, and in one case it reached 82 mm.[7-10,21]

Shape
A short cs had the length of a phalanx of a finger (7% of the cases); a cs of medium length with its cylindrical form corresponded to two phalanges in 74% of the cases, and an elongated cs exhibited a tubular extended form and was as long as three phalanges of a finger in 18% of the cases.

The cs and the great cardiac vein formed a gentle curve in the left coronary sulcus, nearly parallel to the attachment of the posterior (mural) leaflet of the mitral valve. (Fig. 2.2) This curvature described one quarter of a circle (33% of the cases), one eighth of a circle (29%) or had an almost straight course (38%) (Fig. 2.3). In one quarter of the cases there was a sharp

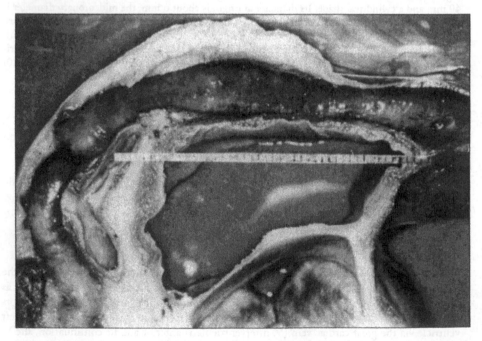

Fig. 2.2. Inferior aspect of an opened cs, which has a length of about 55 mm and shows a gentle curvature in its course. At the ostium (right side) there is a remarkable ostial angle of the cs (arrow). (1) atrial ostium of the coronary sinus; location of the ; (2) coronary sinus; (3) great cardiac vein (V. coronaria sinistra); (9) valve of Vieussens.

bend and an obtuse angle, in 5% a right angle of the terminal cs shortly before it opened into the right atrium.[7] The diameter of the atrial ostium ranged between 7–16 (9.7) mm, the cross-sectional area of the atrium between 20–154 mm^2, and the volume of the cs between 0.67–2.09 mm^3.[20,21] In 1% of the cases there was a sinus coronarius duplex (Fig. 2.4).

Position

The widely postulated location of the cs in the left posterior coronary sulcus was found in only 12% of the cases studied (Fig. 2.5). In most specimens the cs was in a displaced position towards the posterior wall of the left atrium. That displacement or elevation was slight (1-3 mm) in 16% of the cases, moderate (4-7 mm) in 50%, and extreme (8-15 mm) in 22%[7] (Fig. 2.6). An elevation of the cs is demonstrated in a computer-assisted tomogram of the heart (Fig. 2.7). An extreme elevation of the cs, as found here, may enhance the ostial angle through which a catheter tip has to pass on its way into the cs.

The Myocardial Coverage and the External Boundaries of the Coronary Sinus

In all specimens, the cs was completely enclosed by a thin myocardial coat which was part of the posterior wall of the left atrium. The length of that coat was not the same as the length of the cs. In most cases it was longer. At its origin, the seam of the coat was often irregularly formed. In some cases it spread over the origin of the cs to the terminal part of the great cardiac vein (V. coronaria sinistra). Here it developed a myocardial cuff, or one or two myocardial belts, which surrounded the terminal portion of the great cardiac vein. In other cases the seam had an ill-defined edge with a splitting of the myocardial fibers[8] (Fig. 2.7).

At the terminal (right) part of the cs there was no conspicuous landmark in the posterior portion of the coronary sulcus. It was difficult to determine the exact location of the entrance of the cs into the right atrium on the epicardial surface. In most cases the fibers of the myocardial coverage continued regularly into the collageneous fibers of the epicardium on the posterior wall of the right atrium.[8,19]

In rare cases the fibers of the myocardial coverage of the cs formed a wrapping for the terminal (oblique) part of the middle cardiac vein (V. interventricularis posterior) (Fig. 2.8).

The Internal Boundaries and Valves of the Coronary Sinus

The beginning of the cs was marked by the ostial terminal valve of the great cardiac vein, the valve of Vieussens.[24] Opposite the entrance of the great cardiac vein there was the termination of the oblique vein of Marshall[11] which also indicated the beginning of the cs.

The valve of Vieussens[24] firmly established the origin of the cs or marked the end of the great cardiac vein in an average of 87% of the cases. In 62% it was a unicuspid, in 25% a

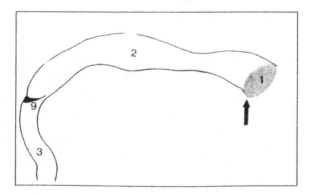

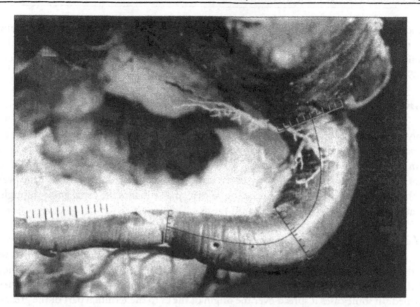

Fig. 2.3. Cranial aspect of a corrosion cast of the cs of a human heart. The cs shows an expressive curvature, which conforms to a quarter circle. Its length is about 40 mm, the shape is narrow and cylindrical, the diameter at origin is about 5.5 mm, the midcoronary diameter is about 10 mm and the ostial diameter about 1 mm. In this case there is no ostial angle of the cs.

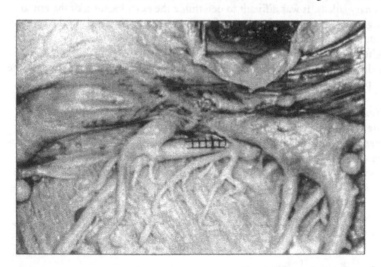

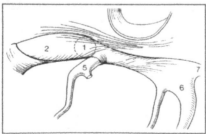

Fig. 2.4. Posterior surface of a human heart specimen with a so called sinus coronarius duplex (double coronary sinus) in the posterior part of the coronary sulcus. The "right" coronary sinus is formed by the widened confluence of the middle and small cardiac veins. (1) atrial ostium of the coronary sinus; location of the valve of Thebesius; (2) coronary sinus; (5) posterior left ventricular; (6) middle cardiac vein (V. interventricularis posterior); (7) small cardiac vein.

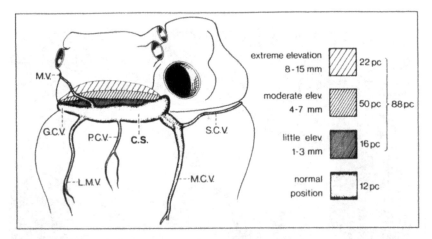

Fig. 2.5. Frequency of grade of elevation of the cs from the posterior coronary sulcus to the posterior wall of the left atrium. Abbreviations: CS:coronary sinus; GCV:great cardiac vein; LMV:left marginal vein; MV: Marshall's vein, oblique vein of the left atrium; MCV:middle cardiac vein; PCV: posterior cardiac vein, posterior vein of the left ventricle; SCV:small cardiac vein.

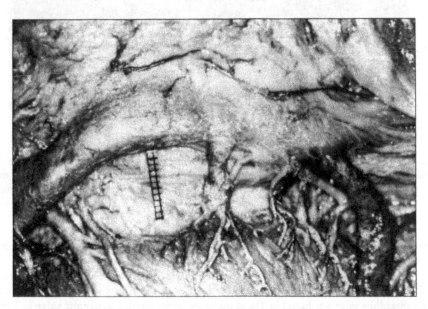

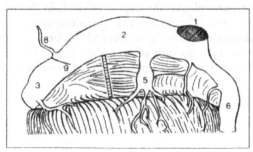

Fig. 2.6. Posterior surface of a human heart specimen with severe elevation of the cs to a high position of about 14 mm about the posterior coronary sulcus. (1) atrial ostium of the coronary sinus; location of the valve of Thebesius; (2) coronary sinus; (3) great cardiac vein (V. coronaria sinistra); (5) posterior left ventricular; (6) middle cardiac vein (V. interventricularis posterior); (8) left atrial oblique vein of Marshall; (9) valve of Vieussens.

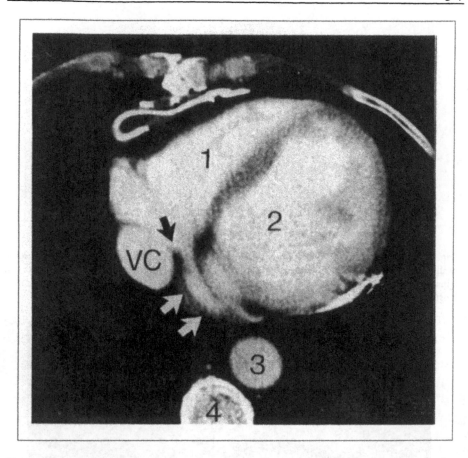

Fig. 2.7. Computer-assisted tomogram of a heart showing the cs (white arrows) with a severe eleva-tion. There is also an acute angle (black arrow) between the inferior vena cava (VC) and the cs. Additionally marked (1) the right ventricle, (2) left ventricle, (3) aorta and (4) body of a vertebra.

bicuspid valve. In 2% of the cases we found a tricuspid valve; in 1% there was a valve-complex with two unicuspid valves following one another (Figs. 2.9–2.12).[7]

The entrance of the cs into the right atrium was guarded by a more or less complete and sufficient fold, the Thebesian valve. In 19% of the cases the ostium was valveless. An incom-plete threadlike valve was found in 2% of the cases, an incomplete crescentic valve in 34%, an incomplete semilunar valve in 7%, an incomplete cribrate valve (Figs. 2.13–2.14) in 7% and a complete circular and membranous valve in 31%[1,7,13,21] In very rare cases a congenital com-plete ostial occlusion (atresia) of the cs has been reported by the authors and by others. In these cases a left vena cava was persistent.[5] In most cases the ostia of the middle cardiac vein and posterior vein of the left ventricle, when these terminate in the cs, were secured by well-formed unicuspid valves.[7]

The Cardiac Veins

Variations in the Distribution, Pattern Occurrence of the Cardiac Veins and Reperfusion Techniques

Given that the tip of a balloon catheter is correctly positioned in the terminal (right) half of the cs, the prospect of successful reperfusion of many cardiac veins is still limited by specific anatomical conditions. Therefore, the area which can be reperfused may be smaller than hitherto predicted (Fig. 2.15).

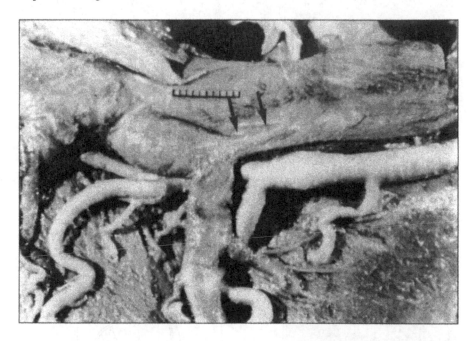

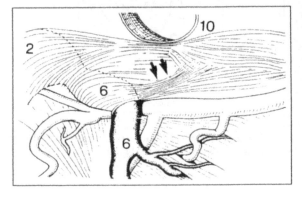

Fig. 2.8. In the middle of the posterior coronary sulcus the myocardial covering of the cs continues into the posterior interventricular sulcus. Therefore a sleeve of atrial muscle extends from the left atrial wall to the oblique terminal part of the middle cardiac vein. Consequently this vein is fixed by myocardial cords at the posterior wall of the right atrium (arrows). The right coronary artery has a pale surface. (2) coronary sinus; (6) middle cardiac vein (V. interventricularis posterior); (10) right atrium.

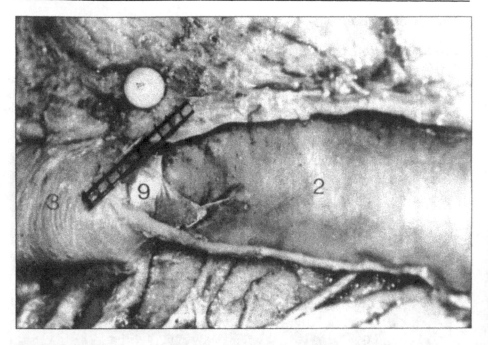

Fig. 2.9. Univalvular Vieussenian valve—marked by a scale and a pinhead—at the junction of the great cardiac vein and the cs. (2) coronary sinus; (3) great cardiac vein (V. coronaria sinistra); (9) valve of Vieussens.

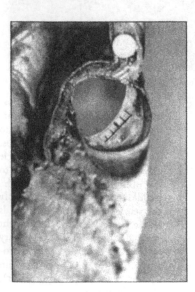

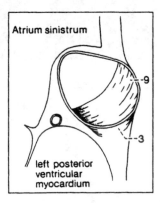

Fig. 2.10. Univalvular (unicuspid) Vieussenian valve on a cross section of the terminal great cardiac vein.

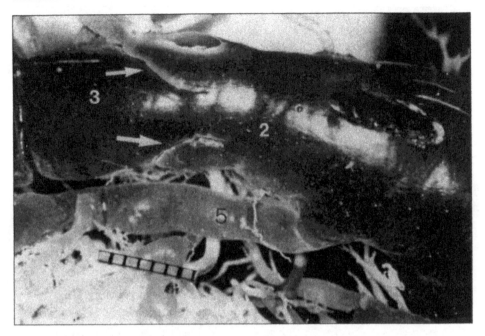

Fig. 2.11. Corrosion cast of the cardiac veins; at the entrance of the cs there are impressions of two endothelial folds; bicuspid formation of the ostial valve (arrows) of the great cardiac vein (Vieussenian valve). (2) coronary sinus; (3) great cardiac vein (V. coronaria sinistra); (5) posterior left ventricular.

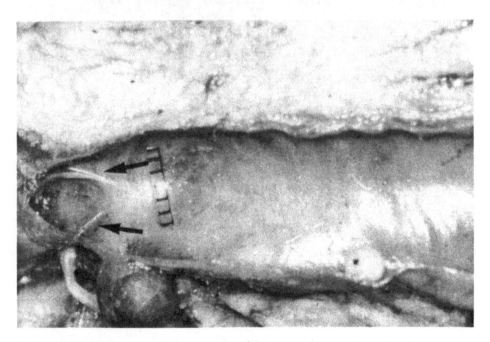

Fig. 2.12. Bicuspid formation of the ostial valve of the great cardiac vein (arrows) at the entrance to the cs., i.e., Valve of Vieussens.

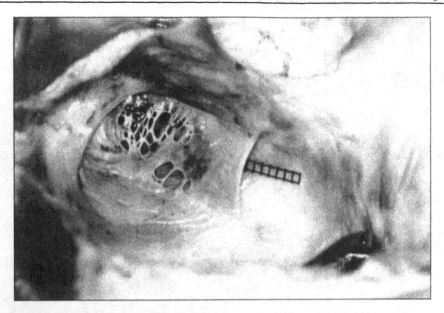

Fig. 2.13. Cribrate valve at the atrial ostium of the of the coronary sinus, valve of Thebesius.

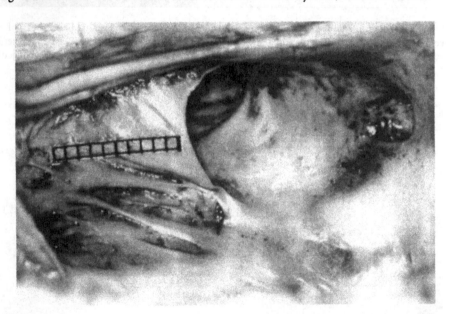

Fig. 2.14. Incomplete semilunar valve at the atrial ostium of the coronary sinus, valve of Thebesius.

Perfused vessel	Reperfused myocardium
V. interventricularis anterior and V. coronaria sinistra = V. cardiaca magna (great cardiac vein)	Anterior half of the inter-anterior and V. ventricular septum; anterior wall of the ventricle; posterior wall of the left atrium; left auricle.

Comment: Prospect of success 85 to 95%. The procedure is limited in single cases by extensive compression of the vein by an intramural segment or by a sclerosed and calcified crossing artery[4] (Figs. 2.16, 2.17); in rare cases the vein has an unusual course and opening into the right atrium[6] (Fig. 2.18). Selective cannulation of the great cardiac vein may also be difficult if there is an S-shaped (sigmoid) course of the terminal portion.[7]

Perfused vessel	Reperfused myocardium
V. marginalis ventriculi sinistri (left marginal vein)	lateral wall of the left ventricle

Comment: Prospect of success 62%. In the remaining percentage a significant left marginal vein does not exist and the myocardium is supplied by small venous branches from the adjacent venous stems.

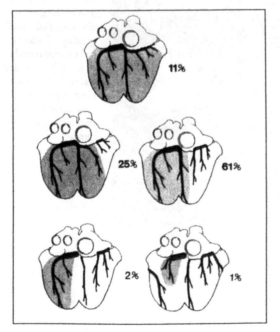

Fig. 2.15. Scheme of the distribution pattern of the cardiac veins and their relationship to the coronary sinus.

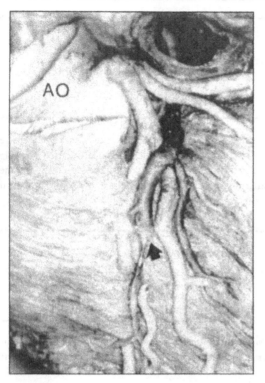

Fig. 2.16. Diaphragmatic surface of a heart with the anterior interventricular groove and its vessels. A short intramural course of the anterior interventricular vein (great cardiac vein) (dark vessel) is marked by an arrow. Two intramural courses of the anterior interventricular branch of the left coronary artery (pale vessel). Ao = Aorta.

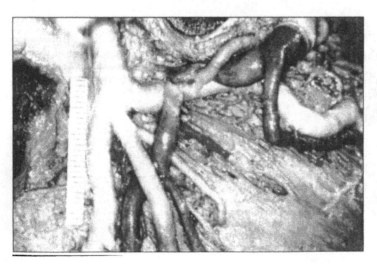

Fig. 2.17. Compression of the great cardiac vein (dark vessel) crossing of sclerosed and calcified branches of the left coronary artery (pale vessel). Catheterization and reperfusion of that vein may be complicated.

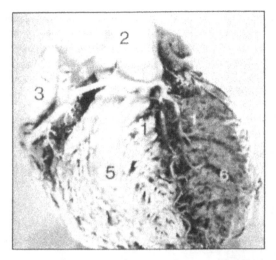

Fig. 2.18. Anterior aspect of a corrosion cast of a heart with aberrant course of the anterior interventricular part (1) of the great cardiac vein, originating in the distal anterior interventricular sulcus, leaving that groove to the right, passing the atrial conus and root of the pulmonary trunk (2), and finally emptying into the right atrium (3). Aorta (4), right ventricle (5), left ventricle (6).

Perfused vessel	Reperfused myocardium
V. posterior ventriculi sinistri (posterior vein of the left ventricle)	Posterior (diaphragmatic) wall of the left ventricle

Comment: Prospect of success 58%. The vein is only well developed in 67% of the cases. In one-third of them it may empty into the terminal great cardiac vein, in the second third into the initial (left) part of the cs and in the last third into the terminal (right) part of the cs (Fig. 2.19). In the last cases the opening of that vein is occluded by the balloon catheter, as are the ostia of the middle and small cardiac veins (Figs. 2.20, 2.21).[4,23]

The posterior vein of the left ventricle which empties into the terminal (right) half of the cs, the posterior interventricular vein (V. cardiaca media) and the small cardiac vein (V. cardiaca parva) can only be selectively perfused by direct cannulation. The reperfusion of these veins by coronary sinus intervention alone is anatomically impossible.

Veins and Myocardium Which Cannot Be Perfused by the Methods of Coronary Sinus Intervention

The cardiologist should be aware that only the parts described above but not the following parts or wall of the atrii and ventricles may be directly perfused by methods of the intervention of the cs[4,7,8] (Figs. 2.20–2.22):

- the posterior half of the posterior interventricular septum and the posterior wall of the right ventricle which are drained by the middle and small cardiac vein (when the latter exists).
- the anterolateral wall of the right ventricle which is drained by the anterior cardiac veins.
- the superior part of the interventricular septum which is drained by superior septal veins. These variably sized veins empty directly into the right auricle or the sinus of the right atrium.
- the entire right atrium and its sinus node which in most parts are drained by the smallest cardiac veins, the Thebesian veins.

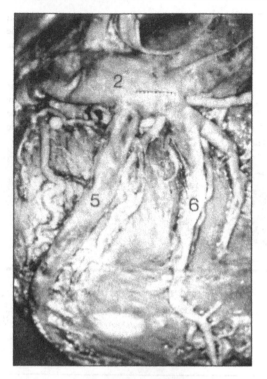

Fig. 2.19. Diaphragmatic surface of the heart with a strong posterior vein of the left ventricle emptying into the terminal (right) third of the cs. (2) coronary sinus; (5) posterior left ventricular; (6) middle cardiac vein (V. interventricularis posterior).

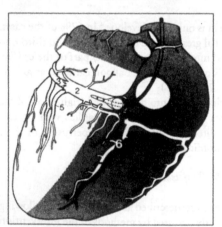

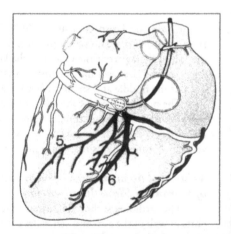

Fig. 2.20. Schematic drawing of the diaphragmatic surface of a heart with translucent catheter of the cs. In correct position the balloon may occlude the ostias of the middle and small cardiac vein. The pale surface of the heart indicates the area of perfusion; the dark zones are the areas of nonperfusion. (2) coronary sinus; (3) great cardiac vein (V. coronaria sinistra); (5) posterior left ventricular; (6) middle cardiac vein (V. interventricularis posterior).

Fig. 2.21. Corresponding to Fig. 2.20 the schematic drawing is showing a left posterior ventricular vein emptying into the terminal (right) third of the cs. In a case like that the balloon catheter will occlude the ostias of that vein as well as of the middle and small cardiac veins. The area of nonperfusion is larger than in Fig. 2.20.

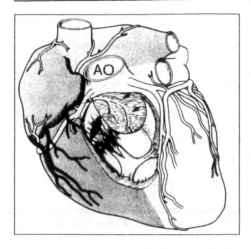

Fig. 2.22. Schematic drawing of the sternocostal surface of a heart showing the superior (basal) part of the interventricular septum and its venous drainage (arrows) through a window of the anterior wall of the right ventricle. The pale and dark zones correspond to legend of Fig. 2.20. Ao = Aorta.

- the interatrial septum and its atrioventricular node which are drained by small atrial veins emptying into the right atrium.
- the anterior and septal walls of the left atrium are drained by veins emptying into the right atrium or into the terminal superior vena cava.

In one-third of cases the roof of the left atrium is drained by special additional veins which open into the left atrium itself or into one of the stems of the pulmonary veins. A few of these veins are even connected to bronchial or mediastinal veins.

Technical Difficulties of Coronary Sinus Catheterization

In general, methods of coronary sinus intervention are facilitated by the obviously insufficient nature of the terminal (Thebesian) and initial (Vieussenian) valves of the cs.

However, these valves may be torn by a catheter tip. Valvular lesions may induce subendocardial and subendothelial hemorrhages and even intraluminal thrombosis. In about 15% of the cases the catheter tip has to pass a sharp angle at the atrial ostium of the cs. This passage may be anatomically impossible.

Selective cannulation of the great cardiac vein and reperfusion may be further complicated by s-shaped, intramural, and ectopic courses as described above.

References

1. Hellerstein HK, Orbison JL. Anatomic variations of the orifice of the human coronary sinus. Circulation 1961; 3:523-524.
2. Hood WB. Regional venous drainage of te human heart. Br Heart J 1968; 30:105-109.
3. James TH, Sherf L, Schlant RC, Silverman ME. Anatomy of the heart. In: Hurst JW, ed. The Heart. 5th ed. New York: McGraw-Hill, 1982:22-74.
4. v. Lüdinghausen M. Clinical anatomy of cardiac veins, Vv. cardiacae. Surg Radiol Anat 1987; 9:159-168.
5. v. Lüdinghausen M, Lechleuthner A. Atresia of the right atrial ostium of the coronary sinus. Acta Anat 1988; 131:81-83.
6. v. Lüdinghausen M. Aberrant course of the anterior interventricular part of the great cardiac vein in the human heart. Gegenbaurs morphol Jahrb, Leipzig 1989; 135,3: 475-478.
7. v. Lüdinghausen M, Schott C. Microanatomy of the human coronary sinus and its major tributaries. Ed S Meerbaum, Darmstadt: Steinkopff 1990:93-122.
8. v. Lüdinghausen M. Myocardial coverage of the coronary sinus and related veins. Clinical Anatomy 1992; 5:1-15.

9. Malhotra VK, Tewari SP, Tewari PS, Agarwa SK. Coronary sinus and its tributaries. Anat Anz (Jena) 1980; 148:331-332.

10. Maros TN, Racz L, Plugor TG. Contribution to the morphology of the human coronary sinus. Anat Anz (Jena) 1983; 154: 133-144.

11. Marshall J. In: Dorland's Illustrated Medical Dictionary. 26th ed, Philadelphia: WB Saunders 1985.

12. McAlpine WA. Heart and coronary arteries. New York: Springer 1975:206-207.

13. Mechanik N. Das Venensystem der Herzwände. Zschr Anat Entw Gesch 1934; 103:813-843.

14. Meerbaum S. The Beck Era: A springboard for renewed research of coronary venous retroperfusion aimed at treatment of myocardial ischemia. In: Mohl W, Wolner E, Glogar D, eds. The Coronary Sinus. New York: Springer 1984:320-327.

15. Meerbaum S. Myocardial perfusion, reperfusion, coronary venous retroperfusion. Darmstadt: Steinkopff 1990:6-16.

16. Mochizuki S. Vv. cordis. In: Adachi B, ed. In: Das Venensystem der Japaner. Rokyo: Kenkyusha 1933:41-64.

17. Mohl W. The development and rationale of pressure controlled intermittent coronary sinus occlusion—a new approach to protect ischemic myocardium. Wiener klin Wschr 1984; 96:537-548.

18. Mohl W. Pressure controlled intermittent coronary sinus occlusion—an alternative to retrograde perfusion of arterial blood. In: Mohl W, Wolner E, Glogar D, eds. The Coronary Sinus. Darmstadt: Steinkopff 1984:418-423.

19. Platzer W. Atlas der topographischen Anatomie. Stuttgart: Thieme 1982:108-109.

20. Potkin BN, Roberts WC. Size of coronary sinus at necropsy in subjects without cardiac disease and in patients with various cardiac conditions. Am J Cardiol 1988; 60:1418-1421.

21. Silver MA, Rowley NE. The functional anatomy of the human coronary sinus. Am Heart J 1988; 115:1080-1084.

22. Thebesius AC. In: Dorland's illustrated medical dictionary. 26th ed. Philadelphia: WB Saunders 1985.

23. Tschabitscher M. The so-called silent zone of the coronary sinus. In: Mohl W, Faxon D, Wolner E, eds. Progress in Coronary Interventions. Darmstadt: Steinkopff 1986:11-14.

24. Vieussens R. In Dorland's illustrated medical dictionary. 26th ed, Philadelphia: WB Saunders 1985.

CHAPTER 3

The Anatomical Basis of Coronary Sinus Reperfusion

Michael von Lüdinghausen, Masahiro Miura

Introduction

The venous drainage system of the myocardium is divided in two parts (Fig. 3.1):

A. The great (major) cardiac venous drainage system (GCVDS) extends over the surface of the ventricular and atrial myocardium. The distribution patterns of these veins are highly variable; however, the strongest veins drain the left ventricular myocardium and empty into the coronary sinus (cs).

B. The small (minor) cardiac venous drainage system (SCVDS) is found in a subendocardial location in the innermost myocardial layers of the cardiac walls. These very short cardiac veins have an ostial diameter of less than 1 mm; in the adult they represent the primitive supply and drainage system of the spongeous myocardium that was carried out by endocardialy-sinusoidal vessels usually connected to the next chamber in the embryo.

A. The GCVDS consists of six intercommunicating parts (Fig. 3.2a,b):
1. the cs and its ventricular tributaries
2. the cs and its left atrial tributaries
3. the remaining left atrial veins
4. the superior septal veins (including the venous drainage of the atrioventricular node)
5. the anterior cardiac venous system
6. the right atrial veins (including the venous drainage of the sinus node)

B. The SCVDS consists of four types of (Thebesian) vessels (Figs. 3.3, 3.4) extending from a subendocaridal origin:
1. the arterio-sinusoidal vessels
2. the arterio-luminal vessels
3. veno-sinusoidal vessels
4. veno-luminal vessels

Characteristic morphology of tributaries of the GCVDS: the veins frequently cross interventricular, coronary and interatrial sulcuses; they exhibit intramurally-widened terminal spaces, collectors, or sinuses; the venous openings into the right and left atrium have ostial valves.[7,11] The characteristic pattern of the Thebesian vessels will be described in a further report.

The tributaries of A1; 4; and 5 drain the myocardium. However, uncertainty exists as to what extent the veins of groups 1 and 2 drain the left ventricular myocardium and can be reached by catheterization of the cs.[5,7,16,17,19]

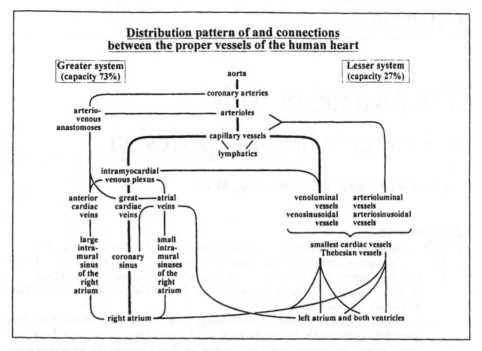

Fig. 3.1. Distribution pattern of, and connections between, the proper vessels of the human heart; physiological investigations reveal that the great (major) cardiac venous system has a capacity to transport blood of 73%, while that of the small (minor) cardiac venous system is 27%.

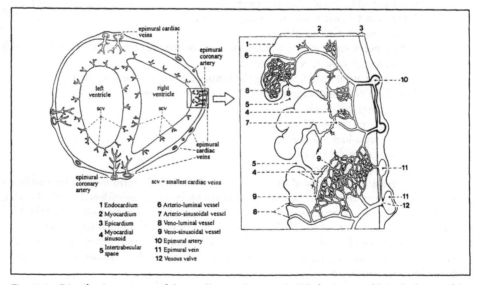

Fig. 3.2a. Distribution pattern of the smallest cardiac vessels (Thebesian vessels) in the layers of the ventricular walls and their relation to the coronary arteries and cardiac veins. The Thebesian vessels constitute the small (minor) cardiac venous drainage system, the coronary arteries and cardiac veins constitute the great (major) cardiac venous drainage system.

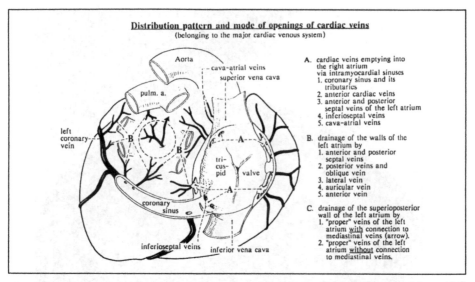

Distribution pattern and mode of openings of cardiac veins
(belonging to the major cardiac venous system)

A. cardiac veins emptying into
   the right atrium
   via intramyocardial sinuses
   1. coronary sinus and its
      tributaries
   2. anterior cardiac veins
   3. anterior and posterior
      septal veins of the left atrium
   4. inferioseptal veins
   5. cava-atrial veins

B. drainage of the walls of the
   left atrium by
   1. anterior and posterior
      septal veins
   2. posterior veins and
      oblique vein
   3. lateral vein
   4. auricular vein
   5. anterior vein

C. drainage of the superioposterior
   wall of the left atrium by
   1. "proper" veins of the left
      atrium with connection to
      mediastinal veins (arrow).
   2. "proper" veins of the left
      atrium without connection
      to mediastinal veins.

Fig. 3.2b. Distribution pattern of the cardiac veins and their mode of opening into the right and left atria of the heart. In the myocardial walls of the atria the veins form smaller or larger intramural venous sinuses or spaces for the collection of blood. The coronary sinus also belongs to this system.

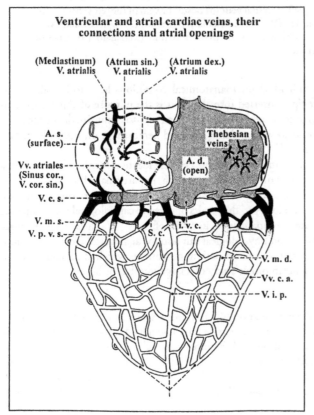

Ventricular and atrial cardiac veins, their connections and atrial openings

Fig. 3.3. Three-dimensional illustration of the ventricular and atrial cardiac veins, their interconnections and atrial openings. It can once more be seen that most of these veins empty via intramyocardial sinuses into the atria.

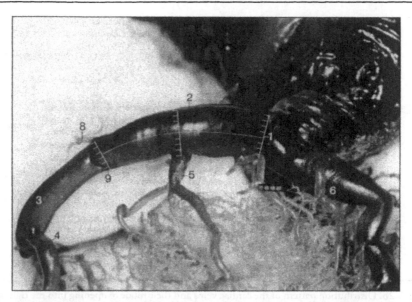

Fig. 3.4. Posterior surface of a corrosion cast of the cs of a human heart. The cs has a length of about 40 mm and is cylindrical in shape. Its diameter at its origin is about 6 mm; the midcoronary diameter is about 8 mm, as is also the ostial diameter. (1) atrial ostium of the cs; location of the valve of Thebesius (2) cs (3) left coronary vein (V. coronaria sinistra) (4) left marginal vein (5) posterior vein of the left ventricle (6) posterior interventricular vein (V. interventricularis posterior) (7) right coronary vein (V. coronaria dextra) (8) oblique vein of the left atrium (Marshall) (9) valve of Vieussens (10) right atrium.

In view of the fact that individual microanatomical conditions have to be taken into consideration when a catheter-tip is inserted into the cs, it is the purpose of this Chapter to clarify the anatomical situation of the cs and its tributaries in order to minimize the instances of failure of the technical procedure, as well as damage to and hemorrhage of, the endocardial-myocardial-endothelial complex.[5,7,14]

On grounds of its morphology the cs is the best possible location for the placement of a balloon catheter for retrograde perfusion or revascularization, in particular of the vessels of the left ventricular myocardium, in a case of severe stenosing coronary heart disease and an ischemia-threatened myocardium. However, the results of invasive cardiological procedures via the cs are not satisfactory and are even inadequate in 1-5% of cases.[16,17] These cases reinforce the need not only for biochemical and physiological but also for anatomical reexamination. It was naturally impossible to carry out such examinations on patients who had undergone treatment; therefore we undertook a postmortem study of a large number of hearts.

Material and Methods

This study was based on the examination of 140 human hearts from the dissection room, from individuals aged between 64 and 88 years at death, of which 64 were male and 76 female. After routine fixation the arteries and veins of the heart specimens were injected with red and blue gelatin, respectively. Microdissections were performed using a stereomicroscope (C. Zeiss, Oberkochen, Germany). Photographs were taken with a Nikon AS camera fitted with a Medical Nikkor C Auto lens 1:5.6, f = 200, using Kodachome 64 films. All scales in the figures are given in millimeters. The nomenclature is based on the Nomina Anatomica, fifth edition, Mexico city, 1980 and sixth edition, Tokyo 1989.

Results and Discussion

The Coronary Sinus

The Significance of the CS and the Most Frequent Tributaries
Among the venous collectors, the cs constitutes the main structure in the left posterior part of the coronary sulcus. The tributaries of the cs carry out, almost exclusively, the drainage of the left ventricular myocardial mass, i.e., the sternocostal, diaphragmatic and lateral walls of the left ventricle and interventricular septum.

In most of the cases studied the cs is as wide and as long as one to three phalanges of the little finger and may be either slightly or strongly curved. It collects the following major cardiac veins: the great vein (which consists initially of the anterior interventricular and later on of the left coronary vein), the left marginal vein, the posterior vein of the left ventricle and the middle (the posterior interventricular vein) and the small cardiac vein (the right coronary vein) (Fig. 3.4).

In this way the cs effects the drainage of the lateral and posterior walls of the left ventricle via the left marginal and septum via the middle cardiac vein.

In addition there are the oblique and posterior veins of the left drainage of atrium, both of which empty into the cs (Fig. 3.4). In one third of the cases either a left marginal or a posterior vein exists.[7,25]

In 55% of the cases the left marginal vein terminates in the V. coronaria sinistra.

In half of the 67% of cases where a posterior vein of the left ventricle exists, it appears either as a very strong vein or a group of small vessels. These may empty either into the left coronary vein or into cs.[7,25]

In addition the oblique vein and the posterior vein of the left atrium drain into the cs.[9,10]

Length, Shape and Position of the CS
The cs resembles a little finger, or part of it, in length and shape.

Length
The length was measured between the entrance of the oblique vein of Marshall[13] and the base of the Thebesian valve.[24] There were numerous variations in both length and shape. The average length was between 15-70 (37.0) mm, and in one case it reached 82 mm.[9,12,23]

A short cs had the length of a phalanx of a finger (7% of the cases); a cs of medium length with its cylindrical form corresponded to two phalanges in 74% of the cases, and an elongated cs had a length of three phalanges and exhibited a tubular, extended form in 18% of the cases.

Shape
The cs and the left coronary vein described a gentle curve in the left coronary sulcus; the cs lies almost parallel to the attachment of the posterior (mural) leaflet of the mitral valve (Fig. 3.5). The curvature of the cs and the left coronary vein either described on quarter of a circle (33% of the cases), one eighth of a circle (29%), or had an almost straight course (38%) (Fig. 3.6).

In one quarter of the cases there was a sharp bend and an obtuse angle and, in 5% of the cases, a right angle of the terminal cs shortly before it opened into the right atrium.[9] The diameter of the atrial ostium ranged between 7-16 (9.7) mm, the cross-sectional area of the cs between 0.67-2.09 mm^3.[22,23] In 1% of the cases there was a sinus coronarius duplex (Fig. 3.7).

Position

The widely-postulated location of the cs in the left posterior coronary sulcus was found in only 12% of the cases studied (Fig. 3.8). In most specimens the cs was in a displaced position towards the posterior wall of the left atrium. That displacement or elevation was slight (1-3 mm) in 16% of the cases, moderate (4-7 mm) in 50%, and extreme (8-15 mm) in 22%[9] (Figs. 3.9, 3.10). An elevation of the cs is demonstrated in a computer-assisted tomogram of the heart (Fig. 3.10). An extreme elevation of the cs, as found here, may enhance the ostial angle through which a catheter tip has to pass on its way into the cs.

The Myocardial Coverage, Myocardial Coat and Belts of the CS and their Relations to the External Boundaries of the CS

In all specimens, the cs was completely enclosed by a thin myocardial coat which was part of the posterior wall of the left atrium. The length of that coat was not the same as the length of the cs. In some cases it was longer and covered the terminal left coronary vein. Here, at its origin, the seam of the coat was often irregularly formed, for instance as a myocardial cuff, with one or two myocardial belts, which surrounded the terminal portion of the great cardiac vein. In other cases the seam had an ill-defined edge with a splitting of the myocardial fibers (Fig. 3.10).[10] The terminal (right) part of the cs was situated in the posterior portion of the coronary sulcus, without any significant topographical landmark. It was difficult to determine the exact location of the entrance of the cs into the right atrium on the epicardial surface. In most cases

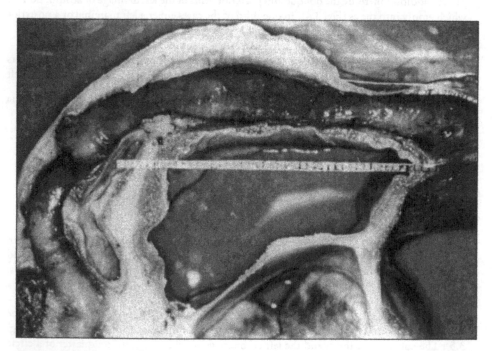

Fig. 3.5. Inferior aspect of an opened cs, which has a length of about 55 mm; its course exhibits a gentle curvature. When it reaches the ostium, the cs forms a remarkable ostial angle (arrow). 1) atrial ostium of the cs; location of the valve of Thebesius; 2) cs; 3) left coronary vein (V. coronaria sinistra); 9) valve of vieussens.

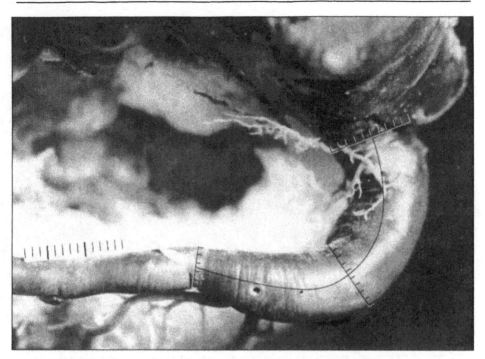

Fig. 3.6. Cranial aspect of a corrosion cast of the cs of a human heart. The cs exhibits a marked curvature, which conforms to a quarter circle. It is about 40 mm in length, and has the shape of a narrow cylinder. It is about 5.5 mm in diameter at origin, with midcoronary and ostial diameters of around 10 mm. In this case there is no ostial angle of the cs.

the fibers of the myocardial coverage continued regularly into the collagenous fibers of the epicardium on the posterior wall of the right atrium.[10,21]

In rare cases the fibers of the myocardial coverage of the cs formed a wrapping for the terminal part of the posterior interventricular vein, which is often enlarged. Thus a so-called cs duplex had developed (Fig. 3.11).

The Valves of the CS and their Relations to the Internal Boundaries of the CS

The beginning of the cs was marked by the ostial terminal valve of the great cardiac vein, the valve of Vieussens.[26] Opposite the openings of the great cardiac vein into cs there was the termination of the oblique vein of Marshall[13] which also indicated the beginning of the cs (Fig. 3.12).

The valve of Vieussens[26] firmly established the origin of the cs or marked the end of the great cardiac vein in an average of 87% of the cases. In 62% it was a unicuspid, in 25% a bicuspid valve. In two cases we found a tricuspid valve; one heart specimen showed a valve-complex with two unicuspid valves one after the other (Figs. 3.13, 3.14, 3.15).[9]

The entrance of the cs into the right atrium was guarded by a more or less complete and sufficient fold, the Thebesian valve. In 19% of the cases the ostium was valveless. An incomplete threadlike valve was found in 2% of the cases, an incomplete crescentic valve in 34%, an incomplete semilunar valve in 7%, an incomplete cribriform valve (Figs. 3.15, 3.17) in 7%, and a complete circular and membranous valve in 31%.[3,9,15,23]

In very rare cases a congenital, complete ostial occlusion (atresia) of the cs has been observed by the authors and by others.[3,4,15] In these cases a left vena cava was persistent.[7] In most

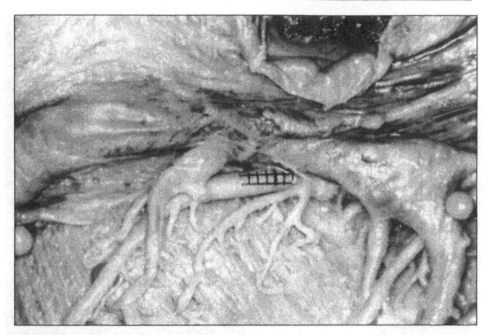

Fig. 3.7. Posterior surface of a human heart specimen with a so-called sinus coronarius duplex (double cs). The right coronary sinus is constituted by the widened confluence of the middle and small cardiac veins.

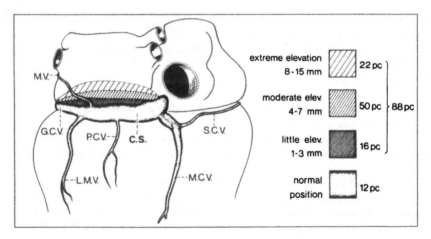

Fig. 3.8. Degree of elevation of the cs from the posterior coronary sulcus to the posterior wall of the left atrium. Abbreviations: CS; coronary sinus; GCV: great cardiac vein; LMV: left marginal vein; MV: Marshall's vein, oblique vein of the left atrium; MCV: middle cardiac vein; PCV: posterior vein of the left ventricle; SCV: small cardiac vein.

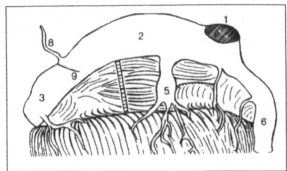

Fig. 3.9. Posterior surface of a human heart with acute elevation of the cs to a position of about 14 mm above the posterior coronary sulcus. 1) atrial ostium of the cs; location of the valve of Thebesius; 2) cs; 3) left coronary vein (V. coronaria sinistra). 5) posterior vein of the left ventricle; 6) posterior interventricular vein (V. interventricularis posterior); 8) oblique vein of the left atrium (Marshall); 9) valve of Vieussens.

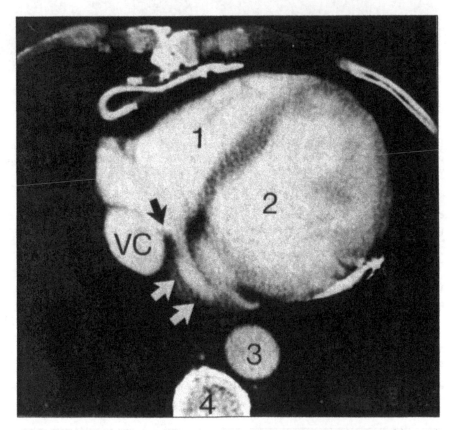

Fig. 3.10. CT- image of a heart showing the cs (white arrows) with an acute elevation of the cs. There is also an acute angle (black arrow) between the inferior vena cava (VC) and the cs. 1) the right ventricle; 2) left ventricle; 3) thoracic aorta; 4) body of a thoracic vertebra.

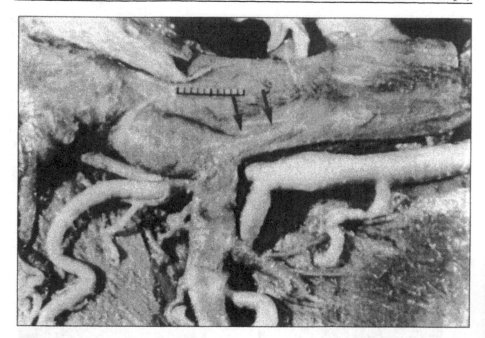

Fig. 3.11. In this case the myocardial coat of the cs covers also the terminal (oblique) part of the posterior interventricular vein. This vein is subsequently fixed by myocardial cords at the posterior wall of the right atrium (arrows). The right coronary artery has a pale-colored surface.

cases the ostia of the middle cardiac vein and posterior vein of the left ventricle, when these terminate in the cs, were secured by well-formed unicuspid valves.[9]

The Cardiac Veins

Variations in the Distribution and Pattern of Occurrence of the Cardiac Veins, and Reperfusion Techniques

Given that the tip of a balloon catheter is correctly positioned in the terminal (right) half of the cs, the prospect of successful reperfusion of many cardiac veins is still limited by specific anatomical conditions. Therefore, the area which can be reperfused may be smaller that hitherto predicted (Fig. 3.18).

Perfused vessel	Reperfused myocardium
V. interventricularis ant. and V. coronaria sinistra = V. cardiaca magna (great cardiac vein)	Anterior half of interventricular septum; anterior wall of left ventricle; anterior and posterior wall of left atrium; left auricle

Comment: Prospect of success 85-95%. The procedure would be limited in individual cases by extensive compression of the vein by an intramural segment or by a sclerosed and calcified crossing artery[6] (Fig. 3.19); in rare cases the vein had an unusual course and opening into the right atrium[8] (Fig. 3.21).

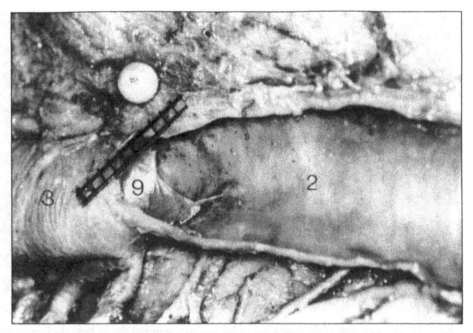

Fig. 3.12. Univalvular Vieussenian valve—marked by a scale and pinhead—at the junction of the left coronary vein and the cs. 2) opened cs; 3) left coronary vein; 9) valve of Vieussens.

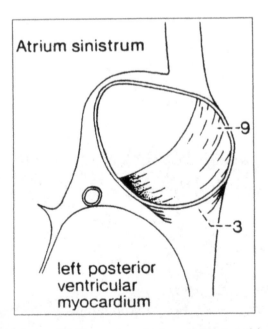

Fig. 3.13. Univalvular (unicuspid) Vieussenian valve in a cross-section of the terminal left coronary vein.

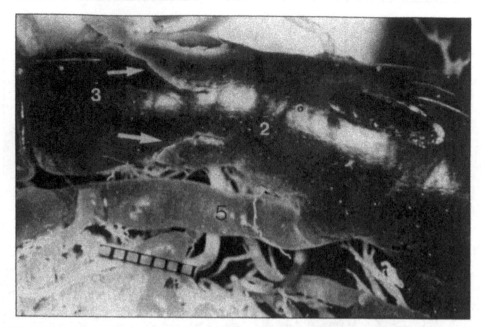

Fig. 3.14. Corrosion cast of the confluence of left coronary vein and the cs; here, the impressions made by two endothelial folds can be seen. Bicuspid formation of the ostial valve (Vieussenian valve) of the great cardiac vein (arrows). 2) cs; 3) left coronary vein (V. coronaria sinistra); 5) posterior vein of the left ventricle.

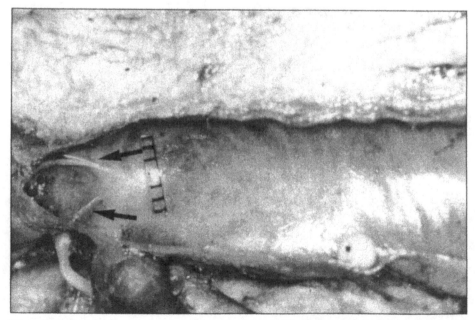

Fig. 3.15. Specimen showing an opened cs with a bicuspid formation of the ostial valve of the left coronary vein (arrows).

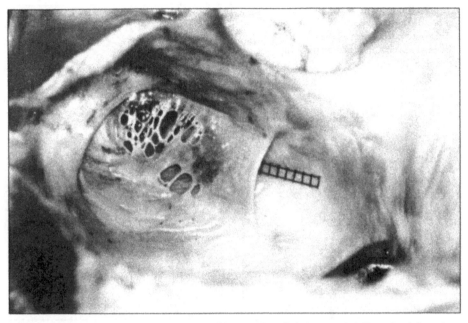

Fig. 3.16. Cribrate valve at the atrial ostium of the cs, valve of Thebesius; view from the right atrium.

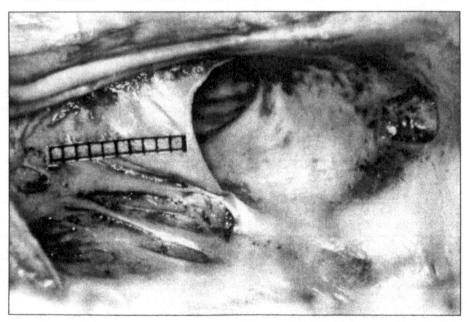

Fig. 3.17. Semilunar valve at the atrial ostium of the cs, valve of Thebesius; view from the right atrium.

Fig. 3.18. Diagram of the entire surface of the heart demonstrating the
distribution pattern of all the ventricular cardiac veins and their relationship
to the cs.

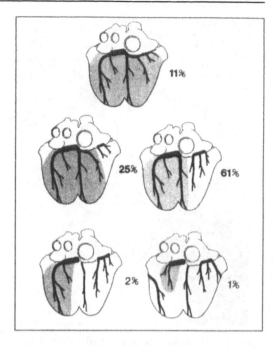

Selective cannulation of the left coronary vein may also be difficult if there is an S-shaped (sigmoid) course of the terminal portion.[9]

Perfused vessel	Reperfused myocardium
V. marginalis ventriculi sinistri (left marginal vein)	lateral wall of the left ventricle

Comment: Prospect of success 62%. In the remaining percentage of our cases a significant left marginal vein does not exist and the myocardium is drained by a great number of small veins emptying into the terminal left part of the coronary vein or initial part of the cs. In these cases a distinct posterior vein of the left ventricle is well-developed (see next paragraph).

Perfused vessel	Reperfused myocardium
sinistri (posterior vein of the left ventricle)	wall of the left ventricle

Comment: The vein is well-developed in 67% of the cases. In the same cases the left marginal vein is underdeveloped. In one-third of the cases the posterior vein of the left ventricle empties into the terminal great cardiac vein, in the second third into the initial (left) part of the cs and in the final third into the terminal (right) part of the cs (Fig. 3.22).

The posterior interventricular and right coronary veins may not be perfused when a balloon-catheter is in a normal position in cs. These veins (Figs. 3.23, 3.24)[6,25] can only be selectively perfused by direct cannulation. The use of the reperfusion method alone is anatomically and functionally impossible.

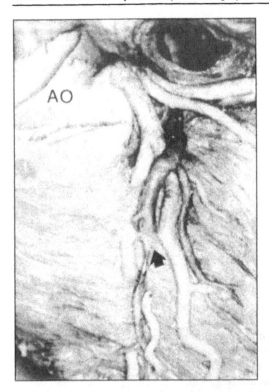

Fig. 3.19. Sternocostal surface of a heart with the anterior interventricular groove and its vessels. A short intramural course of the anterior interventricular vein (dark vessel) is marked by an arrow. Two intramural courses of the anterior interventricular branch of the left coronary artery (pale colored vessel) are shown. Ao = Aorta

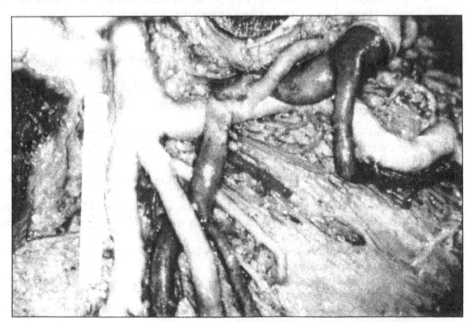

Fig. 3.20. Compression of the great cardiac vein (dark vessel) by sclerosed and calcified branches of the left coronary artery (pale-colored vessel). The catheterization and reperfusion of this vein may be a complicated procedure.

Fig. 3.21. Anterior aspect of a corrosion cast of a heart with aberrant course of the anterior interventricular vein originating in the distal anterior interventricular sulcus, leaving it to the right, passing the arterial conus and root of the pulmonary trunk, then and finally emptying into the right atrium. 1) anterior interventricular vein; 2) pulmonary trunk; 3) right atrium; 4) aorta; 5) right ventricle; 6) left ventricle.

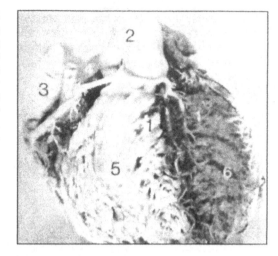

Peculiarities

1. The distribution pattern and the mode of opening of the tributaries of the cs are highly variable (Fig. 3.6).
2. Superior ventricular septal veins may drain into the terminal cs, directly into the right atrium, or into the system of anterior cardiac veins (Fig. 3.7).
3. The left atrial veins empty into the left atrium (Fig. 3.8) and the anterior cardiac or the right atrial veins into the right atrium (Fig. 3.8).
4. Quite frequently, left atrial veins empty into the right atrium or are interconnected with mediastinal veins after they have crossed the bare area at the epipericardial reflection (Fig. 3.9).

Veins and Myocardium which Cannot be Perfused by the Methods of Coronary Sinus Intervention

The cardiologist should be aware that only the parts described above but not the following walls of the heart chambers may be directly perfused by methods of intervention in the cs[6,9,10] (Figs. 3.23-3.25):

- the posterior half of the posterior interventricular septum and the posterior wall of the right ventricle which are drained by the posterior interventricular and right coronary veins (when the latter exist).
- the anterolateral wall of the right ventricle which is drained by the anterior cardiac veins.
- the superior part of the interventricular septum which is drained by superior septal veins. These variably-sized veins empty directly into the right auricle or the sinus of the atrium.
- the entire right atrium and its sinus node which in most of their parts are drained by the smallest cardiac (Thebesian) veins.
- the interatrial septum and its atrioventricular node which are drained by small atrial veins emptying into the right atrium.
- the anterior and septal walls of the left atrium are drained by veins emptying into the right atrium or into the terminal superior vena cava.

In one third of cases the roof of the left atrium is drained by special additional veins which open into the left atrium itself or into one of the stems of the pulmonary veins. A few of these veins are even connected to bronchial or mediastinal veins.

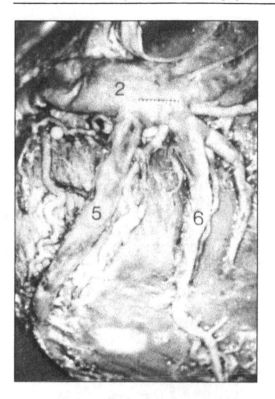

Fig. 3.22. Diaphragmatic surface of the heart with a strong posterior vein of the left ventricle emptying into the terminal (right) third of the cs. 2) cs; 5) posterior vein of the left ventricle; 6) posterior interventricular vein.

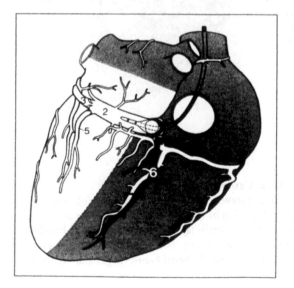

Fig. 3.23. Schematic drawing of the diaphragmatic surface of a heart showing a translucent catheter inserted into the cs. In correct position the balloon will occlude the ostias of the posterior interventricular and right coronary veins. The pale-colored surface of the heart indicates the area of perfusion; the dark zones are the areas on nonperfusion. 2) cs; 3) left coronary vein; 5) posterior vein of the left ventricle; 6) posterior interventricular vein.

Fig. 3.24. This schematic drawing corresponds to that in Fig. 3.23, but shows a left posterior ventricular vein which empties into the terminal (right) third of the cs. In a case such as this the balloon-catheter will occlude the ostias of most cardiac veins except the left coronary vein. The area of nonperfusion is larger than that in Fig. 3.23.

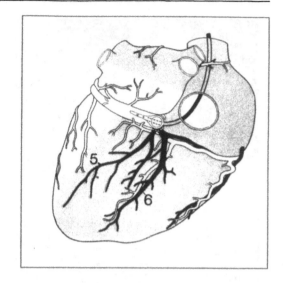

Fig. 3.25. Schematic drawing of the sternocostal surface of a heart showing the superior (basal) part of the interventricular septum and its venous drainage (arrows) through a window in the anterior wall of the right ventricle. The superior part of the interventricular septum in 20% of the cases is drained by veins which belong to the group of anterior cardiac veins and empty directly into the right atrium. The pale and dark zones correspond to those of Fig. 3.24. Ao = Aorta

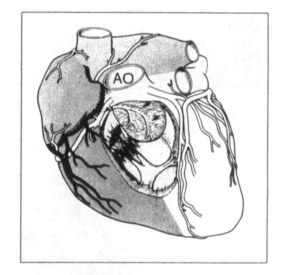

Technical Difficulties of Coronary Sinus Catheterization

In general, methods of coronary sinus intervention are facilitated by the obviously insufficient nature of the terminal (Thebesian) and initial (Vieussenian) valves of the cs.

However, these valves may be thick, may contain layers of myocardial fiber bundles, be inflexible and therefore be torn by a protruding catheter tip. Subsequently, valvular lesions may occur which could induce subendocardial and subendothelial hemorrhages and even intraluminal thrombosis.

Selective cannulation and reperfusion of the left coronary and anterior intraventricular veins may be further complicated by s-shaped, intramural, and ectopic course.

Cannulation of the posterior interventricular vein may be difficult because of an almost right angle between the terminal oblique and straight parts in the posterior interventricular sulcus. The turning point of that angle is sometimes protected by a unicuspid valve (instead of an ostial valve). In one third of the cases we found distinct unicuspid ostial valves at the openings of the posterior septal veins. These valves appeared to be insufficient because they occluded almost one or two thirds of the ostial diameter.

References

1. Bankl H. Congenital malformation of the heart and great vessels. Synopsis of pathology, embryology, and natural history. Baltimore, Munich: Urban & Schwarzenberg, 312-324.
2. Bankl H, Kretschmer G. Residuen embryonaler Strukturen in den Vorhöfen des menschlichen Herzens. Beitr Path Anat 1968; 138:1-35.
3. Hellerestein HK, Orbison JL. Anatomic variations of the orifice of the human coronary sinus. Circulation 1961; 3:523-524.
4. Hood WB. Regional venous drainage of the human heart. Br Heart J 1968; 30:105-109.
5. James TH, Sherf L, Schlant RC, Silverman ME. Anatomy of the heart. In: Hurst JW, ed. The Heart. 5th ed. New York: McGraw-Hill 1982:22-74.
6. v. Lüdinghausen M. Clinical anatomy of cardiac veins, Vv. cardiacae. Surg Radiol Anat 1987; 9:159-168.
7. v. Lüdinghausen M, Lechleuthner A. Atresia of the right atrial ostium of the coronary sinus. acta Anat 1988; 131:81-83.
8. v. Lüdinghausen M. Aberrant course of the anterior interventricular part of the great cardiac vein in the human heart. Gegenbaurs Morphol Jahrb, Leipzig 1989; 135:475-478.
9. v. Lüdinghausen M, Schott C. Microanatomy of the human coronary sinus and its major tributaries. Meerbaum S, ed. Darmstadt: Steinkopff 1990:93-122.
10. v. Lüdinghausen M. Myocardial coverage of the coronary sinus and related veins. Clin Anat 1992; 5:1-15.
11. v. Lüdinghausen M, Ohmachi N, Besch S, Mettenleiter A. Atrial veins of the human heart. Clin Anat 1995; 8:169-189.
12. Malhotra VK, Tewari SP, Tewari PS, Agarwa SK. Coronary sinus and its tributaries. Anat Anz (Jena) 1980; 148:331-332.
13. Mantini E, Grondin CM, Lillehei CW, Edwards JE. Congenital anomalies involving the coronary sinus. Circulation 1966; 33:317-327.
14. Maros TM, Racz L, Plugor TG. Contriction to the morphology of the human coronary sinus. Anat Anz (Jena) 1983; 154:133-144.
15. Marshall J. On the development of the great anterior veins in man and mammalia; including an account of certain remnants of foetal structure found in the adult, a comparative view of these great veins in the different mammalia, and an analysis of their occasional peculiarities in the human subject. Philos Trans R Soc Lond 1950; 140:133-170.
16. McAlpine WA. Heart and coronary arteries. New York: Springer 1975:26-207.
17. Mechanik N. Das Venensystem der Herzwände. Zachr Anat Entw Gexch 1934; 103:813-843.
18. Meerbaum S. The Beck Era: A springboard for renewed research of coronary venous retroperfusion aimed at treatment of myocardial ischemia. In: Mohl W, Wolner E, Glogar D, eds. The Coronary Sinus. New York 1984:320-327.
19. Meerbaum S. Myocardial perfusion, reperfusion, coronary venous retroperfusion. Darmstadt: Steinkopff 1990:6-16.
20. Mochizuki S. Vv. cordis. In: Adachi B, ed. In: Das Venensystem der Japaner. Tokyo: Kenkyusha 1933:41-64.
21. Mohl W. The development and rationale of pressure controlled intermittent coronary sinus occlusion—A new approach to protect ischemic myocardium. Wien klin Wschr 1984; 96:537-548.
22. Mohl W. Pressure controlled intermittent coronary sinus occlusion—An alternative to retrograde perfusion of arterial blood. In: Mohl W, Wolner E, Glogar D, eds. The Coronary Sinus. Darmstadt: Steinkopff 1984:418-423.
23. Platzer W. Atlas der topographischen Anatomie. Stuttgart: Thieme 1982:108-109.

24. Potkin BN, Roberts WC. Size of coronary sinus at necropsy in subjects without cardiac disease and in patients with various cardiac conditions. Am J Cardiol 1988; 60:1418-1421.
25. Silver MA, Rowley NE. The functional anatomy of the human coronary sinus. Am Heart J 1988; 115:1080-1084.
26. Thebesius AC. De circulo sanuinis in corde. Lugduni Batavorum 1708.
27. Tschabitscher M. The so-called silent zone of the coronary sinus. In: Mohl W, Faxon D, Wolner E, eds. Progress in Coronary Sinus Interventions. Darmstadt: Steinkopff 1986:11-14.
28. Vieussens R. In: Dorland's Illustrated Medical Dictionary. 26th ed., Philadelphia: WB Saunders 1985.

CHAPTER 4

Structure and Function of the Cardiac Lymphatic System

Hubert Schad

The physiology of the lymphatic system lives like Cinderella at the side of her attractive sisters the physiology of the heart and of the circulation. Lymphatic vessels, however, have been observed in classical antiquity. Hippocrates (460-377 B.C.) reported vessels draining "white blood" and Aristoteles (384-322 B.C.) described vessels containing a colorless fluid.[1] But this knowledge fell into oblivion until the lymphatic system was newly discovered in the 17th century by Asellius (1581-1626).[1] His studies have stimulated a number of investigations on the lymphatic system and in 1651 on October 30, the cardiac lymphatic system was discovered by the Swedish anatomist Olaf Rudbeck. On this day he has observed "... in a dog lymphatic glands receiving large afferents from the heart ...".[2] Famous names associated with the investigation of the anatomy of the cardiac lymphatic system in the last century are His, Henle, and Ranvier.[3] Aagaard[4] presented in 1924 a detailed description of the mammalian cardiac lymphatic system including lymphatics in atrioventricular valves. The most comprehensive studies on the structure of the cardiac lymphatic system, however, were given by Patek in 1939, and he established the intercommunicating network of lymphatic capillaries in the subendo-, myo-, and subepicardium.[5] Stimulated by the anatomical studies of Patek, Cecil K. Drinker cannulated in 1940 a cardiac lymphatic main trunk in dogs to collect the total amount of cardiac lymphatic drainage and to analyze the composition of cardiac lymph.[6] Studies on the functional significance of the cardiac lymphatic drainage, however, were started as late as in the fifties by the Budapest group of Rusznyak, Földi, and Szabo.[1]

The Anatomy of the Cardiac Lymphatic System[3,7]

The cardiac lymphatic system does not differ in principal from that in most other tissues. It originates from the interstitium as closed, blind-ended, finger-like vessels. These terminal lymphatics or lymphatic capillaries, join and build up collecting lymphatics, which in turn form larger lymphatic vessels ending in a few main trunks, which run on the epicardial surface of the heart, and finally drain into mediastinal lymph nodes.

Lymphatic Capillaries

Lymphatic capillaries have a diameter of 20-100 mm. They consist of a single layer of endothelial cells on a discontinuous basal lamina of various thickness. The endothelial cells show pinocytotic vesicles. The cell-to-cell relationships are variable including cellular overlapping. In these regions open intercellular clefts are present, which enable a free communication of the lumen of the terminal lymphatics and the interstitial space thus facilitating the uptake of fluid and molecules including proteins into the lymphatic capillaries. The lymphatic capillaries

---

Coronary Sinus Interventions in Cardiac Surgery, Second Edition edited by Werner Mohl.
©2000 Eurekah.com.

are fixed in the surrounding tissue by *anchoring filaments* which arise from the outer surface of the endothelial cells. These anchoring filaments do not only prevent compression of the lymphatic capillaries when interstitial fluid volume increases, which would impede the drainage of the tissue and promote edema formation, but they even pull open the intercellular clefts facilitating the influx of interstitial fluid into the terminal lymphatics.[8]

Lymphatics of the Ventricles

The ventricular walls of the heart are provided with three lymphatic plexuses, which are connected to form a functional unit. The *subendocardial plexus* is localized in the subendocardial connective tissue. It is a well developed two dimensional network of lymphatic capillaries, which do not build up collecting ducts. The *myocardial plexus* intersperses uniformly throughout the ventricular walls as a loosely meshed three-dimensional network. The lymphatic vessels contain a few valves, nevertheless the entire plexus is considered to be composed of only lymphatic capillaries. The myocardial plexus is connected by short vessels both to the subendocardial and to the *subepicardial plexus*. The latter also consists of lymphatic capillaries and is located in the connective tissue between the myocardium and the epicardium. It covers both ventricles, but leaves open the anterior and posterior interventricular sulcus. The lymphatic capillaries converge to form collecting lymphatics. The larger subepicardial lymphatics build up the superficial efferent drainage vessels which are richly supplied with smooth muscle cells and with valves. The smooth muscle cells enable the lymphatics to contract and the valves ensure lymph flow in a centripetal direction. The large superficial lymphatic vessels follow the coronary arteries, converge, and usually form a right and left main trunk. These join into one supracardiac channel, which runs dorsal of the pulmonary artery and aorta. It drains into the cardiac lymph node which is situated between the superior vena cava and the brachiocephalic. The efferent lymphatics of this node run into the right lymph duct which empties into the venous system at the right angulus venosus formed by the subclavian and internal jugular vein. Occasionally, connections of the cardiac lymphatic system and the thoracic duct have been observed. The epicardial lymph vessels and the cardiac lymphatics entering mediastinal lymph nodes can be visualized easily by injection of Evans blue into the myocardium.

Lymphatics of the Atria

Previous studies on the existence of a lymphatic system in the atrial walls yielded contradictory results. Today, however, there is general agreement that the atria possess a lymphatic system, which was also demonstrated for man by dye injection into the atrial myocardium.[9] It is less extensive than in the ventricles. The atrial lymphatic capillaries form a rather scanty network. It extends throughout the subepicardium of both atria. Early studies in dogs have also shown subendocardial lymphatics,[4] but this was not confirmed by subsequent studies in rabbits.[10] These different results are possibly due to differences in species or in the methods to study atrial lymphatics. In human atria, a superficial epicardial and a deeper subepicardial network have been demonstrated.[11]

Lymphatics of Cardiac Valves

Cardiac valves also have lymphatic vessels. This is very surprising because the valves are not supplied by blood vessels—and this raises the question the origin of the fluid—which they drain. This is not known. Nevertheless, lymphatic capillaries have been observed in the triscupid and the mitral valves of different species including man. It was not possible, however, to demonstrate lymphatics for the pulmonary and aortic valves. The lymphatics of the atrio-ventricular valves drain into the atrial lymphatic system.

Lymphatics of the Conduction System[11,12]

Lymphatic vessels have been described repeatedly in close vicinity to the conduction system of the heart. For the conduction system of the human heart, lymphatic capillary networks have been demonstrated in the sinoatrial node, in the atrioventricular node, and in the His bundle. The lymphatics from the sinoatrial node usually drain into the right cardiac main trunk, and those from the atrioventricular node and from the His bundle into the left main trunk.

Lympho-Venous Anastomoses

In previous animal studies,[13,14] lympho-venous anastomoses were not observed in physiological conditions, but they could be demonstrated following ligation of the cardiac lymphatics. Recently, however, lympho-venous anastomoses were demonstrated for papillary muscles of human hearts with intact lymphatic drainage.[15] Possibly, direct connections of the lymphatic and the coronary system are a normal feature of the human heart and may be of significance above all when cardiac lymph drainage is impeded.

Innervation of Lymphatics

The great lymph ducts and the lymphatics in various tissues are supplied by adrenergic, cholinergic, and peptidergic nerves.[16,17] Studies on the innervation of the cardiac lymphatic system, however, are not available to my knowledge.

Formation of Lymph

The formation of lymph comprises transvascular flow of fluid and solutes in the microcirculation and the uptake of the microvascular filtrate by the lymphatics. The principal mechanisms are the same for different tissues.

Microvascular Fluid Exchange[18-20]

The driving force of fluid exchange in the microvascular bed is the transvascular pressure difference which depends on the hydrostatic and colloid osmotic pressure of the blood and the interstitial fluid. The effective filtration pressure (Peff) is given by the microvascular blood pressure (Pmv), the interstitial fluid pressure (Pif), and plasma and interstitial fluid oncotic pressure (ppl, pif). The microvascular walls, however, are not perfectly impermeable to proteins. They do not represent an ideal semipermeable membrane and thus the oncotic pressure of the plasma proteins and the proteins in the interstitial fluid becomes not entirely effective across the vessel walls. This is taken into account by the reflection coefficient s. It gives the fraction of the maximal oncotic pressure across an ideal semipermeable membrane which becomes effective across the microvascular barrier (s = peff/pmax). s varies from 0-1 and depends on the radius of macromolecules and on the permeability of the microvasculature. p decreases with decreasing molecular radius and with increasing microvascular permeability.

Table 4.1. Lymph composition

Reflection coefficients		Prot	Alb	IgG	Fib	IgM	Ref
molecular radius (nm)			3.7	5.3	10.0	12.0	
reflection coefficient *s*							
skin, subcutis	(dog)	0.90	0.87	0.91	0.96	0.97	[21]
intestine	(cat)	0.83	0.80	——	0.89	0.95	[22]
heart	**(dog)**	**0.67**	**0.59**	**0.70**	——	**0.87**	[23]
lung	(sheep)	0.65	0.59	0.72	——	0.84	[24]
liver	(cat)	0.20	0.10	——	0.44	0.53	[25]

Prot = total protein; Alb = albumin; IgG, IgM = immunoglobulin G, M; Fib = fibrinogen

Furthermore, the transvascular fluid exchange depends on the permeability of the microvessels to water, i.e., the hydraulic conductivity $LH2O$, and on the area of exchange S. These two parameters are frequently combined and denoted as the *capillary filtration coefficient* CFC, which gives the volume filtered by 1mmHg of effective filtration pressure during 1 minute in 100 g (or 100 ml) of tissue. Thus, the microvascular filtration rate Jv is given by

$$Jv = LH_2O \bullet S \bullet [(Pmv\text{-}Pif)\text{-} s \bullet (ppl\text{-}pif)] = CFC \bullet Peff$$

When hydrostatic and oncotic forces are in balance, no transvascular net-displacement of fluid occurs. When the transvascular plasma oncotic pressure [the sum of transvascular hydrostatic and interstitial fluid oncotic pressures *(s • ppl > (Pmv-Pif)+ spif)* is high], then fluid will be reabsorbed from the extravascular compartment into the blood. Physiologically, the microvascular blood pressure exceeds the filtration opposing pressure *Po*, i.e., the sum of the transvascular oncotic pressure difference and the interstitial fluid pressure *(Pmv > Po = s • (ppl-pif) + Pif)*, and filtration takes place in the microcirculation. In the steady state, the filtrate is returned to the blood by the lymphatic system, i.e., the filtration rate in a given tissue equals the lymph flow *Qly* out of this tissue:

Jv = Qly.

Transvascular fluid net movement in the coronary circulation was shown by an arteriocoronary sinus difference in blood density Δr.[26] Δr was positive during physiological conditions indicating net filtration; it increased during elevation of coronary sinus pressure by partial coronary sinus occlusion according to a rise in net filtration. Negative Dr was observed during intermittent coronary sinus occlusion by a balloon corresponding to microvascular fluid reabsorption from the myocardium, probably because *Pmv* fell transiently below *Po* during deflation of the balloon.

The Microvascular Blood Pressure (Pmv)

The blood pressure in the microcirculation was analyzed extensively in various tissues and species including capillary blood pressure in human skin.[27] Studies on the blood pressure in the coronary microcirculation in the beating heart are limited due to technical difficulties. In cat left and in rabbit right ventricular epicardial arterioles of about 100 μm in diameter pressures, of 50-60% of aortic pressures were observed,[28,29] and a pressure of about 10% of aortic pressure was noted in similar-sized epicardial venules of feline left ventricles were.[28]

Changes in arterial pressure have only little effects on the pressure in exchange vessels[30,31] reflecting the myogenic autoregulation. Changes in venous pressure, however, are transmitted by about 85% to the microvascular pressure in skin and muscle.[27,32] Therefore, small increases in venous pressure are very effective in enhancing *Peff* and thus microvascular filtration and lymph flow. Measurements of the transmission of changes in coronary venous pressure on *Peff* in the myocardium are not available, but it is well known that elevation of coronary sinus pressure is accompanied by a many-fold increase in cardiac lymph flow.[23,33-35]

The Interstitial Fluid Pressure (Pif)

Today, there is no doubt that the interstitial fluid pressure is subatmospheric in some tissues.[18] For the canine heart, however, a left ventricular end-diastolic interstitial fluid pressure of +15 mm Hg has been reported repeatedly.[33,34,36,37] Myocardial *Pif* increases during systole in parallel with the ventricular pressure.[33,38] Possibly there exists a transmural gradient of *Pif*,[38] as well documented for the intramyocardial solid tissue pressure,[38] with a systolic *Pif* of about 50% of left ventricular pressure in the subepicardium and equal to ventricular pressure in the subendocardium.[38] Other investigators,[33] however, have described uniform transmural distribution of the interstitial fluid pressure. That would indicate hydraulic continuity of the interstitial fluid and equilibrium of the interstitial fluid pressure during the cardiac cycle.[33] In consequence of the pulsatile nature of the interstitial fluid pressure, effective filtration pressure and microvascular filtration should also vary with the cardiac cycle being maximal at the end of diastole, and possibly, no filtration occurs during systole.

The interstitial fluid pressure of right ventricular myocardium was not yet determined to my knowledge. Systolic right ventricular *Pif* can be assumed to be lower than left ventricular *Pif* according to the differences in the developed pressure during contraction. Enddiastolic right ventricular *Pif*, however, may be as high as in the left ventricular wall, because end-diastolic *Pif* reflects properties of the tissue but not the ventricular pressure.

Interstitial fluid pressure opposes microvascular filtration and a negative feedback mechanism can be assumed: increased filtration enhances interstitial fluid and thus interstitial fluid pressure, which then in turn reduces filtration. Indeed, this hypothesis got support recently from animal experiments indicating a reduced microvascular filtration rate when myocardial *Pif* was elevated by obstruction of the cardiac lymphatic drainage.[37]

The Colloid Osmotic Pressure (p)

The colloid osmotic pressure of plasma and interstitial fluid does not correlate linearly with the protein concentration C ($g \bullet d\text{-}1$), but increases steeper than protein concentration. The relation was empirically determined by a number of investigators and is well described by

$$p = 2.1\ C + 0.16\ C2 + 0.009\ C3\ (C\ in\ g \bullet dl\text{-}1,\ p\ in\ mm\ Hg)^{39}$$

Colloid osmotic pressure, however, not only depends on total protein concentration but also on the protein pattern. Appropriate corrections for pathological albumin to globulin ratios are available in the literature.[40]

The colloid osmotic pressure of interstitial fluid is significantly lower than that of plasma. It is reflected by the lymph, but lymph colloid osmotic pressure is probably different from interstitial fluid p. The difference in p of plasma and prenodal lymph in normal canine hearts during baseline conditions has been found to be about 6 mm Hg.[33] Increased microvascular filtration during elevated coronary sinus pressure increased this difference which in turn reduced effective filtration pressure thus counteracting filtration.[33]

The Capillary Filtration Coefficient CFC (ml • min-1 • mmHg-1 • 100g-1)

As mentioned above, the *CFC* reflects the permeability to water and the filtering area of the microcirculation. Data of cardiac *CFC* in man are not available. In isolated, crystalloid perfused rabbit hearts, a *CFC* of 0.35 has been determined.[41] This value is very high as compared to 0.030 for rat skeletal muscle.[42] The difference can be attributed in part to a somewhat higher permeability of exchange vessels in the heart than in skeletal muscle, but it is undoubtedly related to the generally accepted 5-10 fold capillary surface area in myocardium as compared to skeletal muscle.[28,43]

Microvascular Exchange of Solutes (Js)[18,19,44]

The principal mechanisms of transvascular solute exchange are diffusion, convection (= solvent drag), and vesicular transport. Small molecules move across the microvascular barrier almost exclusively by diffusion. The transvascular transport of macromolecules is described by

$$Js = PS \bullet DC + Jv \bullet (1\text{-}s) \bullet Cpl + Qv \bullet a \bullet DC$$

[PS • DC] denotes diffusion, which depends on the microvascular permeability *P*, the available surface area *S* , and the transvascular concentration difference *DC* for a given molecule. Permeability to macromolecules varies greatly for different organs with the "tightest" microvessels in the brain, and the most permeable exchange vessels in territories with discontinuous capillaries or sinusoids, e.g., the liver. A relative estimate of the permeability is given by the reflection coefficient *s* (see above). Microvascular solute permeability (and hydraulic conductivity), however, is not uniform along the microvessels, but increases from the arteriolar to the venous end.[45,46] And it is generally accepted that microvascular filtration takes place above all in the postcapillary venules. Furthermore, the transvascular transport of similar-sized proteins depends on their electrical charge. Less negatively or more positively charged molecules penetrate the microvascular barrier better.[44] This phenomenon is related to negative charges in the glycolcalyx of the basal membrane.[44] The permeability of cardiac microvessels to small molecules is greater than this in skeletal muscle.[43] Similar permeability to albumin, however, has been found in isolated venules from hearts and skeletal muscles.[47] The permeability-surface product PS varies with changes in coronary blood flow[48-50] in consequence of capillary recruitment and derecruitment, i.e., the positive correlation of *PS* and coronary perfusion reflects changes in surface area. On the other hand, cardiac microvascular permeability to macromolecules is significantly increased following transient ischemia as evidenced, for example, by the myocardial accumulation of radiolabeled protein[51] or by the leakage of fluorescent dextran, which can be observed by in vivo microscopy.[52]

[Jv • (1-s) • Cpl] gives the amount of solute transport by convection across the microvascular wall, i.e., how many solutes are carried by the volume flow. Solute concentration in the filtrate decreases with increasing molecular size, which is taken into account by the solvent drag coefficient *(1-s)*, and it also decreases with increasing filtration, because the movement of solutes across the microvascular wall is impeded as compared to plasma water. These features are reflected by the lymph to plasma ratio *Cly/Cpl* of protein concentration as illustrated by the following data[23]:

Jv = Qly (μl • min⁻¹)   Cly/Cpl

molecular radius (nm)		total protein	albumin	IgG	IgM
			3.7	5.3	12.0
	6	0.78	—	—	—
	38	0.48	—	—	—
	118	0.33	0.41	0.30	0.13

[Qv • α • ΔC] describes the transvascular solute transport by vesicles. The transported amount depends on the vesicular volume transport *Qv*, the transvascular concentration difference ΔC of the transported solutes, and the partition coefficient α of the molecules between plasma and vesicle. However, the quantity and physiological significance of this mechanism is uncertain. Possibly, transcytosis is of minor importance for the transvascular transport of plasma proteins, but may be a highly selective transport mechanism e.g., for lipoproteins or macromolecular hormones.[44]

The contribution of diffusion (+ transcytosis) and convection to transvascular protein transport depends on the transvascular volume flow. The convective fraction increases with increasing filtration.[47,53,54] In isolated coronary venules, convective transport of albumin rose from < 40% at a net filtration pressure of 3-4 mmHg to nearly 70% at 11 mm Hg.[47]

Uptake of the Microvascular Filtrate by the Lymphatic Capillaries

The interstitial fluid may be assumed to flow due to a hydrostatic pressure gradient from the interstitial space with a high fluid pressure into the terminal lymphatics with a lower intravascular pressure. The pressure in cardiac terminal lymphatics is not known. The uptake of the interstitial fluid by the terminal lymphatics is readily explained, however, by their structure and the periodic cardiac contraction: muscular contraction compresses the terminal lymphatics and pushes the lymph centripetally, whereas closure of the interendothelial clefts of the terminal lymphatics prevents backflow of the lymph into the interstitium; during muscular relaxation, the interendothelial clefts are pulled open by the anchoring filaments and interstitial fluid is sucked into the lymphatic capillaries.[55] Furthermore, the endothelial cells of the terminal lymphatics in the heart show plasmalemmal vesicles,[56] which may additionally contribute to the lymphatic uptake of interstitial fluid and proteins.

The Cardiac Lymph

Flow and composition of cardiac lymph depend not only on the effective filtration pressure and the sieving properties of the coronary microcirculation. Cardiac lymph drainage is accomplished by the combined action of several propulsive forces and cardiac lymph carries as well as filtered plasma proteins, macromolecules of the interstitial matrix, and proteins of intracellular origin.

Driving Forces of Cardiac Lymph Flow

Cardiac lymph is propelled from the subendocardial plexus to the cardiac lymph node by several factors. The significance of each for the outflow of lymph from the myocardium is different, however.

Myocardial Contractions

The main force of cardiac lymph propulsion is undoubtedly the myocardial contraction. During systole, the myocardium is squeezed and the lymph is propelled to the superficial lymphatic trunks and forced to flow away from the heart. Accordingly, recent studies have shown a significant decrease in cardiac lymph flow following cardiac arrest during cardiopulmonary bypass.[57,58] During cardiac relaxation, the epicardial surface of the heart and the superficial lymphatic trunks are pressed against the pericardium and lymph is propelled away from the heart due to the valves of the lymphatic vessels. The subendo- to subepicardial gradient of intramyocardial pressure, which is present at least during systole, can be assumed also to promote lymph flow within the lymphatic capillary network of the ventricular wall.

Intrinsic Contractions of Lymphatics

Intrinsic contractions of collecting lymphatics and lymphatic trunks represent a very important basic mechanism of lymphatic transport. These contractions and the lymphatic valves maintain a centripetal lymph flow in different tissues and the thoracic duct.[59-62] The pumping activity of the lymphatics is stimulated by increased filling or distension,[61-65] which occurs with rising interstitial volume. Thus, the transport of lymph is coupled to lymph formation by a positive feed-back mechanism. Furthermore, the intrinsic contractions are affected by vasoactive drugs with respect to the rate (chronotropy) and the force (inotropy) of contraction. For example, (compiled from[18,66,67]):

- positive chronotropic action:
  bradykinin > 5-HT > PGF-2a > noradrenaline > histamin (H-1)
  5-HT = 5-hydroxytryptamine; PGF-2a = prostaglandin F-2a;
- negative chronotropic action: VIP > ANP > isoproterenol > histamine (H-2)
  SVIP = vasoactive intestinal peptide; ANP = atrial natriuretic peptide

- inotropy is increased by noradrenaline and reduced by ANP,
- acetylcholine decreases rate and force of contractions via nitric oxide
- reactive oxygen metabolites as produced in ischemia-reperfusion reduce contraction rate, ejection fraction, and stroke volume of lymphatics

The importance of intrinsic contractions of lymphatics for the lymph drainage of the heart, however, has not been investigated yet.

Respiration

Respiration is presumed to support cardiac lymph flow.[3] The respiratory changes in intrathoracic pressure, however, are only of minor significance for thoracic duct lymph flow.[68] Probably this applies also to cardiac lymphatic drainage.

Vis a tergo

Usually, the *vis a tergo*, i.e., the interstitial pressure, which is built up by the microvascular filtration, is considered to contribute of lymph propulsion. Accordingly, a linear increase in cardiac lymph flow has been observed with increasing interstitial fluid pressure during elevated microvascular filtration.[33]

Alternatively, it has been suggested that lymph flow is not a function of interstitial fluid pressure but of interstitial fluid volume,[18] because lymphatic drainage has been found to correlate closely with the volume but not with the fluid pressure of the interstitial space.[69,70] An increase in lymph flow in consequence to an enlarged interstitial volume is explained by the above-mentioned stimulation of the intrinsic pumping activity of the lymphatics with increased filling. A recent study[35] has demonstrated a simultaneous increase in lymph driving pressure and lymph flow in the prenodal major left cardiac lymph trunk from 18.5-47.3 mm Hg and from 36-245 μl/min, respectively. Whether or not the intrinsic pumping activity of the lymphatics was activated in these experiments, however, has been not presented.

Cardiac lymph flow at baseline lymph production is nearly abolished in arrested hearts during cardiopulmonary bypass[57,58] as mentioned above. The remaining cardiac lymph drainage, < 30% of baseline, should be maintained by the vis a tergo and intrinsic contractions of lymphatics. These driving forces may be more important, however, when lymph formation is increased.

The Amount of Cardiac Lymph Flow

Information on the amount of lymph draining the whole heart are limited. The available data were obtained in dogs[71-77] and range from 0.5-5.5 ml/h^{-1}. Interestingly, Miller[75] did not found a correlation between cardiac lymph flow and body weight of the studied dogs (16-24 kg). It seems unlikely, however, that this applies generally although cardiac lymph flow certainly shows a great variability. Possibly, the differences in weight and the number of animals were to small too see the expected positive relation.

As already described, cardiac lymph flow shows a many-fold increase when the coronary sinus pressure is elevated,[23,33-35,78] which can be attributed to a rise in microvascular filtration pressure. Increasing coronary perfusion pressure by partial aortic occlusion or intravenous infusion of phenylephrine or angiotensin II was also reported to elevate cardiac lymph flow as a consequence of an enhanced microvascular blood pressure.[35,76] Relating the increase in lymph flow to the change in pressure shows a much steeper increase with coronary sinus than with arterial pressure, which reflects the different transmission of changes in venous and arterial pressure on microvascular pressure (see above).

An increase in cardiac lymph flow was observed following short term systemic hypoxia.[72] This was related to an enlarged microvascular filtration area by capillary recruitment, but not to a disturbance of microvascular permeability by the reduced oxygen content of the blood. On the other hand, a decrease in cardiac lymph flow was reported during occlusion of the left circumflex coronary artery up to 75 min,[74,79] which is easily explained by a reduction of the filtering surface. During coronary reperfusion cardiac lymph flow increased transiently above the control level.[74,79] This can be attributed to several factors. During the reactive hyperemia following release of coronary occlusion an increased filtration surface and microvascular blood pressure might be assumed. The microvascular permeability is increased following ischemia as mentioned above[51,52] and, thus, the reflection coefficient for plasma proteins is reduced.[23] Consequently, effective filtration pressure is increased because the effective transvascular colloid osmotic pressure difference is reduced.

The Composition of Cardiac Lymph

The concentration of small molecules in the lymph is similar to that in plasma. Small differences are explained by a Donnan-Gibbs distribution in consequence of the difference in intra- and extravascular protein concentration. The plasma proteins, however, are significantly less concentrated in cardiac lymph than in plasma as reflected by the lymph to plasma ratio Cly/Cpl < 1. Cly and thus Cly/Cpl decreases with increasing molecular radius or molecular weight (see above). Cly/Cpl of total plasma proteins is about 0.80 and decreases with increasing lymph production[23,33-35,37,78] as already mentioned, which reflects the sieving properties of the microvascular exchange vessels.

In contrast to plasma proteins, cellular proteins or interstitial macromolecules are more concentrated in cardiac lymph than in plasma and *Cly/Cpl* > 1. For example, the hyaluronan concentration in cardiac lymph has been found to be 20-30 times of the plasma concentration.[57] Lymph to plasma ratios of 6-8 have been reported for the concentration of cellular enzymes (CK, GOT, LHD, MDH) and these *Cly/Cpl* did increase 10-fold following myocardial ischemia.[80,81]

The protein concentration of lymph changes during passage in the lymphatic system. There has been demonstrated an increase from terminal lymphatics to collecting channels, and from prenodal to postnodal lymph.[82-84] The increase in lymph protein concentration during lymph node passage was shown to be due to fluid reabsorption by the plasma colloid osmotic pressure.[85]

Effects of Imbalanced Formation and Drainage of Cardiac Lymph

An imbalance of lymph formation and drainage is given by an impeded lymph flow at normal lymph formation or by an increased microvascular filtration, which exceeds the drainage capacity of the lymphatic system. Most studies on the functional significance of cardiac lymphatic drainage were performed by obstruction of the cardiac lymphatics. An inadequate cardiac lymph flow can be assumed to affect both myocardial structure and function.

Histopathology

Impaired cardiac lymph drainage inevitably causes myocardial edema as demonstrated by an increase in water content.[34,85] Histological changes include interstitial edema, swelling of myofibrils, myofibrillar derangement, and mitochondrial injury.[14,77,87-89] Additionally, there were described subendocardial and myocardial focal hemorrhages following cardiac lymphatic obstruction.[89,90] But these were observed only occasionally and have not been confirmed in other studies.[77,91] It is conceivable that the ultrastructural changes following insufficient cardiac lymph drainage reduce myocardial performance.

Chronic interstitial edema is well known to cause interstitial fibrosis.[92] Accordingly, the left ventricular myocardial collagen concentration was significantly higher in dogs with chronic myocardial edema in response to pulmonary artery banding (see below) than in normal dogs.[34] With prolonged cardiac lymphatic obstruction, thickening of the endocardium with increased elastic and fibrous tissue,[90,93,94] subendocardial fibrosis and thickened leaflets of the atrioventricular valves[77,91] were observed. These fibrotic changes in consequence of chronically impaired cardiac lymph drainage might also adversely affect cardiac function.

The coronary arteries were also reported to be affected by cardiac lymphatic obstruction.[95] Subendothelial edema, interstitial and intracellular edema of the tunica media, degeneration of vascular smooth muscle cells, swelling of the adventitial space, and an increased content of collagen have been observed.[95] Furthermore, the development of arterio-venous shunts has been described.[95] These observations suggest that an inadequate cardiac lymph drainage contributes to the development and progression of coronary artery disease.

Coronary Blood Flow

Cardiac lymphatic obstruction may be assumed to interfere with myocardial blood flow due to an increase in interstitial pressure, which then enhances coronary flow resistance. Indeed, when cardiac lymphatic outflow pressure was elevated so that lymph flow was abolished, interstitial fluid pressure rose from 15.0-27.5 mm Hg.[37] Baseline coronary blood flow, however, was not significantly affected following cardiac lymphatic obstruction, whereas reactive hyperemia and adenosine induced vasodilation were reduced.[95,96] Obviously, blood flow to the edematous myocardium was maintained on the expense of the coronary flow reserve. Consequently, an increased myocardial oxygen demand should not be met adequately by a rise in blood flow and myocardial ischemia would result.

Electrocardiogram (ECG)

As a consequence to cardiac lymphatic obstruction, alterations have been reported in ECG resembling those observed in "...myocardial hypoxemia..." or in "...grave anoxemia...".[97] Similarly, elevated ST- and negative T-segments have been described in dogs.[98] These pathological changes were attributed to the myocardial dilatation by the edema. Furthermore, cardiac arrhythmias have been reported similar to those found in sick sinus syndrome in man.[87] Other investigators, however, did not observe changes in ECG following interruption of the cardiac lymph drainage.[99,100]

Cardiac Performance

The histological effects of acute and chronic obstruction of the cardiac lymphatic system or of an imbalance of cardiac lymph formation and drainage should impair cardiac performance as mentioned above. Indeed, this has been confirmed repeatedly in the last years.

One of the earlier investigations on the functional importance of intact cardiac lymphatic drainage studied the cardiac output following cardiac lymphatic obstruction in isolated rat hearts.[88] Cardiac output decreased by 33% within 90 min in the lymphostatic hearts, whereas it remained stable in hearts with freely draining lymph. The reduction in cardiac function following lymphatic obstruction was not related to coronary perfusion, which was not different in lymph obstructed and control hearts and did not change during the experiment.

In anaesthetized dogs, interruption of the cardiac lymph drainage by ligation of the epicardial lymphatics, the afferent and efferent lymphatics of the pretracheal and cardiac lymph nodes and of the thoracic duct caused myocardial edema within 3 hours.[86] Simultaneously, the left ventricular function assessed by the preload recruitable stroke work (PRSW) was impaired significantly.[86]

In another study in dogs,[34] cardiac lymph production was promoted by elevation of the coronary sinus pressure and cardiac lymph drainage was almost abolished by elevating the superior vena caval pressure. This maneuver produced 35% increase in myocardial extravascular fluid within 3 hours and a 40% reduction in cardiac output. The impaired myocardial performance was not related to decreased coronary artery blood flow, which was maintained during increased coronary sinus pressure. Thus, the impaired myocardial function probably resulted from the myocardial edema in consequence to an imbalance of lymph formation and drainage.

Enhanced myocardial water content and depressed left ventricular performance was also observed in dogs with chronic elevation of right heart pressure by pulmonary artery banding.[34] In this model, the enhanced right heart pressure affected both left ventricular microvascular filtration and cardiac lymph drainage: coronary sinus and left ventricular microvascular pressure was increased, which promoted cardiac lymph formation, and superior vena caval pressure was elevated, which impeded cardiac lymph drainage. Again, an imbalance of lymph formation and flow was present causing edema and impaired left ventricular function.

Experiments with cardiopulmonary bypass and cardiac arrest[57,58] showed a reduction of cardiac lymph flow to < 30% of baseline during cardiac arrest and myocardial edema developed. Cardiac performance (assessed by PRSW) was significantly impaired after bypass and the depression was closely related to the myocardial water content.

Another experimental study[101] has investigated the effect of increasing coronary sinus pressure and cardiac microvascular permeability on left ventricular dp/dtmax. These interventions caused myocardial edema and a change in dp/dtmax with time, which was closely related to the amount of edema, which had accumulated during the 3 hour experimental period. Cardiac lymphatic drainage was not experimentally impeded in these experiments. Nevertheless, the experimental interventions caused an imbalance of lymph formation and flow as shown by the development of myocardial edema.

As described above, intermittent coronary sinus occlusion (ICSO) was reported to give rise to fluid reabsorption from the myocardium at least during deflation of the coronary sinus balloon.[26] Possibly, reduction of myocardial edema contributes to the functional improvement of ischemic myocardium by ICSO.[102] The effect of ICSO on myocardial interstitial fluid volume, however, remains to be established.

In summary, the studies demonstrate the importance of an adequate drainage of cardiac lymph and normal myocardial water content for the performance of the heart. Acute and chronic cardiac edema impairs cardiac function. Edema develops as a consequence of an imbalance of the formation and drainage of lymph. This occurs when a high venous pressure promotes microvascular filtration and impedes lymph flow, e.g., in congestive heart failure, in pulmonary hypertension, and after a Fontan operation. The cardiac edema and the resulting histological changes including fibrosis possibly contribute to the cardiac dysfunction.

References

1. Rusznyak I, Földi M, Szabo G. Lymphologie. Physiologie und Pathologie der Lymphgefässe und des Lymphkreislaufs. G. Fischer, Stuttgart. 1969.
2. Blair DM. The lymphatics of the heart: A Hunterian memorandum. Glasgow Med J 1925; 103:364-367.
3. Miller AJ. Lymphatics of the heart. New York: Raven Press, 1982.
4. Aagaard OC. Les vaisseaux lymphatique du coeur chez l'homme et chez quelques mammiferes: Levin and Munksgaard, Copenhagen 1924.
5. Patek PR. The morphology of the lymphatics of the mammalian heart. Am J Anat 1939; 64:203-249.
6. Drinker CK, Warren MF, Maurer FW, McCarrell JD. The flow, pressure, and composition of cardiac lymph. Am J Physiol 1940; 130:43-55.
7. Shimada T, Morita T, Oya M, Kitamura H. Morphological studies of the cardiac lymphatic system. Arch Histol Cytol 1990; 53 (suppl):115-126.
8. Leak LV. The structure of lymphatic capillaries in Lymph formation. Fed Proc 1976; 35:1863-1871.

9. Servelle M, Andrieux J, Cornu C, deLoche A, Nussaume O. Les lymphatiques du coeur (injections perioperatoires). Arch Mal Coeur 1967; 60:89-106.
10. Marchetti C, Poggi P, Calligaro A, Casasco A. Lymph vessels of the rabbit heart: Distribution and fine structure in atria. Lymphology 1986; 19:33-37.
11. Eliskova M, Eliska O. Light microscopy of the lymphatics of the human atrial wall and lymphatic drainage of the supraventricular pacemaker. Int Angiol 1989; 8:1-6.
12. Eliska O, Eliskova M. Lymphatic drainage of the ventricular conduction system in man and in dog. Acta Anat Basel 1980; 107:205-213.
13. Eliska O, Eliskova M. Contribution to the solution of the question of lympho-venous anastomoses in heart of dog. Lymphology 1975; 8:11-15.
14. Gavrish AS. Morphological changes in the heart accompanying the lymph flow disturbance. Cor Vasa 1981; 23:366-374.
15. Eliskova M, Oldrich E. How lymph is drained away from the human papillary muscle: Anatomical conditions. Cardiology 1992; 81 371-377.
16. Hukkanen M, Konttinen YT, Terenghi G, Polak JM. Peptide-containing innervation of rat femoral lymphatic vessels. Microvasc Res 1992; 43:7-19.
17. McHale NG. Lymphatic innervation. Blood Vessels 1990; 27:127-136.
18. Aukland K, Reed RK. Interstitial-lymphatic mechanisms in the control of extracellular fluid volume. Physiol Rev 1993; 73:1-78.
19. Renkin EM. Cellular and intercellular transport pathways in exchange vessels. Am Rev Respir Dis 1992; 73:1-78.
20. Levick JR. Fluid exchange across endothelium. Int J Microcirc 1997; 17:241-247.
21. Perry MA, Navia CA, Granger DN, Parker JC, Taylor AE. Calculation of equivalent pore radii in dog hindpaw capillaries using endogenous lymph and plasma proteins. Microvasc Res 1983; 26:250-253.
22. Mortillaro NA, Taylor AE. Microvascular permeability to endogenous plasma proteins in the jejunum. Am J Physiol 1990; 258:H1650-H1654.
23. Pilati CF. Macromolecular transport in canine coronary microvasculature. Am J Physiol 1990; 258:H748-H753.
24. Smith L, Andreasson S, Berglund S, Rippe B, Risberg B. Oleic acid reduces pulmonary microvascular sieving capacity in sheep. J Appl Physiol 1989; 66:2866-2872.
25. Granger DN, Miller T, Allen R, Parker RE, Parker JC, Taylor AE. Permselectivity of the liver blood-lymph barrier to endogenous macromolecules. Gastroenterology 1979; 77:103-109.
26. Kenner T, Moser M, Mohl W. Arteriovenous difference of the blood density in the coronary circulation. J Biomech Eng 1985; 107:34-40.
27. Mahy IR, Tooke JE, Shore AC. Capillary pressure during and after incremental venous pressure elevation in man. J Physiol Lond 1995; 485:213-219.
28. Chilian WM, Eastham CL, Layne SM, Marcus ML. Small vessel phenomena in the coronary microcirculation: Phasic intramyocardial perfusion and coronary micro- vascular dynamics. Prog Cardiovasc Dis 1988; 31:17-38.
29. Nellis SH, Liedtke AJ, Whitesell L. Small coronary vessel pressure and diameter in an intact beating rabbit heart using fixed-position and free-motion techniques. Circ Res 1981; 48:342-353.
30. Ekelund U, Björnberg J, Grande PO, Albert U, Mellander S. Myogenic vascular regulation in skeletal muscle in vivo is not dependent of endothelium-derived nitric oxide. Acta Physiol Scand 1992; 144:199-207.
31. Shore AC, Sandeman DD, Tooke JE. Effect of an increase in systemic blood pressure on nailfold capillary pressure in humans. Am J Physiol 1993; 265:H820-H8239.
32. Diana JN, Shadur C. Effect of arterial and venous pressure on capillary pressure and vascular volume. Am J Physiol 1973; 225:637-650.
33. Laine GA, Granger HJ. Microvascular, interstitial, and lymphatic interactions in normal heart. Am J Physiol 1985; 249:H834-H842.
34. Laine GA, Allen SJ. Left ventricular myocardial edema. Lymph flow, interstitial fibrosis, and cardiac function. Circ Res 1991; 68:1713-1721.

35. Mehlhorn U, Davis KL, Laine GA, Allen SJ, Geissler HJ, Adams DL. Myocardial fluid balance in acute hypertension. Microcirculation 1996; 3:371-378.
36. Rosenkranz ER, Utley JR, Menninger JF, Dembitsky WP, Hargens AR, Peters RM. Interstitial fluid pressure changes during cardiopulmonary bypass. Ann Thorac Surg 1980; 30:536-542.
37. Stewart RH, Rohn DA, Mehlhorn U, Davis KL, Allen SJ, Laine GA. Regulation of microvascular filtration in the myocardium by interstitial fluid pressure. Am J Physiol 1996; 271:R1465-R1469.
38. Rabbany SY, Kresh YJ, Noordergraaf A. Differentiation of intramyocardial fluid pressure from fiber stress. Technol Health Care 1997; 5:145-157.
39. Landis EM, Pappenheimer JR. Exchange of substances through the capillary walls. In: Handbook of Physiology, Vol II, Sect 2, Circulation, 1963; 961-1034.
40. Nitta S, Ohnuki T, Ohkuda K, Nakada T, Staub NC. The corrected protein equation to estimate plasma colloid osmotic pressure and its development on a nomogram. Tohoku J Exp Med 1981; 135:43-49.
41. Vargas F, Johnson JA. An estimate of reflection coefficients of rabbit heart capillaries. J Gen Physiol 1964; 47:667-877.
42. Sexton WL, Poole DC, Mathieu-Costello O. Microcirculatory structure-function relationships in skeletal muscle of diabetic rats. Am J Physiol 1994; 266:H1502-H1511.
43. Parker JC, Perry MA, Taylor AE. Permeability of the microvascular barrier. In: Edema. Edts.: Staub NC, Taylor AE. Raven Press, New York 1984; 143-187.
44. Rippe B, Haraldsson B. Transport of macromolecules across microvascular walls: The two-pore theory. Physiol Rev 1994; 74:163-219.
45. Hauck G. Zur Frage der Existenz eines "Gradient of Vascular Permeability" an der Endstrombahn. Arch Kreislaufforsch 1969; 59:197-227.
46. Qiao RL, Bhattacharya J. Segmentel barriere properties of the pulmonary microvascular bed. J Appl Physiol 1991; 71:2152-2129.
47. Yuan Y, Chilian WM, Granger HJ, Zawieja DC. Permeability to albumin in isolated coronary venules. Am J Physiol 1993; 265:H543-H552.
48. Caldwell JH, Martin GV, Raymond GM, Bassingthwaighte JB. Regional myocardial blood flow and capillary permeability surface area products are nearly proportional. Am J Physiol 1994; 267:H654-H666.
49. Cousineau DF, Goresky CA, Rose CP, Simard A, Schwab AJ. Effects of flow, perfusion pressure, and oxygen consumption on capillary exchange. J Appl Physiol 1995; 78:1350-1359.
50. Harris TR, Gervin CA, Burks D, Custer P. Effects of coronary flow reduction on capillary-myocardial exchange in dogs. Am J Physiol 1978; 234:H679-H689.
51. Horwitz LD, Kaufmann D, Kong Y. An antibody to leukocyte integrins attenuates coronary vascular injury due to ischemia and reperfusion in dogs. Am J Physiol 1997; 272:H618-H624.
52. Tillmanns H, Neumann FJ, Tiefenbacher C, Dorigo O, Parekh N, Waas W, Zimmermann R, Steinhausen M, Kuebler W. Activation of neutrophils in the microvasculature of the ischaemic and reperfused myocardium. Eur Heart J 1993; 14 Suppl I:82-86.
53. Renkin EM, Joyner WL, Sloop CH, Watson PD. Influence of pressure on plasma-lymph transport in the dog paw: Convective and dissapative mechanisms. Microvasc Res 1977; 14:191-204.
54. Watson PD, Wolf MB. Transport parameter estimation from lymph measurements and the Patlak equation. Am J Physiol 1992; 262:H293-H298.
55. Schmid-Schönbein GW. Microlymphatics and lymph flow. Physiol Rev 1990; 70:987-1028.
56. Boucher Y, Roberge S, Roy PE. Ultrastructural comparative study on lymphatic capillaries of the subendocardium, myocardium, and subepicardium of the heart left ventricle. Microvasc Res 1985; 29:305-319.
57. Mehlhorn U, Davis KL, Burke EJ, Adams D, Laine GA, Allen SJ. Impact of cardiopulmonary bypass and cardioplegic arrest on myocardial lymphatic function. Am J Physiol 1995; 268:H178-H183.
58. Mehlhorn U, Allen SJ, Adams DL, Davis KL, Gogola GR, de-Vivie ER, Laine GA. Normothermic continuous antegrade blood cardioplegia does not prevent myocardial edema and cardiac dysfunction. Circulation 1995; 92:1940-1946.

59. Mislin H. Die Motorik der Lymphgefässe und die Regulation der Lymphherzen. In: Handbuch der allgemeinen Pathologie. Springer, Berlin-Heidelberg-NewYork 1972; Vol III/6:219-238.
60. Olszewski WL, Engeset A. Intrinsic contractility of prenodal lymph vessels and lymph flow in human leg. Am J Physiol 1980; 239:H775-H783.
61. Reddy NP, Staub NC. Intrinsic propulsive activity of thoracic duct perfused in anaesthetized dogs. Microvasc Res 1981; 21:183-192.
62. Hargens AR, Zweifach BW. Contractile stimuli in collecting lymph vessels. Am J Physiol 1977; 233:H57-H65.
63. Benoit JN, Zawieja DC, Goodman AH, Granger HJ. Characterization of intact mesenteric lymphatic pump and its responsiveness to edemagenic stress. Am J Physiol 1989; 257:H2059-H2069.
64. McHale NG, Roddie IC. The effect of transmural pressure on pumping activity in isolated bovine lymphatic vessels. J Physiol Lond 1976; 261:255-269.
65. Ohhashi T, Azuma T, Sakaguchi M. Active and passive mechanical characteristics of bovine mesenteric lymphatics. Am J Physiol 1980; 239:H88-H95.
66. Ohhashi T, Yokoyama S. Nitric oxide and the lymph system. Jap J Physiol 1994; 44:327-342.
67. Greiner ST, Davis KL, Zawieja DC. Effects of reactive oxygen metabolites on lymphatic pumping function. In Interstitium, connective tissue and lymphatics. Reed RK, McHale NG, Bert JL, Winlove CP, Laine GA (eds.). Portland Press, London 1995; 191-203.
68. Schad H, Folwaczny H, Brechtelsbauer H, Birkenfeld G. The significance of respiration for thoracic duct flow in relation to other driving forces of lymph flow. Pflügers Arch 1978; 378:121-126.
69. Aarli V, Reed RK, Aukland K. Effect of longstanding venous stasis and hypoproteinemia on lymph flow in the rat tail. Acta Physiol Scand 1991; 142:1-9.
70. Pippard CJ, Roddie IC. Lymph flow in sheep limbs during local exposure to subatmospheric pressure. J Physiol Lond 1989; 419:45-57.
71. Fairman RP, Glauser FL, Falls R. Increases in lung lymph and albumin clearance with ethchlorvynol. J Appl Physiol 1981; 50:1151-115.
72. Fjeld MB, Kluge TH, Stokke KT, Skrede S. The effect of generalized hypoxia upon flow and composition of cardiac lymph in the dog. 1976; 6:255-259.
73. Leeds S, Uhley HN, Sampson JJ, Friedman M. The cardiac lymphatics after ligation of the coronary sinus. Proc Soc Exp Biol Med 1970; 135:59-62.
74. Michael LH, Lewis RM, Brandon TA, Entman ML. Cardiac lymph flow in conscious dogs. Am J Physiol 1979; 237:H311-H317.
75. Miller AJ. The lymphatics of the heart. Arch Int Med 1963; 112:501-511.
76. Reddy HK, Sigusch H, Zhou G, Tyagi SC, Janicki JS, Weber KT. Coronary vascular hyperpermeability and angiotensin II. J Lab Clin Med 1995; 126:307-315.
77. Ullal SR. Cardiac lymph and lymphatics. Experimental observations and clinical significance. Ann Roy Coll Surg Engl 1972; 51:282-298.
78. Laine GA. Microvascular changes in the heart during chronic arterial hypertension. Circ Res 1988; 62:953-960.
79. Michael LH, Hunt JR, Weilbaecher D, Perryman MB, Roberts R, Lewis RM, Entman ML. Creatine kinase and phosphorylase in cardiac lymph: Coronary occlusion and reperfusion. Am J Physiol 1985; 248:H350-H359.
80. Spieckermann PG, Nordbeck H, Knoll D, Kohl FV, Sakai K, Bretschneider HJ. Bedeutung der Herzlymphe für den Enzymtransport ins Blut beim Myokardinfarkt. Dtsch Med Wochenschr 1974; 99:1143-1144.
81. Szabo G, Magyar Z, Reffy A. Lymphatic transport of enzyme after experimental myocardial infarction. Lymphology 1974; 7:37-44.
82. Hargens AR, Zweifach BW. Transport between blood and peripheral lymph in intestine. Microvasc Res 1976; 11:89-101.
83. Knox P, Pflug JJ. The effect of the canine popliteal node on the composition of lymph. J Physiol London 1983; 345:1-14.
84. Quin JW, Shannon AD. The effect of anaestesia and surgery on lymph flow, protein and leukocyte concentration in lymph of the sheep. Lymphology 1975; 8:126-135.

85. Adair TH, Moffat DS, Paulsen AW, Guyton AC. Quantitation of changes in lymph protein concentration during lymph node transit. Am J Physiol 1982; 243:H351-H359.

86. Ludwig LL, Schertel ER, Pratt JW, McClure DE, Ying AJ, Heck CF, Myerowitz PD. Impairment of left ventricular function by acute cardiac lymphatic obstruction. Cardiovasc Res 1997; 33:164-171.

87. Gloviczki P, Solti F, Szlavy L, Jellinek H. Ultrastructural and electrophysiological changes of experimental acute lymphostasis. Lymphology 1983; 16:185-192.

88. Guski H, Buntrock P, Braselmann H, Marx I. The effect of lymphostasis on the isolated working rat heart. 1974; 30:1452-1455.

89. Sun SC, Lie JT. Cardiac lymphatic obstruction; ultrastructure of acute-phase myocardial injury in dogs. Mayo Clin Proc 1977, 52:785-792.

90. Miller AJ, Pick R, Katz LN. Ventricular endomyocardial changes after impairment of cardiac lymph flow in dogs. Br Heart J 1963; 25:182-190.

91. Symbas PN, Schlant RC, Gravanis MB, Shepherd RL. Pathologic and functional effects on the heart following interruption of the cardiac lymph drainage. J Thorac Cardiovasc Surg 1969; 57:577-584.

92. Witte CL, Witte MH, Dumont AE. Pathophysiology of chronic edema, lymphedema, and fibrosis. In: Edema. Edts.: Staub NC, Taylor AE. Raven Press, New York. 1984; 521-542.

93. McKinney B. Endocardial changes produced in Patus monkeys by the ablation of cardiac lymphatics and the administration of a plantain diet. Am Heart J 1976; 91:484-491.

94. Symbas PN, Cooper T, Gantner GA, Willman VL. Lymphatic drainage of the heart: Effects of experimental interruption of lymphatics. Surg Forum 1963; 14:254-256.

95. Solti F, Lengyel E, Jellinek H, Schneider F, Juhasz-Nagy A, Kekesi V. Coronary arteriopathy after lymphatic blockade: An experimental study in dogs. Lymphology 1994; 27:173-180.

96. Solti F, Nemeth V, Juhasz-Nagy A. Effect of acute cardiac lymph stasis on metabolic coronary adaptation in the dog. Lymphology 1985; 18:136-142.

97. Földi M, Romhanyi G, Rusznyak I, Solti F, Szabo G. Über die Insuffizienz der Lymphströmung im Herzen. Acta Med Acad Sci Hung 1954; 6:61-75.

98. Jacobs G, Kleinschmidt F, Benesch L, Lenz W, Uhlig G, Huth F. Tierexperimentelle Untersuchungen des kardialen Lymphgefäss-systems. Thoraxchirurgie 1976; 24:453-467.

99. Miller AJ, Pick R, Katz LN. Ventricular endomyocardial pathology produced by chronic cardiac lymphatic obstruction. Circ Res 1960; 8:941-947.

100. Ullal SR, Kluge TH, Gerbode F. Functional and pathologic changes in the heart following chronic cardiac obstruction. Surgery 1972; 71:328-334.

101. Laine GA. Change in (dP/dt)max as an index of myocardial microvascular permeability. Circ Res 1987; 61:203-208.

102. Heimisch W, Mohl W, Mendler N. Intermittent coronary sinus occlusion: effects on regional function of the normal and ischemic myocardium. In: The coronary sinus. Mohl W, Wolner E, Glogar D (eds). Steinkopff, Darmstadt 1984; 465-472.

CHAPTER 5

Regional Differences and Variability in Left Ventricular Wall Motion

Werner Heimisch

Introduction

In our understanding of the mechanical performance of the heart as a pump we mostly rely on the famous studies of Otto Frank[1] and Ernest Starling[2] whose observations have been widely accepted for a century. Thus, the clinical therapeutic regimens contain volume substitution (preload), antihypertensive therapy (afterload), bradycardic agent (heart rate) and positive inotropic agent (contractility) drug administration. All these maneuvers involve the heart as a whole. In most of our patients, however, just parts of the ventricle are injured by insufficient energy supply. Therefore, if we treat the ventricle as a whole we may ask whether all the parts of the ventricle act in unison. When we look at heart preparations for morphological analyses (Fig. 5.1) it becomes obvious from the global as well as local anisotropy that there must be an inhomogeneity in myocardial contraction i) across the ventricular wall, ii) from site to site from apex to the base, and, moreover, iii) at any site along different angular orientations.

Regional blood supply measured by antegrade volume-flow through the coronary arteries may cause differential effects on the dependent myocardium. This will primarily be according to the specific amount of oxygen transported (limited oxygen supply by coronary artery stenosis or reduced oxygen transport due to hemodilution or perfusion with desaturated instead of arterial blood). Additionally the functional response of the myocardium to local impediment of the coronary blood flow might depend on the coronary artery architecture and on the absence or presence of collaterals—genetically preformed or acquired.

Thus, this chapter deals with regional differences in left ventricular performance, with species-related differences of myocardial functional response to coronary artery blood flow restriction, and with variations of oxygen delivery irrespective of blood volume-flow and their effects on myocardial function.

Local Differences in Left Ventricular Wall Motion

When we look directly at the beating heart during surgery or at its intracavitary 'shadow' of the contrast medium during cardiac catheterization, a heterogeneous motion becomes evident even in patients with regular ventricular wall function, i.e., in patients with intact coronary artery circulation. Two major reasons may be responsible for this: First, a twisted common band-like structure of the whole biventricular heart pump introduces a global anisotropy (Fig. 5.1).[3] This has been demonstrated for more than a century by heart preparations for morphological studies which reached an artistic reading by Torrent-Guasp.[4] Second, at any part of this muscle band forming the ventricular wall there is a local anisotropy across the wall which has

Coronary Sinus Interventions in Cardiac Surgery, Second Edition edited by Werner Mohl.
©2000 Eurekah.com.

Fig. 5.1. Biventricular muscle band seen from the apex after removal of the most apical part of the myocardial mass. (Photograph by courtesy of P.P. Lunkenheimer, MD, Experimental Cardiac and Thoracovascular Surgery, Westfälische Wilhelms-Universität, Münster, Germany)

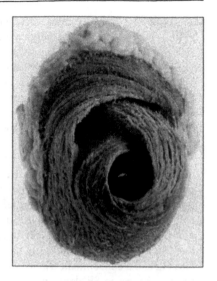

been described by Streeter and Hanna[5] as "a...nested set of fiber shells, with ... a fiber orientation like that of blades of an opened Japanese fan." Although, the morphology of the heart has been extensively studied and the anisotropy has been taken into account in theoretical considerations, the functional consequences of this muscular structure could not be documented for a long time as there were no methods appropriate to assess local myocardial function in the beating heart. The pattern of local left ventricular wall motion could be first recorded continuously and even in chronic animal preparations by an ultrasound transit time technique called 'sonomicrometry'.[6] The method became even more reliable and easier to apply with the development of miniaturized implantable piezoceramic transducers with circular sound radiation which further allowed the study of geometrical changes in size and shape of a well-defined wall area.[7] By using sonomicrometry, a mapping of the cyclic motion at several sites along the major axis of the canine left ventricular anterior free wall has been first performed by LeWinter et al.[8] To do this, they implanted pairs of ultrasonic transducers in parallel to the myocardial fiber orientation into the middle layer of the wall and subepicardially, each near the base, at the midventricular level, and near the apex. In the epicardial segments which were oriented about 20° counter-clockwise to the long axis of the left ventricle there were no regional differences in shortening fraction across the ventricular free wall. When compared to these epicardial segments, an about four-fold shortening fraction of the hoop axis fibers had been observed in the midwall layers. Furthermore, in the middle layer of the ventricular wall, shortening fraction averaged 20% of the end-diastolic length near the apex, significantly more than shortening at the midventricular (13%) or basal (14%) levels. The gradient of shortening fraction became more even from the apex to the base (20%-13%-9%) during transient periods of aortic constriction, i.e., pressure loading of the left ventricle.

In order to obtain more clinically relevant data about regional ventricular wall motion we modified this study in that we implanted the transducers into subendocardial layers in parallel and perpendicular to the major axis of the left ventricle.[9,10] Firstly, dimensional changes of the endocardium determine the shape and size of the instantaneous ventricular cavity and, thus, of the stroke volume, and, secondly, cineventriculographic studies are also based on analyses of the inner ventricular cross-sectional changes without respect to the myocardial fiber orientation. Though we used slightly different criteria for the calculation of shortening fraction (SF), the results from 46 canine experiments fitted well with the previous data from the literature:

$$SF\% = (L_0 - L_c) * 100\% / edL$$

with: SF: shortening fraction of subendocardial left ventricular wall segment;

    L_o: segment length at the time of aortic valve opening;

    L_c: segment length at the time of aortic valve closure;

   edL: segment length at the end of ventricular diastole.

This formula differs slightly from the algorithm used by some investigators who calculate SF from maximal segment length instead of L_o and minimal segment length instead of L_c at control conditions; their criteria, however, become inconsistent as soon as paradoxical systolic dilatation or bulging occurs due to hypoxic injury. This problem is overcome by the use of the above cited formula.

According to our data, SF of the hoop axis declines from 15.2% at the apex to 8.3% at the midventricular level and to 7.9% at the base during 'control conditions' with the dogs anesthetized, mechanically ventilated, and the thorax and pericardium open. The respective SF values from parallel to the major axis of the left ventricle were 6.7%-4.4%-6.9%. Afterload augmentation was performed by graded inflation of a saline-filled balloon catheter with its tip positioned just distal to the aortic arch. An elevation of the peak left ventricular pressure from 125 mm Hg to 151 mm Hg caused an augmentation of the enddiastolic pressure from 7.3-11.4 mm Hg and a concomitant 6% increase in edL along the minor ventricular diameter but no evident changes in SF along any direction at the basal and midventricular site. At the apical site, however, SF decreased by 30% along the hoop axis whereas it increased by 50% along the major heart axis. This resulted in a piston pump-like motion of the pressure loaded ventricle during contraction. A similar contraction pattern was observed after positive inotropic stimulation (10 μg isoproterenol).

The effects of volume loading on regional ventricular wall motion were observed after rapid i.v. infusion of dextran 60 (30 ml/kg body weight). This augmented enddiastolic left ventricular pressure by 104% but increased left ventricular peak pressure moderately by only 14%; the lowered blood viscosity due to hemodilution yielded this primary increase in preload. Volume loading became evident in a 6-8% enlargement of the apical and midventricular end-diastolic dimensions. At the basal site, the segment dilation averaged 9% in parallel to the minor axis but only 3% along the major axis. Irrespective of this, the amount of systolic shortening increased in both directions by about 50% near the base and by about 30% at the equatorial level of the ventricle. Near the apex, changes in SF did not correlate with the extent of segment dilatation: SF changes averaged between -5% and +10%.

According to the data obtained by this functional mapping of the ventricular wall motion, we monitor routinely in our experiments the mechanical function of the ventricular wall region of interest—mostly areas of the anterior free wall supplied either by the circumflex or by the anterior descending branch of the left coronary artery—by measuring the cyclic motion of subendocardial wall segments which are oriented *in parallel to the minor ventricular axis* avoiding the apical third of the left ventricle. The reason for this is: Firstly, the sum of all the local dimensional changes of the endocardium yields the total pump function of the left ventricle. Secondly, the endocardium has been shown to be most sensitive to alterations in the energy demand/supply ratio. Thirdly, the ultrasonic transducers for detection of dimensional changes can be placed accurately in this deep wall layer and stay there in a stable position for hours, for days, or longer. Finally, segments oriented in parallel to the minor heart axis at basal or midventricular wall regions are found to be most representative in their dimensional changes to geometrical alterations of the total left ventricle. Superficially, in subepicardial layers the relative extent of systolic shortening SF amounts to only between 30% and 70% of that obtained in *subendocardial* layers.[8,10,11] Thus, the response to functional alterations is less pronounced in subepicardial wall segments as compared to those of subendocardial layers.

Local ventricular wall function also could be assessed by measuring the cyclic variations in wall thickening.[12] This method requires very accurate transducer alignment to avoid misreadings which might result from transmural shear motion.[13] And, moreover, systematic mapping of the wall thickening patterns across the left ventricle has not yet been performed. As long as no manipulations are made which alter left ventricular wall mass or volume, measurements of either wall thickness or segment length should reveal equivalent statements. In most animal experiments, myocardial mass and volume of the ventricular wall can be assumed to be constant for the investigational period. It might slowly increase by developing edema and is rapidly enlarged by excessive antegrade as well as retrograde coronary artery hyperperfusion. Antegrade coronary artery perfusion with coronary perfusion pressure more than 20% above the aortic pressure results in an expansion of left ventricular wall thickness and in a diminution of the subendocardial wall dimensions.[14] Obviously, with increasing wall thickness an intramural ballooning causes an enlargement of the external ventricular silhouette and a compression of the intraventricular cavity. Similar observations were made during intermittent coronary sinus occlusion in dogs at intact or only moderately impeded antegrade coronary artery perfusion but disappeared in the presence of total occlusion of the left anterior descending coronary artery.[15] An increase in end-diastolic wall thickness which might indicate a ballooning of the wall became evident during coronary venous retroperfusion in pigs when the retrograde flow markedly exceeded the amount of antegrade control flow.[16] As an increase in end-diastolic ventricular wall thickness may indicate a return from ischemic dilation as well as a progressive swelling or ballooning, correct interpretation of the mechanisms calls for additional simultaneous measurements of changes in corresponding wall segments when alterations of the wall volume are to be suspected.

In the past, most studies dealing with local or regional differences in left ventricular wall motion were performed in anesthetized dogs. In the meantime, most experiments concerning the cardiovascular system and its autoregulatory mechanisms are performed in pigs. From my experience, SF of the swine left ventricular free wall in the acute experiment at rest exceeds that of the canine one by up to 70%. Systematical mapping of the contraction pattern of the porcine left ventricle, however, has not yet been performed.

Mapping of the mechanical action of the heart by sonomicrometry is a highly invasive and time-consuming procedure and, unfortunately, the results originate mainly from acute experiments with anesthetized animals. Forthcoming noninvasive techniques like nuclear magnetic resonance imaging with its sophisticated technical and analytical features[3,17] might enable us to institute reference maps of local myocardial function in the healthy human with respect to his physical activities or life style as well as in the ill patient on account of his disease.

Variability in Ventricular Wall Motion Pattern

If one questions now whether a SF of 10% indicates regular or hypokinetic wall motion, you should ask for the circumstances like site and orientation of measurement, species, at rest or during exercise, etc. To classify a ventricular wall segment as a regularly or less efficient contracting part of the ventricle is possible only after the response to variations in pressure load or wall stress, in work and power is analyzed. As soon as ventricular wall regions dilate during systole (dyskinesia) or are almost akinetic for the whole cardiac cycle, physical load variations are in general inappropriate to test the viability of the myocardium; such tests are reserved for methods which are based on the detection of local metabolism, e.g., positron emission tomography.[18] The main problem is to differentiate between regular contraction and little to moderate hypokinesia. In the acute animal experiment, we commonly start from normal myocardial function at control conditions and, thus, we are able to install graded regional impairment of left ventricular function and to model coronary artery disease of well-defined severity. By modeling coronary artery disease we discriminate between 'critical' and 'functionally effective' coronary artery stenosis. A coronary artery stenosis might be defined to be 'critical' or 'sub-critical' when the coronary artery is narrowed to a degree just not affecting the extent of contraction of the dependent myocardial region[19] or when the stenosis reaches a degree where reactive hyperemia following a 15 second coronary artery occlusion is just abolished.[20] 'Functionally effective' coronary artery stenosis always results in an impairment of the mechanical function and in an at least minimal hypokinesia of the afflicted wall region.

There are only weak discriminations between normal and hypokinetic ventricular wall motion unless verified by functional stress tests. If one is familiar with it, the left ventricular pressure-dimension loop may best and easiest inform about the actual functional state of the ventricular wall segment under study.[21,22] It is mentioned that there are some peculiarities in the shape of the pressure-length loop which might indicate an acute ischemic insult (Fig. 5.2). Depending on the site and layer where the ultrasonic transducers are implanted, the recorded tracing may show conformational changes of the ventricle which appear as length changes during the isovolumic contraction and relaxation. Pronounced regional wall shortening during isovolumic ventricular relaxation (postsystolic shortening (PSS)) also has been observed in the acutely ischemic myocardium and has been identified to be a predictor of the early and late recovery of function after coronary artery reperfusion.[23] In addition to PSS, the oxygen-deprived myocardial muscle often dilates during the very early systole which is followed by a seemingly regular shortening for the remaining ejection phase. Such early-systolic dilatation (ESD) might result from inhomogeneous force distribution inside the heart chamber generated by maximal blood acceleration at the onset of ejection.[24] As shown in Figure 6.2, PSS and ESD are immediately recognized in left ventricular pressure-length loops; otherwise cumbersome data analysis would be necessary to detect these signs of hypofunction.

Essentially, pressure-length loops represent local increments of the global pressure-volume diagram and, consequently, changes in size of the pressure-length loop indicate changes in work of the corresponding ventricular wall region. As with to the pressure-volume area, a reduction of the area covered by the pressure-length loop does not necessarily indicate an impairment of the wall region. Mainly heart rate variations cause marked alterations in the pres-

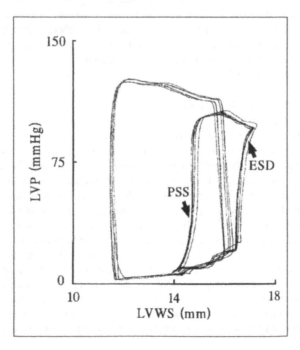

Fig. 5.2. Groups of left ventricular pressure-length loops recorded each for one respiratory period (respiratory rate: 15/min) before (left group) and after myocardial stunning at identical heart rates of 80 beats/min. The jeopardized left ventricular wall segment shows early-systolic dilatation (ESD) as well as postsystolic shortening (PSS). LVP: left ventricular pressure; LVWS: left ventricular wall segment length. (Loops have been recorded by Thermal Array Recorder System TA 6000, generously placed at our disposal by GOULD-Nicolet, Dietzenbach, Germany)

sure-length loop by variations in the extent of shortening of the unimpeded myocardial contraction. Thus, pressure-length loops are the most prominent aid to recognize variations in the functional state and work of the myocardium. However, to validate the energetic situation of myocardial regions heart rate and/or ejection time has to enter into the evaluation. This enables an analysis of myocardial function in terms of physical power and of the amount of local contribution to the total power processed by the heart. The following index of regional myocardial power (RMP) has been proven to be highly sensitive to an unbalance of energy demand/supply ratio.[25]

$$RMP = SF * AoP_{ej} * HR / t_{ej}$$

with: SF: shortening fraction of left ventricular wall segment;

         AoP_{ej} : aortic mean pressure during ventricular ejection;

         HR: heart rate in beats per minute;

         t_{ej} : duration of ventricular ejection from aortic valve opening to closure.

Functional State of the Myocardium and Oxygen Delivery: Rules and Exceptions

The most common way to model myocardial ischemia in acute animal experiments is to narrow a main branch of the coronary artery by a mechanical obstructer. To what degree the blood flow through the coronary artery will be restricted depends on the aim of the study. Although this procedure directly affects the coronary blood flow, other parameters may serve as a measure of impairment. In our experimental studies on ischemic myocardium a branch of the left coronary artery is narrowed by a micrometer-driven snare until the extent of systolic shortening of the dependent ventricular wall area diminishes to the limit set in advance. A retrospective evaluation of the relation between reduction in coronary artery blood flow and myocardial systolic shortening revealed that a 50% decrease in blood flow through the left anterior descending coronary artery (LAD) curtails systolic wall segment shortening by about 50% in dogs but by more than 80% in pigs (Table 5.1). It is assumed that this discrepancy arises from differences in the coronary vascular bed: acute support for energy supply to the oxygen-deprived region can be activated by preformed collaterals which exist in dogs but do not in pigs. In humans, the presence of collaterals may follow genetic orders, collaterals may be acquired by physical activities, or they might have 'grown' to compensate for gradual occlusions of adjoining coronary vessels. Thus, without cardiac catheterization it is uncertain in human individuals whether there are collaterals and to what degree they might be able to support the oxygen supply. Comparable functional consequences to ischemic injury can be expected only from individuals with similar coronary architecture. Presence or absence of collaterals is one factor which determines regional myocardial blood supply. Although the antegrade volume-flow of blood through the coronary artery is commonly measured as representative for myocardial energy supply, the energy delivery is in fact determined by the oxygen dissolved and transported by the fluid.

As shown in Table 8.1, a 50% reduction of systolic shortening in the canine myocardium was achieved by diminishing the coronary blood volume flow and, consequently, by diminishing the oxygen delivery to 50% (Table 5.2A). The oxygen flow to the myocardium, however, can be varied independently from blood volume flow. This has been shown in a study about the effects of hemodilution on myocardial function when the coronary reserve capacity was exhausted.[19] For this reason, a 'subcritical' stenosis of the LAD has been established by narrowing the vessel to a degree which did just not affect the dependent wall motion. This 'subcritical' LAD stenosis restricted the coronary blood flow by less than 15%, but the shortening fraction of anterior wall segments was not influenced. In the presence of this stenosis the hematocrit

Table 5.1. Species-related effects of coronary artery blood flow obstruction on left ventricular wall segment shortening in anesthetized dogs vs. pigs.

Species	Q_{LAD}	(L_{LAD}
Dog		
n = 44	- 51.0 + 3.3%	- 49.0 + 2.4%
Pig		
n = 45	- 46.7 + 2.1%	- 81.7 + 0.9%

Q_{LAD}: blood flow through the left anterior descending coronary artery;
(L_{LAD}: systolic shortening of a wall segment supplied by the LAD.
(Data are given as % changes from control before LAD narrowing; mean + sem)

was lowered from 45% to 15% in steps of 5% by isovolumic exchange of blood for dextran 60. At a hematocrit of 15% the blood flow through the narrowed coronary artery had increased by 47% due to the lowered viscosity. At the same time, however, the oxygen transport capacity of the diluted blood was reduced by 51% which resulted in a concomitant 46% decrease in the amount of systolic shortening (Table 5.2B). When the coronary artery stenosis had been removed, the blood flow increased due to both the lowered viscosity and reactive hyperemia to three-fold the control flow. With respect to oxygen transport this flow augmentation compensated for the lowered hematocrit; the oxygen supply reached again 94% of control and myocardial shortening fraction also returned to 94 + 6% of the control value before hemodilution.

The fact that the myocardial shortening fraction almost linearly follows changes of oxygen delivery is further documented in an experimental model of anomalous origin of left coronary artery from the pulmonary artery—a rare congenital cardiac malformation.[26] To study the effects of antegrade coronary artery perfusion with venous blood in dogs, the LAD has been cannulated and perfused via a flow-controlled pump with either arterial blood from the aorta or venous blood from the pulmonary artery. Oxygen content of the arterial blood was 193 + 7 ml O_2 per liter of blood and it was 145 + 7 ml O_2 per liter of venous blood. From actual coronary blood flow times oxygen content of the perfusate (arterial or venous blood) divided by heart rate, oxygen delivery to the myocardium has been calculated in microliter of oxygen per heart beat. Data corresponding to an oxygen delivery between 45-55% of control perfusion with arterial blood are averaged in Table 6.2C. At half the oxygen delivery, coronary perfusion with venous blood was reduced by only 29% in blood flow; at the same time systolic wall shortening decreased by 42% which was in the order of the averaged 49% reduction in oxygen delivery.

These results demonstrate that the systolic function of the myocardium directly depends on the actual oxygen delivery. On the other hand we know, of course, from many studies that acute improvements in oxygen supply do not always myocardial contraction. This leads to the definitions of hibernating, stunned, or infarcted myocardium.[27] The experimental data presented in Tables 5.1 and 5.2 describe acute responses in the mechanical function of ventricular wall regions to acute reductions in oxygen supply. This close interplay gets lost after a prolonged period of severe oxygen deficiency when myocardial stunning develops. In 44 experiments with domestic pigs, myocardial stunning has been provoked according to the protocol described in detail by Schad et al.[23] After 90 minutes of unimpeded reperfusion with arterial blood the spontaneous coronary blood flow has been recovered to 106 ± 4% of control value whereas systolic shortening of the dependent wall region remained markedly depressed at 36 ± 2%.

In 1978, we presented a clinical study about the acute effects of aortocoronary bypass surgery on left ventricular function and regional myocardial mechanics.[28] At that time, neither the term 'stunning' nor 'hibernation' in myocardial ischemia had been coined. The study was

Table 5.2. Alterations in coronary artery blood volume flow, oxygen delivery, and segmental ventricular wall shortening by different types of intervention in anesthetized dogs.

Intervention	Q_{blood}	Q_{oxygen}	ΔL
A: Coronary artery stenosis			
n = 44	- 51 ± 3%	- 51 ± 3%	- 49 ± 2%
B: Coronary artery stenosis			
+ isovolumic hemodilution	+ 47 ± 10%	- 51 ± 8%	- 46 ± 8%
n = 20			
C: Coronary artery perfusion			
with venous blood	- 29 ± 3%	- 49 ± 2%	- 42 ± 6%
n = 7			

Q_{blood}: changes in blood volume flow; Q_{oxygen}: changes in oxygen delivery;
ΔL: changes in systolic shortening of dependent left ventricular wall segments.
(A and C: data are given as % changes from unrestricted control perfusion with arterial blood; B:
data are given as % changes from perfusion with nondiluted blood through a 'subcritically'
stenosed LAD (for details see the text); (mean ± sem))

performed in 22 men divided into two groups of 11 (Table 5.3). Patients were grouped according to the clinical status: Patients with a short history (< 6 months) of coronary artery disease but rapid progression of symptoms were appointed to the group of 'unstable angina', the others with documented history of previous myocardial infarction but free of symptoms at rest were classified as 'stable angina'. All patients underwent aorto-coronary venous bypass grafting (ACVBG). Intraoperatively, during stable conditions 30 minutes after completion of cardiopulmonary bypass left ventricular pressure, ACVBG flow, and—by sonomicrometry—regional myocardial wall motion were assessed before, during, and after graft cross-clamping. Exclusively in patients (9 of 11 patients) considered to suffer previously from unstable angina, an acute positive functional response to revascularization could be verified. No acute functional improvements were observed in the other patients despite almost regular blood flow through the grafts and at least moderate reactive hyperemic response to graft cross-clamping in six patients. In two patients with intraoperatively continuing contraction disorders, postoperative examination revealed regular ventricular contraction. From these findings it was suggested 20 years ago "that there is some potential for long-term recovery in these hearts".[28] Nowadays, the lack of acute functional improvement might be interpreted as a property of 'stunned myocardium'. In contrast, acute improvement of mechanical function after restoration of blood flow and, thus, energy supply as seen in 9 of 11 patients with unstable angina suggests to 'hibernating myocardium'.

Unfortunately, hypokinesia per se gives no indication whether it is a transient expression to an acute energy deficiency or a lasting sign of previous severe ischemic injury. There are only a few less invasive examination procedures which might be suited in patients to unmask viable hibernating myocardium. Synchronized diastolic coronary venous retroperfusion seems to be one of these techniques.[29,30] Whether this technique is of value to elucidate the anatomic location of viable myocardium depends on whether all the ventricular regions of interest are accessible to the retrograde perfusion in like manner.[31,32]

Table 5.3. Functional response of the myocardium to coronary revascularization in patients with aorto-coronary venous bypass graft (ACVBG) operation

Diagnosis	Pts. n =	Preoperative ventriculogram	ACVBG intraoperatively cross-clamped	unclamped	ΔL
Unstable	2	Normal	Hypokinesia	Normal	± 17%
Angina	7	Hypokinesia	Hypokinesia	Normal	± 62 ± 50%
	2	Dyskinesia	Dyskinesia	Dyskinesia	± 0%
Stable	2	Normal	Normal	Normal	± 0%
Angina	5	Hypokinesia	Hypokinesia	Hypokinesia	+ 1 ± 2%
	4	Dyskinesia	Dys-/Akinesia	Dys-/Akinesia	− 1 ± 2%

(L: % changes in systolic shortening of left ventricular wall segments obtained intraoperatively by ACVBG unclamping (mean (± sd)).

Conclusion

Performance of the heart results from a complex interplay between rate of fiber contraction, the fiber stress-strain relationship, the active state of the muscle, the force-velocity relationship etc. Global pump performance is a function of locally different amount of mechanical wall function. This might be seen as a heterogeneity in myocardial function or as a consequence of "heart structure conditions function and vice versa".[33] In any case, left ventricular wall motion differs from region to region and is modulated by load alterations and by the response to changing metabolic requirements of the peripheral tissue. Thus, there are no definite set values which have to be fulfilled at any time by any part of the ventricle. Temporal and regional differences in left ventricular wall motion have to be validated with respect to their functional reserve. Functional reserve is assessed most reliably by load tests which are quite similar to those performed on an engine test bench. If a sufficient functional reserve can be mobilized we might suppose that the myocardial region under study works highly efficient at rest. If there is no positive response of locally hypokinetic regions to physical stress tests their possible viability might be discovered by studying local metabolism e.g., by PET. Recent developments in magnetic resonance imaging techniques and in three-dimensional echocardiographicy leave us confident that regional differences and variability in left ventricular wall motion will be ascertained in the near future, rapidly, and noninvasively. This should enable us to prepare maps and isograms of the heart with respect to mechanical function and efficiency as a base against which we can discriminate between regular myocardial contraction, apparently normal contraction but marginal energy supply, and ischemic hypokinesia.

Acknowledgment

The reported investigations were performed at the Department of Cardiovascular Surgery (Director: Prof. Fritz Sebening, MD; Prof. Hans Meisner, MD) and in the Cardiovascular Research Laboratory (Head: Prof. Nikolaus Mendler, MD) of the German Heart Center Munich, Germany.

References

1. Frank O. Zur Dynamik des Herzmuskels. Z Biol 1895; 32:370-437.
2. Starling EH. The Arris and Gale lectures on some points in the pathology of the heart disease. Lecture I: On the compensatory mechanisms of the heart. Lancet 1897; 1:569-572.

3. Schmid P, Niederer P, Lunkenheimer PP et al. The anisotropic structure of the human left and right ventricles. Technol Health Care 1997; 5:29-43.
4. Torrent-Guasp F, Whimster WF, Redmann K. A silicone rubber mould of the heart. Technol Health Care 1997; 5:13-20.
5. Streeter DD Jr, Hanna WT. Engineering mechanics for successive states in canine left ventricular myocardium. Circ Res 1973; 33:639-664.
6. Franklin DL, Kemper WS, Patrick T et al. Techniques for continuous measurement of regional myocardial segment dimensions in chronic animal preparations. Fed Proc 1973; 32:343.
7. Heimisch W, Hagl S, Gebhardt K et al. Direct measurement of cyclic changes in regional wall geometry in the left ventricle of the dog. Innov Tech Biol Med 1981; 2:487-501.
8. LeWinter M, Kent RS, Kroener JM et al. Regional differences in myocardial performance in the left ventricle of the dog. Circ Res 1975; 37:191-199.
9. Heimisch W, Hagl S, Janeczka I et al. Regional differences in left ventricular wall motion. Eur Surg Res 1981; 13:85.
10. Heimisch W. Die Sonomikrometrie in der Herz- und Kreislaufforschung (Sonomicrometry in cardiovascular research) [Dr. rer. biol. hum. (PhD)]. Munich - Germany: Ludwig-Maximilians-Universität München, 1989.
11. Heimisch W, Hagl S, Mendler N et al. Ventricular wall thickening determines the endo/epicardial shortening ratio: agreement of experimental results with geometric model. Eur Heart J 1983; 4(suppl E):35.
12. Ross J Jr, Franklin D. Analysis of regional myocardial function, dimensions, and wall thickness in the characterization of myocardial ischemia and infarction. Circulation 1976; 53(Suppl 1):88-92.
13. Osakada G, Sasayama S, Kawai C et al. The analysis of left ventricular wall thickness and shear by an ultrasonic triangulation technique in the dog. Circ Res 1980; 47:173-181.
14. Heimisch W, Schad H, Mendler N. Coronary hyperperfusion in vivo: Effects on left ventricular wall geometry, myocardial performance, and coronary hemodynamics. Phys Med Biol 1994; 39a:200.
15. Heimisch W, Mohl W, Mendler N et al. Intermittent coronary sinus occlusion: Effects on regional function of the normal and ischemic myocardium. In: Mohl W, Wolner E, Glogar D, eds. The Coronary Sinus. Darmstadt NewYork: Steinkopff, Springer-Verlag, 1984:465-472.
16. Oh BH, Volpini M, Kambayashi M et al. Myocardial function and transmural blood flow during coronary venous retroperfusion in pigs. Circulation 1992; 86:1265-1279.
17. Maier SE, Fischer SE, McKinnon GC et al. Evaluation of left ventricular segmental wall motion in hypertrophic cardiomyopathy with myocardial tagging. Circulation 1992; 86:1919-1928.
18. Haas F, Haehnel CJ, Picker W et al. Preoperative positron emission tomographic viability assessment and perioperative and postoperative risk in patients with advanced ischemic heart disease. J Am Coll Cardiol 1997; 30:1693-1700.
19. Hagl S, Heimisch W, Meisner H et al. The effect of hemodilution on regional myocardial function in the presence of coronary stenosis. Basic Res Cardiol 1977; 72:344-364.
20. Schad H, Heimisch W, Mendler N. Models of coronary artery disease: "critical" versus "functional" coronary artery stenosis. Thorac Cardiovasc Surg 1991; 39:13-18.
21. Heimisch W, Mendler N, Schad H et al. The pressure-dimension loop: At-a-glance indicator of the actual functional state of the myocardium. In: Amlaner CJ, Jr., ed. Tenth International Symposium on Biotelemetry. Fayetteville, AR, USA: University of Arkansas Press, Fayetteville London, 1989:633-639.
22. Settergren G. The loop displayed before your eyes could one day tell you the secrets of the heart. J Cardiothorac Vasc Anesth 1991; 5:537-538.
23. Takayama M, Norris RM, Brown MA et al. Postsystolic shortening of acutely ischemic canine myocardium predicts early and late recovery of function after coronary artery reperfusion. Circulation 1988; 78:994-1007.
24. Heimisch W, Schad H, Mendler N et al. Cyclic motion of ischemic ventricular wall area and hydrodynamics of the blood during ejection. Thorac Cardiovasc Surg 1991; 39(suppl):205-210.
25. Schad H, Heimisch W, Eising GP et al. Effect of milrinone and atrial pacing on stunned myocardium. Eur J Cardio-Thorac Surg 1997; 11:1125-1132.
26. Heimisch W, Schad H, Mendler N. Coronary artery perfusion: significance of blood volume-flow, perfusion pressure, and oxygen delivery. Phys Med Biol 1994; 39a:202.
27. Opie LH, ed. Stunning, hibernation, and calcium in myocardial ischemia and reperfusion. Boston Dordrecht London: Kluwer Academic Publ., 1992.

28. Hagl S, Meisner H, Heimisch W et al. Acute effects of aortocoronary bypass surgery on left ventricular function and regional myocardial mechanics: a clinical study. Ann Thorac Surg 1978; 26:548-558.
29. Hajduczki I, Kar S, Areeda J et al. Reversal of chronic regional myocardial dysfunction (hibernating myocardium) by synchronized diastolic coronary venous retroperfusion during coronary angioplasty. J Am Coll Cardiol 1990; 15:238-242.
30. Nienaber CA, Abend M, Rehders TC et al. Synchronized coronary venous retroperfusion: Can retrograde delivery of flow identify "hibernating myocardium"? Z Kardiol 1993; 82:415-424.
31. Feld F, Ekas RD, Felli P et al. Differential effects of synchronized coronary sinus retroperfusion on regional myocardial function during brief occlusion of the left anterior descending and circumflex coronary arteries. Cathet Cardiovasc Diagn 1994; 32:70-78.
32. Wakida Y, Haendchen RV, Kobayashi S et al. Percutaneous cooling of ischemic myocardium by hypothermic retroperfusion of autologous arterial blood: effects on regional myocardial temperature distribution and infarct size. J Am Coll Cardiol 1991; 18:293-300.
33. Lunkenheimer PP. Structure conditions function and vice versa [editorial]. Technol Health Care 1997; 5:1-12.

CHAPTER 6

Computer Simulation and Modeling of the Coronary Circulation

Friederike Neumann, Martin Neumann, Rudolf Karch,
and Wolfgang Schreiner

Computer Simulation in Coronary Physiology

In the large field of physiological processes such as, for instance, transportation and delivery of substances in the circulatory systems of the body, computer experiments and simulation studies can be very effectively applied. In the computer model, significant characteristics (e.g., perfusion pressure and total flow in the circulation, or the bifurcation law of branching vessels) are taken into account in terms of boundary conditions and constraints. After tuning the parameters and validating a model such that measurement data (e.g., pulsatile blood flow) can be quantitatively or at least qualitatively reproduced, the model is ready to be applied to scrutinize a large variety of questions which cannot be addressed experimentally because of ethical reasons, very high costs, or methodological limitations. The possibility of systematic parameter variation in the computer model is a powerful approach to simulate arbitrary "experimental" conditions under which functional relations of the system may be studied and elucidated.

A major field of computer simulation in physiology is the hemodynamics of the cardiovascular system and, in particular, of the coronary circulation. Different parts of the vascular system are represented usually by electrical elements, and a mathematical model is specified with more or less simplifying assumptions in order to obtain the equations to calculate blood flow within the system. If the circulation is modeled by only a few elements representing entire compartments of the vessel tree ("lumped parameter model"), global blood flow can be simulated for each compartment. If hemodynamic simulations are to be based on a spatially more detailed model which accounts for the complexity of real vessel trees, the structure of the model may either be obtained from morphological measurements for a limited number of major vessels, or by computer simulation of a tree of arbitrary resolution. The morphology of a simulated vessel tree depends largely on the conceptual approach of tree generation.

Models of the Coronary Circulation

In a lumped parameter model (Fig. 6.1), the highly complex structure of the coronary circulation is reduced to only a few compartments, each of which typically represents an entire class of vessels, such as arteries, capillaries or veins, without any possibility to further differentiate spatially within the compartment (e.g., 1-3). Anatomical models comprising a few dozen segments are based on morphometric parameters, such as lengths and radii of vessel segments. In this approach, the real branching geometry is implemented to specifically represent a certain

Coronary Sinus Interventions in Cardiac Surgery, Second Edition edited by Werner Mohl.
©2000 Eurekah.com.

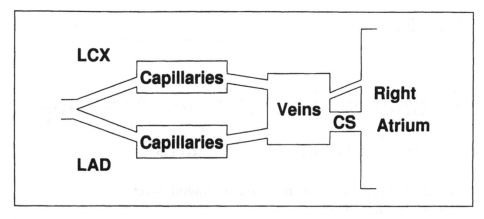

Fig. 6.1. Lumped parameter model of the coronary circulation representing subsystems as individual compartments. The left coronary artery bifurcates into the vascular bed of the left anterior descending (LAD) and the circumflex (LCX) artery. Both their capillary compartments drain into a single coronary venous compartment. Drainage into the right atrium occurs through the coronary sinus (CS) and the Thebesian veins.

vessel and its major branches in detail (e.g., 4). Computer generated fractal models using either deterministic or stochastic laws for the generation of vessel systems, yield self-similar structures in the sense that subareas on a smaller scale repeat the properties already seen on a larger scale. These models incorporate known features of real vessel trees, such as the average shrinkage of segment lengths and radii across successive bifurcations, but the structures of such fractal models need not, in general, be geometrically realizable in space (e.g., 5-8).

In contrast, geometrically arrangeable tree structures can be modeled and generated by computer simulation with the method of "constrained constructive optimization" (CCO[9,10]). In reality, growth and structure of arterial trees are not purely arbitrary but governed by (global) optimality principles.[11] CCO adopts such principles, e.g., blood delivery through arteries in an efficient, cost-effective way,[12] in order to obtain physiologically reasonable model trees, which are still manageable on medium-scale computer facilities. Without the input of any anatomical data, the resulting structures are "realistic" representations of vessels, comparable to corrosion casts of real arterial trees (Fig. 6.2). The spatial arrangement of segments is not only compatible with anatomical and physiological observations but also geometrically realizable, i.e., no two vessels penetrate into each other. In a CCO model tree, spatial and temporal distribution of pressures and flow can be analyzed in detail from the feeding artery down to the level of individual arterial segments.

Hemodynamic Simulations

In the following, two examples will be given for the simulation of blood flow in the coronary vascular system: a compartment model as well as a simulated branching network. Both models yield pulsatile flow curves for the coronary circulation under specified pressure conditions. In either case, a number of simplifying assumptions have to be made some of which apply to both models, whereas some are specific to the particular approach. Most importantly, neither model accounts for the fact that blood is an inhomogeneous, non-Newtonian fluid, and that the vascular tree is not a passive but an active system which reacts spontaneously to changes in the physiological conditions.

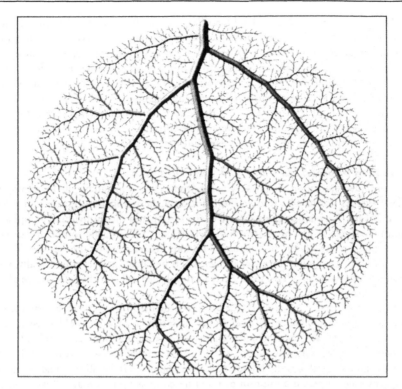

Fig. 6.2. CCO model of a coronary arterial tree with 4000 terminal segments, optimized for mini-mum intravasal volume.

The characteristic shape of flow waves in the coronary arteries is the result of an interplay between two mechanisms: a driving pressure, or pressure gradient between the aortic pressure and the pressure level at the (microcirculatory) terminals of the arterial tree; and the variation of vascular resistance due to intramyocardial compression. It is the temporal relation between aortic driving pressure and intramyocardial pressure, their respective amplitudes, and the vascular compliance which determine systolic flow impediment and diastolic perfusion of the myocardium. In the following modeling approaches, aortic pressure (AoP) and left ventricular pressure (LVP) are represented by Fourier-synthesis using digitized textbook curves.[13] The pulsatile driving pressure is taken to be AoP at a heart rate of 60 bpm. The system is also subject to an intramyocardial squeezing pressure (IMP) proportional to the Fourier-synthesized LVP.

Simulation of Blood Flow in a Compartment Model

In the compartment model (cf. Fig. 6.1), pulsatile perfusion pressure (AoP) applied to the main left coronary artery pumps blood into the two major arteries. The corresponding capillary beds are modeled as distensible compartments, subjected to intramyocardial squeezing pressure (IMP) and draining into a single (compliant) venous compartment. Venous egress occurs via the coronary sinus and an extra outlet for coronary veno-venous shunting and for Thebesian channels. Pulsatile time courses of all coronary hemodynamic characteristics can be obtained by numerical integration of the differential equations used to describe the balance between change in volume, inflow and egress of blood for each compartment. A periodic solution is obtained after an equilibration phase of 20s.[14]

Using the compartment model, blood flow can be simulated for the arterial and for the venous coronary bed. Therefore, the model suggested itself for studying flow under different pressure conditions in the venous system, such as occurring, for instance, during coronary sinus interventions.[1,15] Figure 6.3 displays an example of arterial and venous flow during coronary sinus blockade as performed by "pressure-controlled coronary sinus occlusion" (PICSO, e.g.,16-18). The area between the baseline and the negative portion of the solid curve reflects the volume of blood redistributed from the coronary venous system toward the capillaries within each heartbeat. This blood volume may be considered an important quantity characterizing the degree of "washout" of toxic metabolites by PICSO.

Simulation of Blood Flow in CCO Tree Models

Computer simulation of coronary hemodynamics in a hierarchically branching network of elastic vessels has to take into account not only the particular pressure dynamics in the myocardial arteries, but also the structure of the system and the (individual) compliance of its constituent vessels. In case of a network model such as CCO, usually comprising several thousand vessel segments (cf. Fig. 6.2), practical limitations are given by the fact that in any simulation only a finite number of vessel segments can be taken into account. Finally, CCO and hemodynamic simulations have so far been accomplished only for the arterial tree of the coronary circulation.

In our approach, the arterial CCO tree is represented by a network of nonlinear electric elements. For the compliance of vessel segments, a simple adhoc model has been developed, which was based on an experimentally established relationship between vessel radius and wall thickness.[19] The pulsatile driving pressure (AoP) is applied to the proximal end of the root segment, and the distal pressure is kept constant at 60 mm Hg for all terminal segments. After a transient stage, a periodic solution of pulsatile coronary pressure and flow is obtained by integrating the differential equations for about five heart beats.[20]

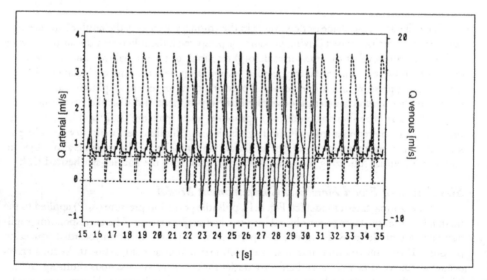

Fig. 6.3. Coronary arterial (solid line) and venous flow (dashed line) in the normal state (5 seconds each at left and right tails of the curves) and during coronary sinus occlusion (PICSO) at $20 < t < 30$ s. (Reprinted with permission from: Schreiner W, Neumann F, Mohl W. Simulation of coronary circulation with special regard to the venous bed and coronary sinus occlusion. J Biomed Eng 1990;12:429-43. ©1990 Butterworth Scientific Ltd.)

Figure 6.4 provides an example which demonstrates that the present approach yields very realistic flow-wave forms for the coronary arteries. This is achieved with a minimum of adjustable parameters and in spite of the drastic approximations made in formulating a simple mathematical relationship for the vascular compliance. Figure 6.4 shows the pulsatile flow in the root segment and every 2 cm downstream along the main vessel of a two-dimensional CCO tree with 4000 terminal segments. (The main vessel is the set of segments obtained by starting at the root and always choosing the larger daughter segment at successive bifurcations.) The curves exhibit the wave form typical of coronary flow and a progressive damping as one moves from the root towards the terminal segment.

In simulation experiments of coronary hemodynamics in a CCO tree, redistribution of flow resulting from changes in the geometrical and functional properties of the tree, in the elastic properties of the segments, or from variations in the way intramyocardial squeezing is applied, may be investigated in arbitrary detail. Figure 6.5 is an example of coronary artery flow at regional variations of intramyocardial pressure in a two-dimensional model tree, representing various degrees of reduced left ventricular function.

Simulation Studies in Coronary Surgery

After validating a computer model of the coronary vascular system, simulation studies may be successfully introduced into the clinical practice of cardiology and cardiac surgery. According to the clinical requirements, either a compartment model or a branching pattern model may be chosen to address a particular clinical question. In order to put some light into the behavior of a whole subsystem of the circulation such as, for instance, the reaction of the venous vasculature to therapeutically manipulated pressure conditions in the coronary sinus, a compartment model would suffice to reproduce the corresponding effects on arterial and venous flow. In other words, the efficacy of different techniques of coronary sinus interventions, such as PICSO, "synchronized retroperfusion" (SRP, e.g., 21,22), etc., may be studied

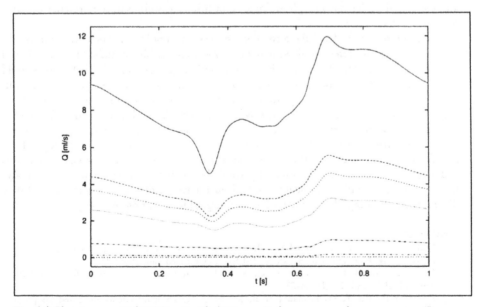

Fig. 6.4. Flow in an arterial CCO tree with 4000 terminal segments, at the root segment ("coronary artery flow", solid line), every 2 cm along its course, and at the terminal segment of the main path (from top to bottom).

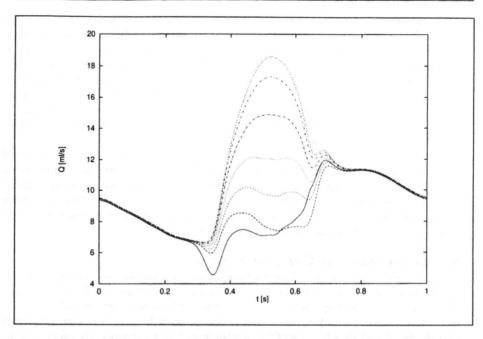

Fig. 6.5. Flow in the root segment at "normal" ventricular squeezing conditions (solid line) and increasing spatial extension of "myocardial dysfunction." The top curve shows flow without intramyocardial pressure and represents total loss of contraction.

and compared under various "physiologic" conditions as well as in the presence of coronary artery disease.[23,24]

In contrast, if more detailed information on the spatial resolution of hemodynamic conditions is required, pressures and flows may much more reasonably be studied in a tree-shaped vascular structure. One of the most important clinical applications of CCO models could certainly be the large field of coronary bypass planning. In this case, the real geometry (coordinates) of a patient's major coronary arteries and the locations of stenoses and lesions would be fed into the model. The network of the smaller arteries could be obtained from CCO modeling, realistically representing the properties of the dense vasculature of the coronary artery system. The result is a full CCO tree, adjusted to the morphometry and pathology of the patient's coronary anatomy. Perfusing the model tree under appropriate pressure conditions and varying the number and location of possible bypass sites in a systematic way, hemodynamic simulation would yield qualitative and quantitative estimates of the myocardial flow distribution, providing a basis of diagnosis and surgical intervention planning.

References

1. Schreiner W, Neumann F, Mohl W. The role of intramyocardial pressure during coronary sinus interventions: A computer model study. IEEE Trans Biomed Eng 1990; 37:956-67.
2. Sun Y, Gewirtz H. Estimation of intramyocardial pressure and coronary blood flow distribution. Am J Physiol 1988; 255:H664-72.
3. Bruinsma P, Arts T, Dankelman J et al. Model of the coronary circulation based on pressure dependence of coronary resistance and compliance. Bas Res Cardiol 1988; 83:510-24.

4. Rooz E, Wiesner TF, Nerem RM. Epicardial coronary blood flow including the presence of steno-sis and aorto-coronary bypasses—I: Model and numerical method. ASME J Biomech Eng 1985; 107:361-7.
5. West BJ, Goldberger AL. Physiology in fractal dimensions. Am Sci 1987; 75:354-64.
6. Pelosi G, Saviozzi G, Trivella MG et al. Small artery occlusion: A theoretical approach to the definition of coronary architecture and resistance by a branching tree model. Microvasc Res 1987; 34:318-35.
7. Dawant B, Levin M, Popel AS. Effect of dispersion of vessel diameters and lengths in stochastic networks I. Modeling of microcirculatory flow. Microvasc Res 1985; 31:203-22.
8. Levin M, Dawant B, Popel AS. Effect of dispersion of vessel diameters and lengths in stochastic networks II. Modeling of microvascular hematocrit distribution. Microvasc Res 1986; 31:223-34.
9. Schreiner W. Computer generation of complex arterial tree models. J Biomed Eng 1993; 15:148-50.
10. Schreiner W, Buxbaum PF. Computer-optimization of vascular trees. IEEE Trans Biomed Eng 1993; 40:482-91.
11. Zamir M. Optimality principles in arterial branching. J Theor Biol 1976; 62:227-51.
12. Thompson DW. On growth and form. Cambridge: University Press, 1942.
13. Milnor WR. Hemodynamics. Baltimore, Hong Kong, London, Sydney: Williams & Wilkins, 1989.
14. Schreiner W, Neumann F, Mohl W. Simulation of coronary circulation with special regard to the venous bed and coronary sinus occlusion. J Biomed Eng 1990; 12:429-43.
15. Schreiner W, Neumann F, Mohl W. Coronary perfusion pressure and inflow resistance have differ-ent influence on intramyocardial flows during coronary sinus interventions. Med Phys 1990; 17:1023-31.
16. Mohl W. The development and rationale of pressure-controlled intermittent coronary sinus occlu-sion—a new approach to protect ischemic myocardium. Wien Klin Wochenschr 1984; 96:20-5.
17. Mohl W. Coronary sinus interventions: From concepts to clinics. J Cardiac Surg 1987; 2:467-93.
18. Mohl W. The momentum of coronary sinus interventions clinically. Circulation 1988; 77:6-12.
19. Podesser B, Neumann F, Neumann M et al. Outer radius—wall thickness—ratio, a quantitative histology of the human coronary arteries. J Vasc Res 1997; in press.
20. Neumann M, Neumann F, Karch R et al. Spatially resolved simulation of coronary hemodynam-ics. In: Cerrolaza M, Jugo D, Brebbia CA, eds. Simulation Modelling in Bioengineering. Southampton Boston: Computational Mechanics Publications, 1996:39-51.
21. Meerbaum S, Lang TW, Osher JV. Diastolic retroperfusion of acutely ischemic myocardium. Am J Cardiol 1976; 37:588-98.
22. Gore JM, Weiner BH, Benotti JR. Preliminary experience with synchronized coronary sinus retroperfusion in humans. Circulation 1984; 74:381.
23. Schreiner W, Neumann F, Nanninga C et al. A computer model of myocardial squeezing and intramyocardial flow during graded coronary artery stenosis in the presence of coronary sinus inter-ventions. Cybernetics and Syst 1989; 20:453-87.
24. Schreiner W, Simon P, Nanninga C et al. Synchronized retroperfusion combined with coronary sinus occlusion: Experimental measurements compared with simulation results and model predic-tions. Cybernetics and Syst 1990; 21:389-421.

CHAPTER 7

The Hazards of Ischemia/Reperfusion Injury During Revascularization Procedures in Acute Myocardial Ischemia

Katharina Palisek, Günter Steurer, and Werner Mohl

E normous advances in surgical, pharmacological, and interventional techniques resulting in early restoration of infarct artery patency significantly improved outcome in patients with acute coronary syndromes.[1] However, time-consuming preparations in patients with acute myocardial ischemia scheduled for emergency bypass surgery, prolonged interventional procedures in patients with complex coronary lesions, and early reestablishment of coronary blood flow in acute myocardial infarction and cardiogenic shock by means of thrombolytic agents or primary angioplasty may result in myocardial tissue damage partly related to reperfusion of oxygenated blood into ischemia-damaged myocardial areas.[2]

Myocardial Ischemia/Reperfusion Injury

Coronary reperfusion within a critical period is essential for survival of ischemic myocardium. In experimental conditions coronary occlusion followed by reperfusion revealed progression of irreversible injury of the ischemic myocardium from the endocardium towards the subepicardium with potentially salvageable myocardium for up to 3-6 hours.[3] The course of events is similar in man depending on the degree of coronary stenosis, size of the ischemic area, size and number of preexisting collateral vessels, and hemodynamic complications. The observation of myocardial stunning,[4] ventricular arrhythmias,[5] or even lethal cell injury in the sequel of successful reperfusion therapy[6] confirmed the clinical relevance of reperfusion injury in acute myocardial ischemia.

Tissue Hypoxia and Anaerobic Metabolism in Acute Myocardial Ischemia

Onset of ischemia is related to significant changes in high energy phosphate state.[7] A rapid catabolism of creatinine phosphokinase and ATP occurs, leading to a loss of degradation products into the extracellular space. ADP and ATP levels are significantly lower after ischemia and stay at a low level for several hours. Lactate levels increase because of heart muscle ischemia. Similarly a calcium triggered, protease dependent conversion of the xanthine dehydrogenase to a superoxide-producing xanthine oxidase occurs. The catabolic degradation of ATP during ischemia leads to an increase in the oxidizable substrate, hypoxanthine.[8]

Coronary Sinus Interventions in Cardiac Surgery, Second Edition edited by Werner Mohl.
©2000 Eurekah.com.

Pathophysiology of Ischemia/Reperfusion Injury

Early reperfusion damages vascular endothelium and capillary structures of the coronary microcirculation by

1. activation of the complement system[9-12]
2. formation of oxygen-derived free radicals,[13-17]
3. disturbance of calcium homeostasis,[5] and
4. apoptosis[21-24] and protects ischemia-induced damaged myocardium by production of heat shock proteins.[25-28] In addition, activation of the adrenergic system may aggravate the occurrence of myocardial ischemia/reperfusion injury.[29]

Ischemia and reperfusion cause inflammation in the affected myocardium, leading to the activation of the complement system and a cascade of factors bringing further threat to the already jeopardized myocardium.[30] Neutrophils migrate in and around the ischemic area, releasing free oxygen-derived radicals and lysozyme enzymes. It has also been suggested, that neutrophils contribute to reperfusion injury by intravascular aggregation in the myocardial capillary system causing inadequate flow.[31] Those neutrophils start their migration into the ischemic areas shortly after the onset of ischemia and increase progressively in number during the following hours so that there is a direct relationship between number of neutrophils in the injured area and length of ischemia. In the meantime the mediator of complement system-related cytotoxicity, the membrane attack complex (MAC), is formed. This complex leads to the lysis of the attacked cell by inserting a pore into the cell membrane, though enabling the cell to control homeostasis and finally leading to rupture of the membrane and cell lysis.

Mitochondria, xanthine oxidase, and prostaglandin biosynthesis are considered possible sources of oxygen-derived free radicals following the infiltration of neutrophil and monocyte cells. The finding of oxygen-derived free radicals in the venous coronary blood after reperfusion of the occluded vessel leads to the conclusion that free radicals are strongly involved in reperfusion injury. Grech et al showed that vessel patency resulted in a significant increase in free radical signal 15 minutes after restoration of coronary flow with a second peak after 24 hours without further angiographic evidence of reocclusion. This leads to the conclusion, that in spite the fact that coronary perfusion has been restored, myocardial damage is still taking place. Finally edema occurs as a result of inflammation, causing mechanical inhibition of diffusion.

A disturbance of the calcium and magnesium homeostasis might contribute to reperfusion injury and myocardial stunning as well. Coronary artery disease and myocardial ischemia increase catecholamines in the serum. This increase is directly related to the severity of coronary artery disease and can be considered a compensatory mechanism of the body to increase perfusion pressure of the vital organs and to improve myocardial contractility. The increase in catecholamines triggers a relative loss of myocardial magnesium, as cellular requirements increase to maintain intracellular metabolic processes. When the support with extracellular magnesium is not sufficient, the steady state might become a vicious circle where catecholamines cause a movement from the intracellular to the extracellular matrix. This decrease of intracellular magnesium leads to an uptake of extracellular calcium ions into the cell. That transient intracellular calcium overload is likely to cause excitation-contraction uncoupling and membrane instability, leading to myocardial dysfunction and arrhythmia. Perfusion of stunned myocardium with low calcium perfusate improved left ventricular function and reperfusion recovery, whereas exposure to high calcium loads resulted in contractile dysfunction. Also magnesium therapy showed beneficial effects in patient with ischemic heart disease.

Activated by myocardial ischemia apoptosis, the programmed death of the cell which follows coronary vessel occlusion due to natural or iatrogenic causes occurs. The process of apoptosis might contribute independently from necrosis to myocyte cell death, and is continues even during and after coronary reperfusion. Extensive apoptotic cardiomyocytes were observed especially at the borders of infarcted myocardium, whereas very few apoptic cells were found in the rest of vital, noninfarcted myocardium. These findings implicate a second, independent factor for myocardial death besides normal cell necrosis due to ischemia. Apoptosis is seemingly not influenced by the restoration of coronary bloodflow.

The production of heat shock proteins (HSP) is triggered by myocardial ischemia as well and is believed to be a rescue mechanism of the jeopardized cell. HSP are known to be expressed after myocardial ischemia and reperfusion, or after preconditioning by heat shock prior to treatment. They are chaperones associating with malfolded proteins preventing their aggregation and seem to protect the myocardial muscle from recurrent ischemia. One can distinguish different types of HSPs expressed such as the inducible HSP 70, the mitochondrial heat shock protein 60 and the small HSP 27. Previous investigations showed that myocardial protection can be achieved by preconditioning of the heart by increasing the body temperature over 40°C for 30 minutes and than returning to normal temperature levels. Rats treated in this way showed significantly smaller infarct areas after 30 min of ligation of a major coronary vessel than the control group. Dillmann et al showed that in transgenetic mice overexpressing HSP 70 the zone of infarction was reduced by 40% and that efflux off creatinine kinase was reduced by 50%, though indicating that this subtype of HSP mediates protection against ischemic injury.

The Possible Role of Coronary Vein Retroperfusion in the Prevention of Ischemia/Reperfusion Injury During Cardiogenic Shock and Acute Coronary Revascularization Procedures

Patients with multiple coronary artery disease, previous myocardial infarction, severely decreased left ventricular function, and prolonged myocardial ischemia undergoing acute coronary interventional procedures are at risk for cardiovascular complications due to myocardial ischemia/reperfusion injury.

Evidence of beneficial effects of coronary sinus interventions in experimental ischemia and clinical studies renewed interest in coronary sinus retroperfusion to protect ischemic myocardium from irreversible damage due to ischemia/reperfusion injury in patients with acute ischemia or cardiogenic shock by extension of the filling capacity of the smallest cardiac veins (SCV) and through improvement of myocardial perfusion.[32] Today's role of coronary sinus intervention in the therapy of coronary artery disease is based on the theory of temporary protection of jeopardized myocardium in patients with acute coronary syndromes undergoing early revascularization procedures.

Since the end of the late 80s coronary angioplasty has entered the daily routine in cardiology. Starting with balloon angioplasty, more and more complex techniques such as coronary stenting, rotational and directional atherectomy and excimer laser have been introduced.[33] Stent implantation started a new area of treatment in interventional cardiology.[34] The restenosis rate was reduced from 30-50% to as low as 20% in elective stent implantation,[5] complications such as acute occlusion of the treated vessel due to complex dissection after balloon angioplasty can be treated by coronary stenting with good clinical and angiographic outcome. Likewise the need for coronary revascularization procedures has increased constantly during the last ten years. The development of new interventional techniques as described above has widened the indications for PTCA immensely so those new concepts for patients with severe coronary artery disease and myocardial infarction had to be worked out.

Coronary Sinus Interventions in Cardiogenic Shock

Cardiogenic shock caused either by necrosis of more than 40% of the left ventricular wall, right heart infarction or rupture of main structures of the heart is the major factor in postinfarction mortality.[37] Hemodynamic stabilization of the patient can be achieved by either pharmacological interventions increase cardiac output or by mechanical support systems such as intraaortic balloon pump or extracorporeal circulation. Treatment is only possible by acute revascularization procedures or acute surgical interventions. The main revascularization techniques include PTCA and thrombolysis therapy, of which thrombolysis is less effective.[38] Coronary sinus interventions could bridge symptomatic and causal treatment. Acute PTCA establishes vessel patency earlier than thrombolysis if the immediate access to a catheterization laboratory is available and yielded better results in immediate and long term results.[39] In patients with severe multivessel disease bypass surgery (CABG), the results are excellent.[40]

Cardiogenic shock, emergency operation, severe left ventricular dysfunction and finally increasing age are reliable predictors of negative outcome in coronary artery surgery.[41] Rescue PTCA is effective in patients with cardiogenic shock diminishing hospital mortality from approximately 80% down to 40-45%.[42] In deaths after extensive myocardial infarction and primary angioplasty, cardiogenic shock is still the most common cause. It has been suggested, that patients with risk factors might profit from additional myocardial salvage or revascularization efforts in the early post infarct period.[43]

Coronary Sinus Interventions in High Risk PTCA

In patients with several risk factors and a complex coronary anatomy, pose a severe problem in revascularization.[44] High risk lesions are defined as significant stenosis in the proximal left anterior descending or left main stem arteries, in which even the slightest disturbance of the remaining minimal blood flow can lead to severe hemodynamic instability. In those patients balloon inflation for balloon angioplasty or stent implantation can lead to intolerable ischemia and cardiogenic shock. PTCA is only undertaken in those patients at the moment if bypass surgery is refused by the surgeon or the patient himself, or as a "bridging" procedure if acute bypass surgery is not available. Recent data suggests that acute PTCA in left main coronary arteries can be of high procedural successful in patients with prohibitive surgical risks.[45-46] During those high risk interventions, retrograde perfusion of the poststenotic, ischemic myocardium protects the heart muscle during those periods of ischemia.[47]

Based on experimental data and results of preliminary clinical studies, coronary vein intervention is used to study the alteration of myocardial metabolism in acute myocardial infarction and to evaluate the effects of retrograde coronary perfusion on myocardial ischemia/reperfusion injury in patients with acute coronary syndromes undergoing coronary interventional procedures or coronary bypass grafting.[48,49]

SSR-Selective Suction and Retroperfusion of Coronary Veins

The SSR device has been developed by Boekstegers and coworkers and is based on a selective approach to the coronary vein via the coronary sinus. The concept of SSR is the pressure-regulated retroinfusion of arterial blood adapted to the coronary venous occlusion pressure. This individual pressure level is determined before ischemia introduced by balloon inflation or other interventional procedures.[50] Oxygenated blood enters the vein through a valve in the balloon-tipped end of the four-lumen catheter and allows retrograde perfusion during periods of ischemia. The main indication for this device is the protection of a circumscribed area of ischemic myocardium, as occurs in coronary interventions such as balloon angioplasty or coronary stenting.

Pressure-Controlled Intermittent Coronary Sinus Occlusion (PICSO)

The technique of PICSO developed by Mohl and coworkers[51] is based on a forced redistribution of venous blood flow into the coronary beds in the setting of coronary artery occlusion to reduce infarct size, improve regional myocardial function, and enhance washout of ischemic metabolic byproducts.

The PICSO system redistributes coronary venous blood flow by changes in pressure gradients throughout the coronary venous system in the setting of coronary artery occlusion. The pump automatically inflates/deflates the balloon according to the occlusion/release timing obtained from the closed-loop feedback algorithm of the system. During balloon inflation there is a slow increase in systolic and diastolic coronary sinus pressure with the effect of redistribution of the coronary venous blood flow from normal to underperfused, ischemic areas (redistribution period). The gradual rise of systolic coronary sinus pressure to a plateau and a concomitant increase of systolic pressure in the perfusion area of the infarct-related coronary artery results in exchange of toxic metabolic products (equilibrium period). The occlusion period is automatically terminated when the exponential curve fitted to the systolic coronary sinus pressure peaks 95% of its predicted plateau value.

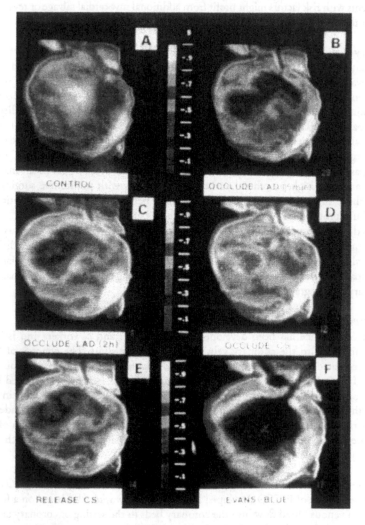

Fig. 7.1. A thermographics study of retrograde myocardial blood supply during coronary sinus intervention in experimented ischemia.

In healthy controls, plateau values of 60-80 mm Hg are usually observed, and occlusion times range approximately from 6-10 seconds. In patients with myocardial infarction, due to the loss of myocardial contractility, however, the slope of the peak values will be drastically reduced resulting in decreased plateau values and substantially prolonged occlusion times. Following termination of the PICSO cycle by deflation of the balloon, coronary sinus pressure abruptly decreases and coronary sinus flow is released, facilitating enhanced drainage of the venous system and reestablishing flow currents that promote washout of accumulated toxic wastes in the ischemic area (washout phase, Fig. 7.1)

Figure 7.1 illustrates a thermographic study of retrograde myocardial blood supply during coronary sinus intervention in experimental ischemia. Note the disappearance of the bluish color during coronary sinus occlusion (D) determining improved perfusion. During coronary sinus release (E) washout takes place (recurrence of bluish color).

After a release period of approximately 6-7 heartbeats and complete return of coronary sinus pressure to baseline levels, the balloon is automatically inflated in order to initiate the next PICSO cycle. The intermittent nature of the inflation/deflation cycle prevents potential complications of hemorrhage, edema, thrombosis, arrhythmia, or conduction disturbances in spite an individual peak coronary sinus pressure of 60 mm Hg or more.[52-55]

Figure 7.3 schematically illustrates a PICSO cycle during acute ischemia and depicts the increase in venous perfusion in relation to the coronary sinus pressure.

Additionally the application of PICSO in patients undergoing bypass surgery led to decreased levels of high energy phosphates (HEP) due to enhanced washout effects and the increased catabolism of nucleotides. Although HEP levels were found to be lower in areas reperfused with PICSO than in the control group, myocardial function was increased. Those effects are probably due to the reutilization of hypoxanthine and adenosine by phosphorylation in the case of adenosine or use of a cosubstrate in the case of hypoxanthine by the purine salvage pathways.[56]

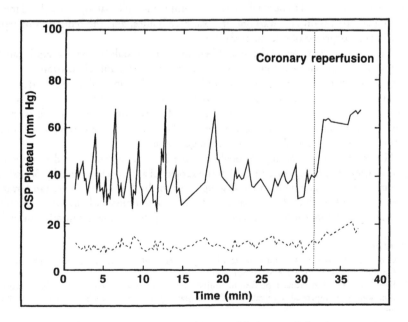

Fig. 7.2. Myocardial blood supply under normal conditions and during acute ischemia.

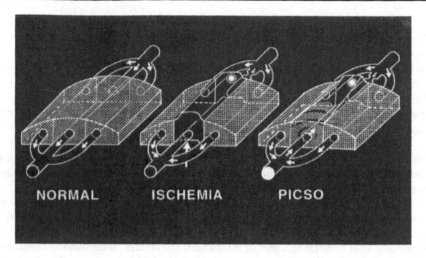

NORMAL   ISCHEMIA   PICSO

Fig. 7.3.

Future Directions

Based on the positive effects of PICSO and SSR in experimental myocardial ischemia and clinical studies randomized clinical studies are elaborated to evaluate the safety and efficacy of PICSO in patients with unstable angina or emerging myocardial infarction, patients with cardiogenic shock symptoms, during high-risk interventional procedures, and during cardiac arrest in bypass surgery.

One of the main assumptions for the treatment with PICSO is the improvement of global myocardial function and decrease of the effects of ischemia on the jeopardized myocardium. This effect is understood to be reached by the maintenance of basal myocardial cell metabolism by retrograde perfusion and washout of toxic metabolites, and the reduction of reperfusion injury in areas deprived of arterial perfusion.

Patients with cardiogenic shock and hemodynamic instability have a significantly worse prognosis for revascularization procedures than patients with stable circulation status. By using retrograde access to the venous system and by the installation of the PICSO device, the left ventricular ejection fraction could be improved and hemodynamic parameters could be stabilized. A single center pilot trial by Mohl and coworkers will determine the effects and benefits of PICSO in unstable patients with cardiogenic shock in intensive care units with respect to global vitality of myocardial muscle and final outcome.

The concept of preventing regional ischemia in patients randomized to undergo either bypass surgery or SSR-supported PTCA is the subject of a study elaborated by Boekstegers et al at the moment. Patients with an equally high risk for both procedures are randomized. As a single center study with SSR in 47 patients showed good results without major complications, the advantages of either technique will now be investigated in a larger number of patients.[57]

References

1. Grover A, Rihal CS. The importance of early patency after acute myocardial infarction. Current Opinion in Cardiology 1995; 10:361-366.
2. Braunwald E. Myocardial reperfusion, limitation of infarct size, reduction of left ventricular dysfunction, and improved survival. Should the paradigm be expanded? Circulation 1989; 79:441-444.

3. Reimer KA, Lowe JE, Ramussen MM, Jennings RB. The wave front phenomenon of ischemia cell death: Myocardial infarct size vs. duration of coronary occlusion in dogs. Circulation 1977; 56:786-794.
4. Bolli R. Myocardial stunning in man. Circulation 1992; 86:1671-1691.
5. Kusama Y, Bernier M, Hearse DJ. Exacerbation of reperfusion arrhythmias by sudden oxidant stress. Circulation Research 1990; 67:481-489.
6. Ambrosio G, Becker LC, Hutchins GM, Weisman HF, Weisfeldt ML. Reduction in experimental infarct size by recombinant human superoxide dismutase: Insights into the pathophysiology of reperfusion injury. Circulation 1986; 74:1424-1433.
7. Fossel ET, Morgan HE, Ingwall JS. Measurements of changes in high-energy phosphates in the cardiac cycle using gated P-31 nuclear magnetic resonance. Proc Nat Acad Sci USA 1980; 77:3654.
8. McCord JM, Roy RS, Schaffer SW. Free radicals and myocardial ischemia. The role of xanthine oxidase. Adv Myocardiol 1985; 5:183-9.
9. Black SC, Schasteen CS, Weiss RH et al. Complement activation and inhibition a myocardial ischemia and reperfusion injury. Annu Rev Pharmacol Toxicol 1994; 270:17-40.
10. Lucchesi BR. Complement, Neutrophils and Free Radicals: Mediators to Reperfusion Injury. Drug research 1994; 44(I), Nr.3a.
11. Pinckard RN, Olson MS, Kelley RE et al. Antibody-independent activation of human C1 after interaction with heart subcellular membranes. J Immunol 1973; 110:1376-82.
12. Hillis LD, Braunwald E. Myocardial Ischemia. N Engl J Med 1977; 110:1376-82.
13. Grech ED, Nicholas JF, Dodd MA et al. Evidence for free radical generation after primary percutaneous transluminal coronary recanalisation in acute myocardial infarction. Am J Card 1996; 77:122-27.
14. Coghlan JG, Flitter WD, Holley AE. Detection of free radicals and cholesterol hydroperoxides in blood taken from the coronary sinus of man during percutaneous transluminal coronary. Free Rad Res Commun 1991; 14:409-417.
15. Baker JE, Felix CC, OlingerGN et al. Myocardial ischemia and reperfusion: direct evidence for free radical generation by electro spin resonance spectroscopy. Proc Natl Acad Sci USA 1988; 85:2786-2789.
16. Lucchesi BR. Myocardial ischemia, reperfusion and free radical injury. Am J Cardiol 1990; 65:14I-23I.
17. McCord JM. Oxygen derived free radicals in postischemic tissue injury. N Engl J Med 1985; 312:159-63.
18. Kusoka H, Koretsune Y, Chacko et al. Excitation-contraction coupling in postischemic myocardium: Does failure of activator Ca transients underline stunning? Circ Res 1990; 66:1268-76.
19. Du Toit EF, Opie LH. Modulation of severity of reperfusion stunning in the isolated rat heart by agents altering calcium flux at onset of reperfusion. Circ Res 1992; 70:960-7.
20. Smetana R, Brochette A, Glover D. Stress and magnesium metabolism in coronary artery disease. Magnesium Bull 1991; 13:125-7.
21. Veinot JP, Gattinger DA, Fliss H. Early Apoptosis in Human Myocardial Infarcts. Hum Path 1997; 28:485-92.
22. Saraste A, Pulkki K, Kallajoki M. Apoptosis in human myocardial infarction. Circulation 1997; 95:320-3.
23. Kajstura J, Cheng W, Reiss K. Apoptotic and necrotic myocyte cell deaths are independent contributing variables of infarct size in rats. Lab Invest 1996; 74:86-107.
24. Olivetti G, Quaini F, Sala R et al. Acute myocardial infarction in humans is associated with activation of programmed myocyte cell death in the surviving portion of the heart. J Moll Cell Cardiol 1996; 28:2005-16.
25. Hendrick J, Hartl F-U. Molecular chaperone function of the heat-shock proteins. Annu Rev Biochem 1993; 62:349-384.
26. Samali A, Cotter TG. Heat shock proteins increase resistance to apoptosis. Exp Cell Res 1996; 223:163-70.
27. Dillmann WH, Mestril R. Heat shock proteins in myocardial stress. Z Kardiol 1995; 84 Suppl 4:87-90.
28. Marber MS, Mestril R, Chi S-H et al. Overexpression of the rat inducible 70-kD heat stress protein in a transgenic mouse increases the resistance of the heart to ischemic injury. J Clin Invest 1995; 95:1446-1456.

30. Meerbaum S, Lang TW, Osher JV et al. Diastolic retroperfusion of acutely ischemic myocardium. Am J Cardiol 1976; 37:588-598.
31. Engler RD, Dahlgren MD, Morris DD et al. Role of leukocytes in response to acute myocardial ischemia and reflow in dogs. Am J Physiol 1986; 251:H314-23.
32. Pratt H. Nutrition of the heart through the vessels of Thebsius and coronary veins. Am J Physiol 1898; 1:86-103.
33. Reifart N. PTCA or second generation devices? Reappraisal of the balloon. Z Kardiol 1995; 84 Suppl 2:43-52.
34. Foley DP, Melkert R, Umans VA. Differences in restenosis propensity of devices for transluminal coronary intervention. Europ Heart J 1995; 16:1331-1346.
35. Goldberg SI, Colombo A, Maiello L. Intracoronary stent insertion after balloon angioplasty of chronic total occlusions.
36. Colombo A, Ferraro M, Itoh A. Results of coronary stenting for restenosis. JACC 1996; 28:830-6.
37. Görge G, Haude M, Baumgart D. Therapy of cardiogenic shock in acute myocardial infarction. Herz 1994; 19:360-70.
38. Meyer J. Intracoronary interventions in the early infarct period. Z Kardiol 1994; 83 Suppl 6.111-9.
39. Holmes DR, Bates ER, Kleiman NS. Contemporary reperfusion therapy for cardiogenic shock: The GUSTO-I Trial experience. JACC 1995; 26 No.3:668-74.
40. Antoniucci D, Santoro GM, Bolognese L. Primary coronary angioplasty for acute myocardial infarction associated with severe left ventricular dysfunction. Results in 50 patients. G Ital Cardiol 1995; 25:1265-71.
41. Magovern JA, Sakert T, Magovern GJ. A model that predicts morbidity and mortality after coronary artery bypass graft surgery. JACC 1996; 29:1147-53.
42. Fontanelli A, Bernardi G, Di Chiara A. Primary percutaneous transluminal coronary in acute myocardial infarction: Immediate and short-term results. Cardiologia 1994; 29:427-34.
43. Krikorian RK, Vacek JL, Baechamp GD. Timing, mode, and predictors of death after direct angioplasty for acute myocardial infarction. Cath Cardiovasc Diagn 1995; 35:192-6.
44. Hamm W et al. A randomized study of coronary angioplasty compared with bypass surgery in patients with symptomatic multivessel coronary disease. N Engl J Med 1994; 331:1037-43.
45. Chauhan A, Zubaid M, Ricci DR. Left main interventions revisited: early and late outcome of PTCA and stenting. Cathet Cardiovasc Diagn 1997; 29:21-9.
46. Gaspardone et al. A comparison of coronary artery stenting with angioplasty for isolated stenosis of the proximal left anterior descending coronary artery. N Engl J Med 1997; 336:817-22.
47. Lincoff AM, Popma JJ, Ellis SG et al. Percutaneous support devices for high risk or complicated coronary angioplasty. JACC 1991; 17:770-80.
48. Mohl W, Glogar HD, Mary H et al. Reduction of infarct size induced by pressure controlled intermittent coronary sinus occlusion. Am J Cardiol 1984; 53:923-28.
49. Boekstegers P, Peter W, Degenfeld G et al. Preservation of regional myocardial function and myocardial oxygen tension during acute ischemia in pigs: Comparison of selective synchronized coronary venous retroperfusion. JACC 1994; 23:459-69.
50. Boekstegers P et al. Selective ECG synchronized suction and retroinfusion of coronary veins: First results of studies in acute ischemia in dogs. Cardiovasc Res 1990; 24:456-64.
51. Mohl W. The development and rationale of pressure controlled intermittent coronary sinus occlusion: A new approach to protect ischemic myocardium. Wi Kli Wo 1984; 96:205-209.
52. Mohl W, Glogar DH, Mary H et al. Reduction of infarct size induced by pressure-controlled intermittent coronary sinus occlusion. Am J Cardiol 1984; 53:923-928.
53. Mohl W, Punzengruber C, Moser. Effects of pressure-controlled intermittent coronary sinus occlusion on regional ischemic myocardial function. J Am Coll Cardiol 1985; 5:939-947.
54. Mohl W, Glogar D, Kenner T. Enhancement of washout induced by PICSO in the canine and human heart. In: W Mohl, W Wolner, and D Glogar, ed. The coronary sinus. New York: Springer-Verlag; 1984:537-548.
55. Jacobs SK, Faxon DP, Coats WD et al. Pressure-controlled, intermittent coronary sinus occlusion (PICSO) during reperfusion markedly reduces infarct size. Clin Res 1985; 33:197A.
56. Boekstegers P et al. High efficacy of a new pressure-regulated and more selective retroinfusion system of coronary veins in patients with normal and high risk PTCA. Circ 1996; 94:94 I-561.

CHAPTER 8

Distribution of Antegrade and Retrograde Cardioplegia-Experimental Results

Gabriel S. Aldea and Richard S. Shemin

Introduction

Previously published clinical series do not reflect the evolution of myocardial protection, anesthetic, and surgical revascularization techniques. Despite the relentless progressive increase in perioperative comorbid risks in patients undergoing CABG, results have remained uniformly excellent.[1-4] This is largely due to experimental advances which resulted in changes in both the composition and the route of delivery of cardioplegic solutions to enhance myocardial protection.

Composition

Previous chapters detailed techniques which enhance myocardial protection by preconditioning the myocardium prior to the ischemic insult and to surgical revascularization. These include GIK, heat shock proteins, and warm induction of cardioplegic arrest.[5,6] In addition, changes in the composition of cardioplegic solution were also demonstrated to enhance myocardial salvage and diminish the risk for postischemic myocardial dysfunction. These include the use of blood cardioplegia, substrate enhancement (aspartate, glutamate), superoxide radical scavengers, and leukocyte depletion.[7-11]

Despite demonstrated efficacy in the laboratory, improved clinical outcome with these techniques, as measured by mortality and residual cardiac function, were only demonstrated in acutely ischemic patients with depressed ventricular function.[12]

Myocardial protection depends on homogeneous distribution of cardioplegic solution to all regions of the heart distal to coronary artery occlusions (CAO) to minimize the potential risk of postischemic myocardial dysfunction and damage. This chapter will focus on experimental studies comparing different routes and methods of delivery to assess: 1) the efficacy of delivery and distribution of cardioplegic solution beyond CAO, 2) measuring cardiac energetic and intracellular pH, and 3) assessing the extent of damage and function following cardioplegic delivery.

Coronary Sinus Interventions in Cardiac Surgery, Second Edition edited by Werner Mohl.
©2000 Eurekah.com.

Delivery

Optimal myocardial protection relies on adequate delivery of cardioplegia to all areas of the heart. The presence of coronary artery obstructions was demonstrated to impair antegrade cardioplegia (AC) delivery.[13-15] Since the coronary venous circulation is free of atherosclerotic disease,[16] this retrograde route provided an ideal conduit and route for delivery of cardioplegia to myocardial regions beyond a coronary artery obstruction. Refinements in coronary sinus (CS) retrograde cardioplegia (RC) techniques have resulted in their widespread clinical application with improvement in clinical outcomes. However, despite these advances, myocardial protection through cardioplegic arrest remain imperfect. Postoperatively, there is evidence of cellular and subcellular alterations even in apparently normal hearts with preserved function.[17-19]

Despite their universal use, patterns of antegrade (AC) and retrograde (RC) cardioplegia delivery to small discrete myocardial regions remains largely unknown. Understanding these patterns may result in improved strategies to enhance myocardial protection. To investigate these patterns, we designed an experimental model to study the distribution of cardioplegia in adult pigs (whose coronary circulation closely resembles that of the human) with unobstructed coronary arteries, using radioactive microsphere methodology. Cardioplegia flow distribution was determined by injecting radioactive microspheres measuring 15 microns in diameter containing one of nine different gamma-emitting nuclides. Absolute flow is calculated in relation to known flow and radioactivity of a reference sample. Other studies use alternative techniques of colored microspheres. Radioactive and colored microsphere methodologies permit precise determination of flow to very small regions of the heart and have the spatial resolution to distinguish variations of flow within and across layers (both horizontally and tangentially). It is the most precise way of quantitating differences between regional subepicardial, mid-wall and subendocardial flows. Other studies use an alternative technique of adding 0.5 mCi of thallium-201 to the cardioplegic solution with regional flow delivery measured by computer planimetry. Although this technique is unable to distinguish subendocardial from subepicardial flow, it is a very useful tool to assess flow regional beyond CAO.

Methods

After induction of warm blood antegrade cardioplegic (AC) arrest (37°C), cardioplegia was administered using a centrifugal pump through a vented multiple perfusion set. Normothermic blood cardioplegic delivery was selected to specifically eliminate the confounding possible effects on regional myocardium distribution at hypothermic conditions and of crystalloid solutions. The AC was administered through a standard 16 Ga. cannula, and the retrograde cardioplegia (RC) through a 15 Fr. cannula with an auto-inflating cuff (DLP Co., Grand Rapids, MI). Aortic root and coronary sinus pressures were simultaneously recorded and cardioplegia flow rates were measured with an in-line electromagnetic flow meter (Carolina Medical Model 701D, Series 600 probe).

Previous work reported significant dislodgment of radiolabeled microspheres entrapped within the myocardial with RC during AC administration, leading to serious errors in regional flow measurements.[13] To prevent this problem, RC flow administration followed AC in all our experimental animals. The sequence of radioactive isotope injection was randomized in each animal.

Validation Studies

In preliminary experimental animals, we determined the proper number of injected radioactive microspheres to result in a minimal entrapment of 400 spheres in greater than 95% of all myocardial regions, for each flow condition. All hearts evaluated in this study fulfilled these criteria.

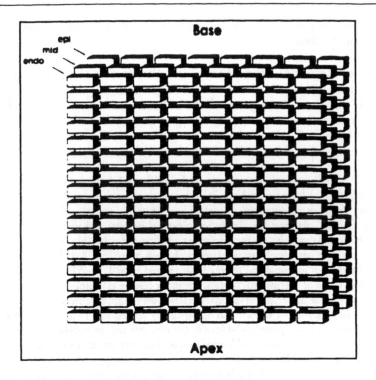

Fig. 8.1. Left ventricular myocardial cutting scheme.

Proper mixing of microspheres and reproducibility of the technique were verified by sequentially injecting two different radiolabeled microspheres for each route of cardioplegia administration. For both AC and RC the correlation coefficients (R2) were greater than 0.84. Consequently, errors resulting from clumping of microspheres, separation, calculation, and random distribution unrelated to flow could be excluded.

We also excluded the possibility that the differences (between AC and RC) in patterns of cardioplegia delivery to discrete myocardial regions were artificially caused by dislodgment of previously entrapped (AC delivered) radioactive microspheres. This was done by collecting the aortic effluent during RC administration, measuring its radioactive content, and comparing it to that of the LV. This confirmed that less than 0.14+0.24 % of LV radioactivity was recovered in the aortic effluent during RC administration which is too small to account for the significant differences in the patterns of cardioplegia flow between AC and RC.

Finally, to exclude the possible effects of edema on the experimental findings, myocardial water content was evaluated in several animals before and after cardioplegic arrest (tissue was desiccated in a vacuum oven for 72 hours). No differences were noted.

Numerical Methods

All comparisons were made by repeated measures of variance and Newman-Keuls, a posterior test of significance. Statistical comparisons of the coefficients of variation (the ratio of the standard deviation of a distribution of measurements to its mean) were performed using the technique of Lewontin, as described by Zar.[20] Correlation coefficients (R2) refer to a "simple" or Pearson product-moment correlation coefficient. All mean values are given plus or minus one standard deviation.

Studies of Regional Blood Flow Distribution in the Beating Heart

It is now well accepted that myocardial perfusion in the normal myocardium is both temporally and spatially heterogeneous.[21,22] This heterogeneity has been observed in the heart of all species studied so far. The work my colleagues and I performed under the direction of Dr. Julien I. E. Hoffman (Cardiovascular Research Institute, UCSF, San Francisco, CA) focused on studying the spatial aspects of the variability of regional myocardial perfusion and its implications.

Austin et al demonstrated the presence of significant inhomogeneity of regional left ventricular myocardial blood flow both at rest and during pharmacologic vasodilation with adenosine[23] in seven experimental animals. These patterns were not related to epicardial gross coronary vascular anatomy (proximity to epicardial vessels) and varied amongst individual animals. We found that although patterns were highly reproducible (Fig. 8.2) resting and maximal flow patterns were completely uncorrelated with each other (Fig. 8.3).[23] Regional reserve, defined as the ratio of maximal and resting flow, ranged from 1.75 (57% of maximum) to 21.9 (resting flow 4.5% of maximum).[23] Thus, coronary reserve is profoundly spatially inhomogeneous. Despite wide dispersion of coronary reserve, we found, by autocorrelation analysis, that the reserve in neighboring regions was significantly correlated. Thus, both resting coronary blood flow and reserve appear to be locally continuous and may define functional zones of vascular control and vulnerability. Normal hearts, therefore, contain small regions that may be relatively more vulnerable to ischemia.

Coggins et al investigated whether coronary vasodilator reserve persists during myocardial ischemia is present in all ventricular regions.[24] Myocardial flow to small discrete regions of the left ventricle were determined using radioactive microsphere methodology, while perfusion pressure was progressively decreased, in eight experimental animals. At each condition, regional flow was assessed at baseline condition and during maximal pharmacologic vasodilation with adenosine. At 70 mm Hg, 100% of left ventricular regions had significant flow reserve, compared to 92%, 55%, and 8% during perfusion at 50, 40, and 30 mmHG (Table 8.1).[27]

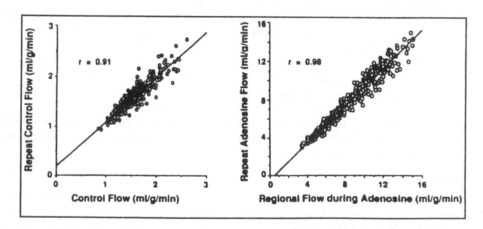

Fig. 8.2. Plots evaluating reproducibility of the distribution of regional blood flow in an individual animal. A second set of microspheres containing a different nuclide was injected 5 minutes after the first. Left panel: comparisons of repeated measurements of regional control coronary flow. Right panel: comparisons of repeated measurements of maximal regional coronary flow (with adenosine).

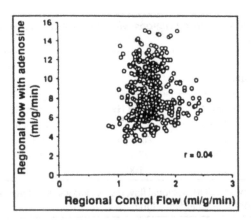

Fig. 8.3. Plots comparing regional myocardial blood flow at rest with regional myocardial blood flow during maximal pharmacological dilation with adenosine in an individual experimental animal.

Absolute flow and the ratio of regions with flow reserve diminished most dramatically in the subendocardium with a progressive decrease in coronary perfusion pressure (Table 8.2).[24]

We concluded that coronary reserve persists in only a subset of left ventricular regions during ischemia, and that the number of regions with persistent reserve diminished with coronary perfusion pressures. These findings may be explained by a model in which regional ischemia is a maximal coronary vasodilator and that persistent pharmacological vasodilator reserve seen when global markers indicate ischemia simply reflect persistent endogenous flow reserve to myocardial regions not yet ischemic, implying that the heart is highly efficient in its metabolic regulation of vascular tone. The persistence of tone during ischemia represents an effort by the heart to shunt blood to areas of the myocardium that need it most. Maximal vasodilation of resistance vessels with pharmacological agents may be deleterious by creating regional steal phenomena. The striking clinical benefit of coronary vasodilators such as nitrates and Ca** channel blockers in the treatment of ischemia probably relies on their ability to reduce myocardial oxygen consumption by decreasing preload and afterload, and on their ability to prevent coronary spasm.

Table 8.1. Mean flow reserve (ml gm/min) in different myocardial layers and mean flow reserve ratio at different perfusion pressures.

LMCA perfusion pressure

	70 mm Hg	50 mm Hg	40 mm Hg	30 mm Hg
Subendocardium	3.86+0.11*	0.51+0.03*	0.14+0.02*	0.02+0.01
Midwall	4.45+0.11*	1.29+0.06*	0.41+0.02*	0.06+0.01
Subepicardium	3.10+0.08*	1.37+0.06*	0.73+0.03*	0.12+0.02*
Endo/epi reserve ratio	1.2	0.37†	0.19†	0.17†

Values are mean +SD. LMCA is left main coronary artery. Endo/epi ratio is the subendocardial/subepicardial flow reserve.*significant flow reserve <0.01, paired t-test, comparing flows before and after adenosine infusion. † significant decrease compared with endo/epi ratio at 70 mm Hg, p <0.05, paired t-test.

Table 8.2. Percent of myocardial regions with significant coronary reserve at different perfusion pressures

LMCA perfusion pressure

	70 mm Hg	50 mm Hg	40 mm Hg	30 mm Hg
Transmural	100	92 + 12	55 + 24	8 + 7
Subendocardium	100	78 + 15	35 + 32	1 + 2
Midwall	100	97 + 5	58 + 20	3 + 3
Subepicardium	100	100	72 + 27	19 + 22

Values are reported as mean + SEM. Regional flow reserve is considered significant if it exceeded twice the total estimated error (95% confidence limit).

These findings may explain the patchy nature of infarction noted with hypoxia or at reduced perfusion pressures. This profound heterogeneity is baseline regional myocardial blood flow and reserve points out the potential difficulties of using global parameters to assess regional "well being".

Experimental Hypotheses

Based on our work in the beating heart model,[23-25] we proposed the following experimental hypotheses: 1) The distribution of cardioplegia may differ with the route of (AC or RC) of cardioplegia delivery; 2) Cardioplegia delivery to small myocardial regions may be significantly inhomogeneous even in the absence of coronary artery disease, and 3) Patterns of AC and RC delivery may be mismatched. To investigate these hypotheses, we designed an experimental model to study the distribution of cardioplegia in adult pigs with unobstructed coronary arteries, using radioactive microsphere methodology.

Studies of Regional Cardioplegia Flow Distributions

We studied the regional flow distribution of antegrade cardioplegia (AC) in nondiseased hearts. Global and regional myocardial flow were measured at different perfusion pressures. Patterns of crystalloid and blood cardioplegia delivery were similar. As coronary perfusion pressure decreased, flow in all layers fell significantly ($p < 0.001$) (Fig. 8.4).[25]

This flow was most dramatic in the subendocardium ($p < 0.05$) (Fig. 8.5). The relationship of pressure and flow with both cardioplegic solutions (blood and crystalloid) was nonlinear. At low coronary perfusion, a given change in pressure resulted in a smaller change in flow than at higher perfusion pressure (Fig. 8.6).[25] In addition, we found that in all the animals and at all perfusion pressures, there was a profound variability in the delivery of cardioplegic solutions to small discrete regions on the left ventricle. At a perfusion pressure of 40 mm Hg, the extremes of regional flow varied on average by 203%. This inhomogeneity increased significantly with decreasing perfusion pressures. At the lowest perfusion pressure measured (20 mm Hg), the extremes of regional flow varied on average by 365%.[25] These findings emphasize the importance of coronary perfusion pressure on the delivery of cardioplegic solutions even in

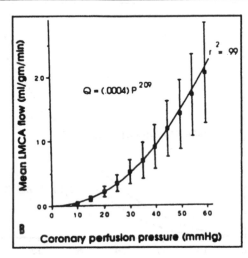

Fig. 8.4. The relationship of left main coronary artery flow (Q) to coronary perfusion pressure (P) mean value for eight experimental animals. Error bars represent standard deviation.

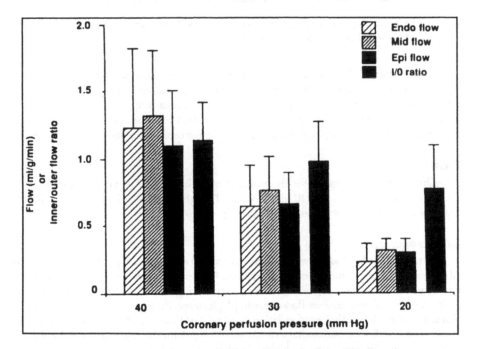

Fig. 8.5. The effect of fall in coronary perfusion pressure on flow within each layer of the heart and on the inner/outer (subendocardial/subepicardial) flow ratio. Each layer had a significantly different flow at each pressure (p < 0.001). The subendocardial/subepicardial ratio was also significantly different at each pressure (p < 0.001). The error bars represent standard deviation.

hearts with unobstructed coronary arteries. Inhomogeneous delivery of cardioplegia will be further accentuated by the presence of coronary artery obstruction, which results in a fall in coronary perfusion pressure beyond such lesions. At low perfusion pressures, not only is the mean flow reduced, but a greater number of regions receive limited amounts of cardioplegia.

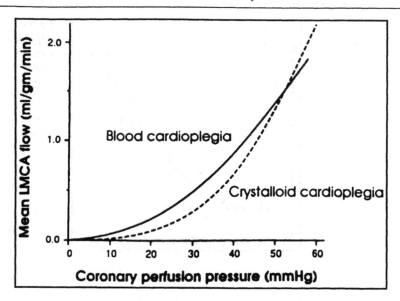

Fig. 8.6. The relationship of coronary perfusion pressure and left main coronary artery flow: comparison of blood and crystalloid cardioplegic formulations.

We investigated the hypothesis that patterns of regional cardioplegia flow delivery may vary with the route (antegrade or retrograde) of cardioplegia delivery. Antegrade and retrograde cardioplegia were delivered at 150 ml/min. In six hearts, the cardioplegia flow delivery to 1152 discrete myocardial regions was determined twice for each route of delivery using one of four different radioactive microspheres for a total of 4608 regional cardioplegia flow measurements

Flow

The mean LV flow for all six experimental animals was $1.37 + 0.31$ ml/gm-min for AC, and $0.39 + 0.09$ ml/gm-min for RC (Fig. 8.7A). This greater than 3-fold difference between routes of administration was highly significant ($p < 0.001$).[26,27]

Inhomogeneity

Patterns of cardioplegia flow to discrete myocardial regions in a representative experimental animal (No. 4) are demonstrated in Figure 8.8. Cardioplegia flow for both routes of delivery was uneven (inhomogeneous), with some regions receiving flows 6-10 fold higher than others. This uneven or inhomogeneous flow of cardioplegia to specific myocardial regions was further characterized by the coefficient of variation (CV(%) = SD/mean x 100). The mean coefficient of variation for all six experimental animals was $48 + 17\%$ for AC and $106 + 16\%$ for RC (Fig. 8.7B).[26,27] This difference was also highly significant ($p < 0.001$).

Correlation

Flows to individual myocardial regions measured with different radioactive microsphere labels were compared. Using linear regression analysis, with each regional flow compared to itself under different experimental conditions, and correlation coefficients ($R2$) were obtained. Correlations of flow in a representative experimental animal (No. 4) are demonstrated in Fig. 8. 9.

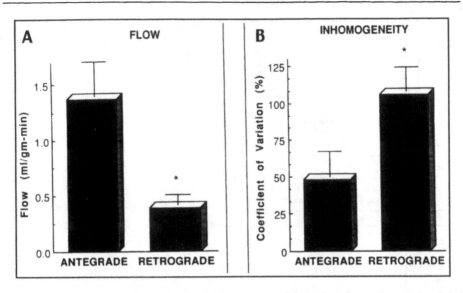

Fig. 8.7. Global left ventricular flow (left) and inhomogeneity of cardioplegia flow to discrete myocardial regions (right) in six experimental animals. Inhomogeneity of regional flow is quantified by the coefficient of variation. *p < 0.001

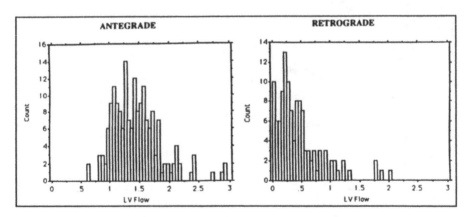

Fig. 8.8. Patterns of antegrade and retrograde cardioplegia flow delivery to discrete myocardial regions in a single animal (No. 4). The number of regions (count) with a characteristic flow (ml/gm-min) is demonstrated by this frequency histogram.

AC and RC flow patterns measured with different radioactive isotopes were highly correlated (R^2 of 0.88 for AC1-AC2, and 0.81 for RC1-RC2).[26,27] Thus, a region with a high flow during a particular route of cardioplegia administration maintained that characteristic high flow when the measurement was repeated, for the same route. However, AC and RC patterns were mismatched ($R^2 = 0.04$). Thus, a region with low flow during AC administration had a different flow profile with RC administration.

　　These findings were consistent in all six experimental animals. The mean correlation coefficients (R^2) were 0.88 + 0.12 for AC1-AC2, 0.84 + 10 for RC1-RC2 , and 0.03+0.04 when AC and RC were compared (Fig. 8.10).[26,27] These highly significant differences ($p < 0.001$) suggest that while patterns of cardioplegia flow are highly reproducible for a given route of

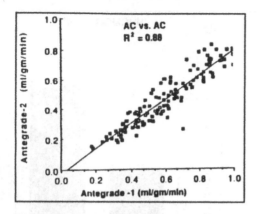

Fig. 8.9. Comparison of correlation of flows to discrete myocardial regions in a single animal (No. 4). R2 is the correlation coefficient.

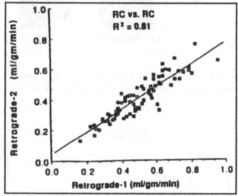

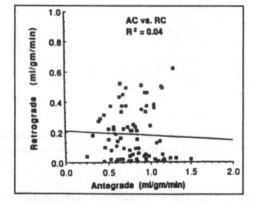

administration, no correlation exists between AC and RC flow patterns confirming they are mismatched.

Other Studies

Studies using colored microspheres in both animal and explanted human hearts have also demonstrated inhomogeneity of cardioplegia delivery even in the absence of coronary artery obstruction. Gates and colleagues have demonstrated that as many as 12.5%-32%

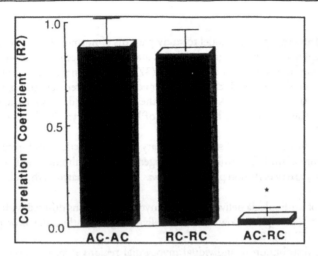

Fig. 8.10. Comparison of mean correlation coefficients of flow to discrete myocardial regions for all six experimental animals. R2 is the correlation coefficient. *p > 0.001.

of all capillary beds are perfused by RC which were not perfused by AC, suggesting that combined AC and RC enhance regional myocardial cardioplegic distribution.[28-30] However, as in our studies, although RC is able to deliver regional cardioplegia to areas beyond coronary artery obstruction not properly protected by AC alone, results in better cooling, and is more effective at evacuating air trapped in the coronary arteries, RC provides significantly less "nutritive" cardioplegic flow is compared with AC (more shunting).[31-34] These and other studies confirm increased inhomogeneity with cardioplegic delivery with RC compared with AC. RC delivery (in isolation) results not only in decreased nutritive flow and increased in inhomogeneous delivery to the left ventricle, but also results in focal areas of hypoperfusion and an even more dramatic decrease in "nutritive" nonshunt flow in the septum and right ventricular free wall. This inhomogeneity is not affected by temperature, increased coronary sinus perfusion pressure, or aortic root venting.[35,36]

Cardiac Energetics

Using 31P Magnetic Resonance Spectroscopy, several studies have demonstrated that RC alone can preserve normal levels of energy metabolites and intracellular pH beyond a LAD coronary artery obstruction.[37-39] However, the efficacy of RC route alone (both with respect to distribution and rate of energy recovery) is lower than AC + RC.[39,40] When RC is administered under normothermic conditions, even in the absence of interrupted flow, ischemic metabolism is established.[40]

Cardiac Function

The clinical significance of adequate regional cardioplegic flow delivery and protection and preservation of cardiac energetics is demonstrated by the ability to attenuate the extent of damage following an acute ischemic injury (long-term) and to preserve regional as well as global myocardial function (short-term). Again, RC has been demonstrated to decrease edema, myocardial water content, and diastolic dysfunction in isolated hearts, but the best preservation of left and right ventricular function is noted when AC and RC are used in a complementary fashion.[26,33,34,38]

Discussion

We designed an experimental model to study patterns of normothermic blood cardioplegia delivery to discrete myocardial regions with AC and RC. We specifically chose to study the regional distribution of warm blood cardioplegia (37°C) to eliminate the potential vasoconstrictive effects of a cold solution which may further accentuate differences (inhomogeneity) in regional flows.[41,42] Although this work centered on the study of blood cardioplegia, our previous work demonstrated similar results when patterns of blood and crystalloid cardioplegia flows were compared.[28]

We concluded that even in the absence of coronary artery obstruction cardioplegia delivery to small discrete regions of the left ventricle is inhomogeneous. This inhomogeneity is profoundly affected by coronary artery perfusion pressure, and was most accentuated in the subendocardium (Fig. 8.11).

The pattern of cardioplegia delivery to small myocardial regions differed with the route of administration.[26,27] For a given flow rate, AC delivers significantly more flow per gram of myocardium than RC (Fig. 8.7A).

Cardioplegia distribution to individual myocardial regions is very uneven (inhomogeneous) for both AC and RC. This inhomogeneity was greatest with RC (Fig. 8.7B).

Differences in the regional delivery of cardioplegia flow did not correlate to the gross coronary vascular anatomy (proximity to epicardial vessels) and varied amongst individual animals. Patterns of regional cardioplegia flow to discrete myocardial regions were highly reproducible for a given route of delivery (Fig. 8.10). However, regional flow patterns with AC were significantly different compared to those with RC. Mismatched patterns of AC and RC cardioplegia delivery suggest that these modalities are complementary.

Even in the absence of coronary artery obstruction, some regions received a 6 to 10 fold higher cardioplegia flow than others (Fig. 8.8). This inhomogeneous delivery may explain the patchy nature of subendocardial infarction noted after ischemic revascularization.[23-26] Measurements inferring "well being" of small discrete myocardial regions from global measurements may be misleading.[24] Inhomogeneous delivery of cardioplegia may be sufficient to result in asynchronous electrical activity and an isoelectric ECG, while individual small regions may have ongoing metabolic activity which may result in postischemic injury. Furthermore, the patchy nature of such damage may go undetected by global measurements of ventricular function, since hypercontractile areas can compensate for small areas of regional dysfunction.

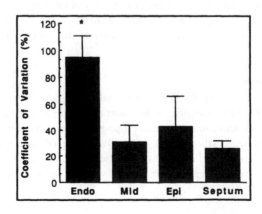

Fig. 8.11. Differences in inhomogeneity of antegrade cardioplegic flow delivery between myocardial layers.

Thus, preserved ventricular function, a normal ECG, or even local metabolic measurements (such as pH or ATP) do not exclude the presence of regional myocardial damage.

Optimal cardioplegia delivery to all myocardial regions is particularly important in the presence of compromised ventricular function.[12,15] Reliance on a single route of cardioplegia delivery may result in inadequate regional myocardial protection. Since the minimal amount of cardioplegia necessary to establish a complete regional metabolic arrest is unknown, in order to best assure protection of the entire myocardium and overcome the cardioplegia flow disparity to small myocardial regions, a generous amount of cardioplegia has to be administered. However, smaller cardioplegia volumes could be used if AC and RC were used as complementary techniques to enhance the regional delivery of cardioplegia. Our findings may explain the experimental and clinical observations of the salutary effect of combining the use of AC and RC in patients with compromised LV function.[27]

Inhomogeneous delivery of cardioplegia to discrete myocardial regions would be further accentuated by the presence of coronary artery obstructions.[13,14] Therefore, based on our experimental results, and those of other studies, we recommend the routine combined use of AC and RC to optimize delivery of cardioplegia to all regions of the heart and minimize the potential of postischemic myocardial dysfunction.

References

1. Fremes SE, Goldman BS, Christakis et al. Current risk of coronary artery bypass surgery for unstable angina. Eur J Cardiothorac Surg 1991; 5:235-243.
2. Naunheim KS, Fiore AC, Arango DC et al. Coronary artery bypass grafting for unstable angina: Risk analysis. Ann Thorac Surg 1989; 47:569-574.
3. Hammermeister KE, Morrison DA. Coronary artery bypass grafting for stable and unstable angina. Cardiol Clinics 199; 9(1):135-155.
4. Lazar HL, Faxon DP, Gunnar RM et al. Changing profile of failed angioplasty; impact on surgical results. Ann Thorac Surg 199; 53:269-273.
5. Gardinac S, Coleman GM, Tagetmeyer H et al. Improved cardiac function with glucose-insulin-potassium after aortocoronary bypass grafting. Ann Thorac Surg 1989; 48:484-489.
6. Knowlton AA, Eberli F, Romo GM et al. Fibronectin expression in the rabbit heart following myocardial infarction. Circulation 1990; 81(Suppl III):289-295.
7. Julia PL, Buckberg GD, Acar C et al. Studies of controlled reperfusion after ischemia. XXI. Reperfusate composition: superiority of blood cardioplegia over crystalloid in limiting reperfusion damage-importance of endogenous oxygen free radical scavengers in red blood cells. J Thorac Cardiovasc Surg 1991; 101(2):303-313.
8. Foglia RP, Partington MT, Buckberg GD et al. Iatrogeneic myocardial edema with crystalloid primes. Effects on left ventricular compliance, performance and perfusion. Current Studies in Hematology and Blood Transfusion 1986; 53:53-63.
9. Rosenkrantz ER, Okamoto F, Buckberg GD et al. Safety of prolonged aortic clamping with blood cardioplegia. III. Aspartate enrichment of glutamate-blood cardioplegia in energy depleted hearts after ischemic reperfusion injury. J Thorac Cardiovasc Surg 1986; 91(3):428-435.
10. Allen BS, Okamoto F, Buckberg GD et al. Reperfusate composition: benefit of marked hypocalcemia and diltiazem of regional recovery. J Thorac Cardiovasc Surg 1986; 92(3):564-572.
11. Kofsy ER, Julia PL, Buckberg GD et al. Studies of controlled reperfusion after ischemia. XXII. Reperfusate composition: effect of leukocyte depletion of blood and blood cardioplegia reperfusates after acute coronary occlusion. J Thorac Cardiovasc Surg 1991; 101(2):350-359.
12. Christakis GT, Fremes SE, Weisel RD et al. Reducing the risk of urgent revascularization for unstable angina: A randomized clinical trial. J Vasc Surg 1986; 3(5):764-772.
13. Partington MT, Acar C, Buckberg GD et al. Studies of retrograde cardioplegia. I. Capillary blood flow distribution to myocardium supplied by open and occluded vessels. J Thorac Cardiovasc Surg 1989; 97(4):606-612.

14. Partington MT, Acar C, Buckberg GD et al. Studies of retrograde cardioplegia. II. Advantages of antegrade/retrograde cardioplegia to optimize distribution to jeopardized myocardium. J Thorac Cardiovasc Surg 1989; 97(4):613-622.

15. Buckberg GD. Recent advances in myocardial protection using antegrade/retrograde blood cardioplegia. E Heart J 1989; 11 suppl H:43-48.

16. Ludenhauser MV. Nomenclature and distribution patterns of cardiac veins in man. In: Mohl W, Faxon DP, eds. Clinics of Coronary Sinus Interventions. Proceedings of the 2nd international symposium on myocardial protection via the coronary sinus. Steinkoff Darmstadt Springer-Verlag, New York 1986:13-29.

17. Ferrans VJ. Morphological methods for evaluating myocardial protection. Ann Thorac Surg 1975; 20:11-20.

18. Flameng W, Borgers M, Dasnen W et al. Ultrastructural and cytochemical correlates of myocardial protection by hypothermia in man. J Thorac Cardiovasc Surg 1980; 79:413-424.

19. Sawa Y, Hijaru M, Shimazaki Y et al. Ultrastructural assessment of infant myocardium receiving crystalloid cardioplegia. Circulation 1986; 76(pt 2):V141-V145.

20. Zar GH. Biostatistical analysis. 2nd ed. Engelwood Cliffs NJ, Prentice-Hall, Inc 1984:122-126.

21. King RB, Bassingthwaighte JB, Hales JRS et al. Stability of heterogeneity of myocardial blood flow in normal awake baboons. Circ Res 1985; 57:285-295.

22. Marcus ML, Kerber RE, Ehrhardt JE et al. Spatial and temporal heterogeneity of left ventricular perfusion in awake dogs. Am Heart J 1977; 94:748-754.

23. Austin RE Jr, Aldea GS, Coggins DL et al. Profound spatial heterogeneity of coronary reserve-discordance between patterns of resting and maximal flow. Circ Res 1990; 67:319-331.

24. Coggins DL, Flynn AE, Austin RE Jr, Aldea GS et al. Nonuniform loss of regional flow reserve during myocardial ischemia in dogs. Circ Res 1990; 67:253-264.

25. Aldea GS, Austin RE Jr, Flynn AE et al. Heterogeneous delivery of cardioplegic solution in the absence of coronary artery disease. J Thorac Cardiovasc Surg 1990; 99(2):345-353.

26. Aldea GS, Hou DI, Fonger JD et al. Inhomogeneous and complementary delivery of antegrade and retrograde cardioplegia in the absence of coronary artery obstruction. Forum Session-73rd Annual Meeting of the American Association for Thoracic Surgery, 1993:56-57.

27. Aldea GS, Hou DI, Fonger JD et al. Inhomogeneous and complementary delivery of antegrade and retrograde cardioplegia in the absence of coronary artery obstruction. J Thorac Cardiovasc Surg; 1993: Publication Pending.

28. Carrier M, Gregoire J, Khalil A et al. Myocardial distribution of cardioplegia administered by antegrade and retrograde routes to ischemic myocardium. Can J Surg 1997; 40(2):108-113.

29. Gates RN, Lee J, Laks H et al. Evidence of improved microvascular perfusion when using antegrade and retrograde cardioplegia. Ann Thorac Surg 1996; 62(5):1388-1391.

30. Lee J, Gates RN, Laks H et al. A comparison of distribution between simultaneous or sequential delivered antegrade/retrograde blood cardioplegia. J Card Surg 1996; 11(2):111-115.

31. Sandhu AA, Spotnitz HM, Dickstein ML et al. Retrograde cardioplegia preserves myocardial function after induced coronary air embolism. J Thorac Cardiovasc Surg 1997; 113:917-922.

32. Dean DA, Jia CX, Cabreriza SE et al. Retrograde coronary perfusion: effect on iatrogenic edema and diastolic properties. Ann Thorac Surg 1998; 449-453.

33. Partington MT, Acar C, Buckberg GD et al. Studies on retrograde cardioplegia. II. Advantages of antegrade/retrograde cardioplegia to optimize distribution in jeopardized myocardium. J Thorac Cardiovasc Surg 1989; 97:613-622.

34. Partington MT, Acar C, Buckberg GD et al. Studies on retrograde cardioplegia. I. Capillary blood flow distribution to myocardium supplied by open and occluded arteries. J Thorac Cardiovasc Surg 1989; 97:605-612.

35. Carrier M, Gregoire J, Khalil A et al. Myocardial distribution of retrograde cardioplegic solution assessed by myocardial thallium 201 uptake. J Thorac Cardiovasc Surg 1994; 108:1115-1118.

36. Huang AH, Sofola IO, Bufkin BL et al. Coronary sinus pressure and arterial venting do not affect retrograde cardioplegia delivery. Ann Thorac Surg 1994; 58:1499-1504.

37. Ye J, Sun J, Shen J et al. Does retrograde warm cardioplegia provide equal protection to both ventricles? A magnetic resonance spectroscopy study in pigs. Circulation 1997; 96(9 suppl): II-II2105.

38. Iannnettoni MD, Rohs TJ Jr, Gallagher KP et al. The regional effect of retrograde cardioplegia in areas of evolving ischemia. Chest 1995; 108:1353-1357.

39. Tiam G, Shen J, Su S et al. Assessment of retrograde cardioplegia with magnetic resonance imaging and localized 31P spectroscopy in isolated pig hearts. J Thorac Cardiovasc Surg 1997; 114:109-116.
40. Hoffenberg EF, Ye J, Sun J et al. Antegrade and retrograde continuous warm cardioplegia: A 31P magnetic resonance study. Ann Thorac Surg 1995; 60:1203-1209.
41. Archie JP, Kirklin JW. Effect of hypothermia in O2 consumption and coronary resistance. Surg Forum 1973; 24:186-188.
42. McDonell DH, Brazier JR, Cooper N et al. Studies on the effect of hypothermia on regional myocardial blood flow. II. Ischemia during moderate hypothermia in continually perfused dogs. J Thorac Cardiovasc Surg 1977; 73:95-101.

CHAPTER 9

The Selection of Antegrade Versus Retrograde Cardioplegia Delivery

Flordeliza S. Villanueva, William D. Spotnitz, and Sanjiv Kaul

Introduction

The optimal delivery of cardioplegia to induce and maintain cardiac arrest is fundamental to myocardial preservation during cardiac surgery. Traditional approaches utilizing intracoronary or intraaortic delivery of cardioplegia rely on antegrade flow through the epicardial coronary arteries to perfuse myocardial tissue. More recently, enthusiasm has grown for venous routes of cardioplegia delivery, relying on retrograde cardioplegia flow through the coronary veins. The common goal of these different approaches is adequate intramyocardial cooling and delivery of nutritive substrate to myocardial cells. Nonetheless, the extent to which basic anatomic and functional differences between the coronary arterial and venous systems result in differences in cooling and nutritive flow between these two techniques has heretofore not been well-defined. Furthermore, there may be differences in the regional distribution of cardioplegia flow as a function of the route of delivery, particularly in the presence of significant coronary artery disease.[1-3] Clinically, such differences in physiology and flow distribution could have important implications for selecting the optimal route of cardioplegia administration.

This Chapter addresses the factors which may influence the selection of the method of cardioplegia delivery: the nutritive capacity and the regional myocardial distribution of retrograde and ntegrade cardioplegia. The first section focuses on recent data from our group,[4,5] and compares the physiology of retrograde and antegrade cardioplegia delivery with respect to microvascular and nutritive flow, and their relation to myocardial cooling. Additionally, because the magnitude and regional distribution of cardioplegia flow may affect the choice of the route of delivery, the second section outlines the role that myocardial contrast echocardiography may have in the intraoperative assessment of cardioplegia flow to the myocardium.

Previous Studies of Retrograde Microvascular Perfusion

Based on studies utilizing gross hemodynamic endpoints after cardiac surgery,[6-9] it has been largely surmised that retrograde administration of cardioplegia results in effective myocardial preservation. There are fewer studies, however, which directly assess the actual extent of microvascular perfusion achieved by retrograde flow through the coronary veins. Previously published experimental studies employing radioactive techniques to quantify capillary perfusion of retrogradely infused solutions have found varying results.[10-14] Solorzano et al found that only 26% of radioactive microspheres were entrapped when delivered retrogradely to excised canine hearts[10] which is in sharp contrast to antegrade perfusion, where nearly 100% of microspheres are entrapped in arterioles.[15,16]

Similarly, measuring volumes of retro-perfusate recovered in the aorta and cardiac chambers, Lolley and colleagues found that coronary sinus retrograde perfusion of excised dog hearts resulted in Thebesian venous drainage that was three-fold greater than capillary flow.[11] Microscopic examination of myocardial specimens stained retrogradely with India-ink in these studies revealed that despite loss of perfusate via Thebesian veins, retrograde infusion can still reach the cellular level. More recently, in an intact canine model, Cohen and coworkers found that only 10% of diffusible radioisotope injected into the great cardiac vein localized to the myocardium,[12] suggesting relatively low retrograde capillary flow even in in vivo models. The data from these studies may partly explain the inability of retrograde perfusion to sustain cardiac metabolism in vivo, and the failure of early strategies to arterialize the coronary venous system for revascularization of patients with coronary artery disease.[17,18]

Retrograde perfusion may have a role, however, in cardioplegic preservation of the nonworking heart during cardiac surgery.[6-9,19] In this context, two in vivo studies using radioactive microspheres have quantified microvascular perfusion by retrograde cardioplegia.[13,14] These studies reported higher microsphere-derived retrograde flow rates and levels of microsphere entrapment than would be predicted from the isolated heart studies described above.[10-12] Such variable results may be due to differences in calculations for microsphere loss, methods for measuring delivered radioactivity, or experimental models. The precise extent of capillary permeation by retrograde cardioplegia and the validity of radioactive microspheres as tracers of nutritive flow in this setting have, therefore, heretofore remained unclear.

Microvascular Perfusion: Antegrade vs. Retrograde Cardioplegia

Radioactive microspheres may not be accurate markers of retrograde cardioplegia flow, as suggested by a series of experiments recently performed by us utilizing the open-chest canine model of cardiopulmonary bypass.[4,5] Dogs were given either antegrade or retrograde cardioplegia through the cross-clamped aortic root or coronary sinus, respectively, at a constant, known flow rate which differed for each dog but was within the same range for both antegrade and retrograde cardioplegia delivery. Radiolabeled microspheres, 11µ in size, were used to determine total microvascular flow. Capillary or nutritive flow beyond the site of 11µ vessels was measured using technetium 99-m Sestamibi and thallium-201, since myocyte extraction of these diffusible radioisotopes denotes capillary perfusion.[20,21] Known activities of these isotopes were injected into the cardioplegia line during cardioplegia infusion, and their extraction by the heart was measured.

The relationship between the rate of cardioplegia delivery and microsphere-derived flow represents total microvascular flow to vessels <11µ in size. If all retrogradely delivered cardioplegia were to ultimately perfuse the capillaries, as with antegrade delivery, this relationship would simulate the line of identity as shown in the figure. In dogs receiving retrograde cardioplegia, although the rate of cardioplegia delivery and microsphere-derived flow were linearly related, there was consistent underestimation of the absolute rate of retrograde cardioplegia delivery to the left ventricle by about 66%. This underestimation is even more pronounced in the right ventricle. These data suggest that, unlike the situation with antegrade cardioplegia where all of it reaches the microvascular level, most of the cardioplegia delivered retrogradely through the coronary sinus does not reach vessels <11µ in size because it is lost from larger venules in the proximal portion of the venous route.

Nutritive Perfusion: Antegrade vs. Retrograde Cardioplegia

Technetium 99-m and thallium-201, which are sequestered by myocytes, were utilized in these experiments as markers of capillary or nutritive flow. As in the warm, beating, blood-perfused heart, the first-pass extraction fractions of these agents are exponentially related to the flow rate[22] in dogs receiving cardioplegia, although because of a lower temperature and thus, a lower metabolic activity, the extraction of these agents is lower in the nonbeating cold heart. Even at comparable levels of myocardial cooling and at similar cardioplegia delivery rates, however, the myocardial extraction fractions of these agents were found to be significantly lower during retrograde than antegrade cardioplegia delivery. Even when the extraction fractions were normalized to microsphere-derived flows to account for reduced availability of the isotopes resulting from cardioplegia loss prior to 11μ venules, when delivered retrogradely, their extractions remained consistently lower. These data suggest that at any given rate of cardioplegia delivery, nutritive flow retrogradely is less than that achieved antegradely and indicate that prior to reaching myocardial cells, retrograde cardioplegia is lost not only through venules $>11\mu$ in size, but also through smaller venules.

Anatomic Basis for Physiologic Differences between Antegrade and Retrograde Cardioplegia

The data presented above may be explained by fundamental differences in the microvascular anatomy of the coronary arterioles and venules. During antegrade flow, there is nearly complete entrapment of all microspheres in precapillary arterioles.[15,16] While arteriovenous and arterio-luminal vessels bypassing capillaries may exist,[23-26] these vessels are few in number, small in size, and probably of little functional significance.[27] Consequently, all cardioplegia traversing the epicardial coronary arteries also negotiates the arterioles and capillaries; microspheres are therefore accurate markers of all levels of antegrade flow: total, arteriolar, and capillary; and these levels of flow are equivalent.

In contradistinction, unique characteristics of the coronary venous anatomy impose a different constraint on microvascular flow during retrograde perfusion. Thebesian veins, veno-luminal vessels shunting blood into cardiac chambers, interpose between veins and capillaries.[23,27-30] When cardioplegia is retrogradely infused through the venous system, some of it drains through Thebesian veins into the cardiac chambers, prior to microsphere entrapment. As such, microsphere-derived flow underestimates whole-organ flow. Additionally, as indicated by the disproportionately low technetium 99-m and thallium-201 extraction relative to microsphere entrapment, retrograde cardioplegia may be lost even beyond sites of microsphere entrapment, prior to the capillaries. In this situation, microsphere-derived flow also overestimates the extent of retrograde nutritive flow.

Thebesian veins are found in relatively small numbers in the ventricles,[31] and under physiologic conditions, Thebesian drainage into cardiac chambers is probably minimal,[32] which is likely due to high intracardiac pressures relative to myocardial venous pressures.[25,30] In the arrested, vented heart, however, Thebesian veins act as low-resistance conduits into the low-pressure cardiac chambers, draining retrograde flow away from venules and capillaries. Additionally, abundant veno-venous anastomoses[27,29] may permit changes in venous flow distribution resulting from alterations in venous pressure[33] to re-route retrograde flow to distantly located veins. Such a phenomenon could explain low retrograde myocardial flow to regions which actually have relatively few Thebesian veins, such as the left ventricle.[34]

Myocardial Cooling: Antegrade vs. Retrograde Cardioplegia

Despite the differences in microvascular and nutritive flow between antegrade and retrograde cardioplegia, both techniques resulted in comparable degrees of cooling of most of the myocardium in these experiments, with the exception of the interventricular septum, which in the dog, receives less perfusion via the retrograde route. The initial lower temperatures of the left ventricular apex, the right ventricular free wall and the interventricular septum during retrograde compared to antegrade cardioplegia delivery was due to 2 min of initial high rate antegrade flow to achieve cardiac arrest in the former group. The rates of cooling, subsequent to cardiac arrest nonetheless, are the same except, as previously stated, for the interventricular septum, which cools at a slower rate. Cardioplegia rate and intramyocardial temperature are inversely related in these experiments. At any given flow rate, maximal cooling of the left ventricular apex, the right ventricular free wall and the interventricular septum by retrograde cardioplegia is similar to that achieved by antegrade cardioplegia. Because, as stated above, the initial myocardial temperature was lower for the dogs receiving retrograde cardioplegia, the interventricular septal temperature at the end of 5 min of retrograde cardioplegia delivery was the same as that achieved for antegrade cardioplegia delivery despite a slower rate of interventricular septal cooling achieved by the former. The extensive venous surface area resulting from venous anastomotic networks far outnumbering that of arterioles,[34] probably enhances the cooling properties of retrograde cardioplegia, despite the low capillary flow achieved by this technique.

Assessment of Cardioplegia Flow Using Myocardial Contrast Echocardiography

Myocardial contrast echocardiography utilizes the intravascular injection of air-filled microbubbles which produce myocardial opacification during simultaneously performed echocardiographic imaging.[35] This technique has been shown to quantify myocardial flow during antegrade infusion of cardioplegia.[36] The myocardial 'wash-in' parameters of these microbubbles, such as time-to-peak contrast effect, have been shown by us to correlate closely with antegrade cardioplegia flow measured using radiolabeled microspheres.[36] We, and others, have also previously shown that myocardial contrast echocardiography performed during retrograde cardioplegia delivery can be used to characterize the intramyocardial distribution of retrograde flow.[37-41] Figure 5.1 is an example of myocardial distribution of retrogradely administered cardioplegia in comparison with radiolabeled microspheres. Myocardial opacification is not noted in regions with <10% of normal flow as determined by radiolabeled microspheres.

In the experiments described above, time-intensity plots were obtained from the myocardium during both antegrade and retrograde cardioplegia delivery. The plots, fit to a general exponential function, appear identical at the same flow rate with the 'wash-in' phase of the curves (time-to-peak contrast effect) being similar for both routes of cardioplegia delivery.

A close linear relationship between the rate of both antegrade and retrograde cardioplegia delivery and the reciprocal of the time-to-peak contrast effect was noted in these experiments, suggesting that myocardial contrast echocardiography can be used to quantify regional myocardial flow irrespective of the route of cardioplegia delivery. Unlike radiolabeled microspheres and diffusible tracers such as technetium 99-m and thallium-201, which must be trapped by the heart to mark the passage of cardioplegia, the passage of microbubbles through the myocardium is registered on real-time echocardiography, regardless of the intramyocardial route the bubbles take or where they ultimately reach. This property of myocardial contrast echocardiography makes it an ideal method of assessing myocardial perfusion during

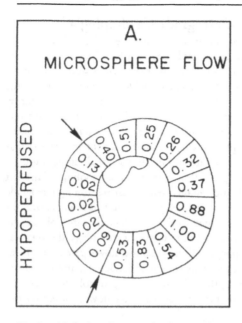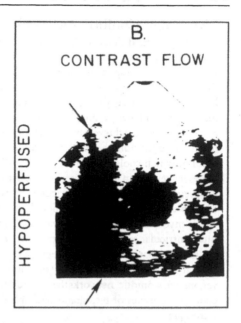

Fig. 5.1 A.) depicts the normalized regional myocardial flow measured using radiolabeled microspheres which were also injected into the cardioplegia line. Regions with less flow in Fig. 5.7A show less contrast enhancement in Fig. 5.7.B.) From Villanueva et al, Surgical Forum 1990;XII:252-254, with permission of the American College of Surgeons. B.) A short-axis image of the left ventricle during myocardial contrast echocardiography where microbubbles of air were injected into the cardioplegia line during retrograde delivery.

retrograde cardioplegia delivery, where the other methods significantly underestimate cardioplegia flow rate to the myocardium.

Summary

There are fundamental physiologic differences in the nutritive characteristics of retrogradely and anterogradely administered cardioplegia. In the nonworking canine heart, at comparable degrees of total flow, the retrograde route results in less cardioplegia delivery to microvessels <11μ in size than does the antegrade route. Moreover, there is further loss of retrogradely delivered cardioplegia between 11μ venules and capillaries, resulting in significantly lower nutritive flow compared to that achieved by antegrade delivery. Thebesian venous drainage is most likely responsible for the precapillary loss of retrogradely delivered cardioplegia.

In spite of the relative paucity of capillary perfusion, cooling of most of the myocardium (except for the interventricular septum) by retrograde cardioplegia is equivalent to that of antegrade cardioplegia, probably due to abundant veno-venous anastomotic networks. The excellent intramyocardial cooling achieved by retrograde cardioplegia may account for the favorable clinical results reported using this technique in the operating room.[6-9,42-45] Furthermore, even the low nutritive flow achievable with retrograde cardioplegia may be sufficient for the decreased metabolic requirements of the hypothermic, nonworking heart. Due to the differences in arterial and venous microcirculatory anatomy, however, intraoperative approaches to metabolic substrate enhancement of cardioplegic solutions may be most effectively applied using the antegrade route.

Finally, myocardial contrast echocardiography has the potential for providing valuable information regarding the regional myocardial distribution and magnitude of flow during both antegrade and retrograde cardioplegia delivery. Such information may assist the surgeon in determining the optimal route of cardioplegia delivery in patients undergoing cardiac surgery, especially in those with significant epicardial coronary artery disease.

Acknowledgment

This work was supported in part by a grant-in-Aid from the Virginia Affiliate of the American Heart Association, Glen Allen, Virginia and a FIRST Award (R29-HL43787) from the National Institutes of Health, Bethesda, Maryland to Dr. Spotnitz, and a grant-in-aid from the National Center of the American Heart Association, Dallas, Texas and a grant (R01-HL48890) from the National Institutes of Health to Dr. Kaul. It was also supported in part by a grant-in-aid from Molecular Biosystems, Inc., San Diego, California and an equipment grant from General Electric Medical Systems, Milwaukee, Wisconsin. Dr. Villanueva was the recipient of a Fellowship Training Grant from the Virginia Affiliate of the American Heart Association and Dr. Kaul is an Established Investigator of the American Heart Association.

References

1. Becker H, Vinten-Johansen J, Buckberg GD et al. Critical importance of ensuring cardioplegic delivery with coronary stenoses. J Thorac Cardiovasc Surg 1981; 81:507-15.
2. Hilton CJ, Teubl W, Acker M et al. Inadequate cardioplegic protection with obstructed coronary arteries. Ann Thorac Surg 1979; 28:323-34.
3. Gundry SR, Kirsh MM. A comparison of retrograde cardioplegia versus antegrade cardioplegia in the presence of coronary artery obstruction. Ann Thorac Surg 1984; 38:124-27.
4. Villanueva FS, Glasheen WP, Dent JM et al. Discrepancy between capillary perfusion and myocardial cooling during retrograde cardioplegia: Comparison with antegrade cardioplegia. Surg Forum 1992; 43:213-215.
5. Villanueva FS, Spotnitz W, Glasheen W et al. Physiology of retrograde cardioplegia delivery: Comparison with antegrade cardioplegia delivery with respect to myocardial cooling and nutrient flow. J Am Coll Cardiol (in press) (abstr).
6. Haan C, Lazar HL, Bernard S et al. Superiority of retrograde cardioplegia after acute coronary occlusion. Ann Thorac Surg 1991; 51:408-12.
7. Menasche P, Subayi J-B, Picnica A. Retrograde coronary sinus cardioplegia for aortic valve operations: A clinical report on 500 patients. Ann Thorac Surg 1990; 49:556-64.
8. Diehl JT, Eichhorn EJ, Konstam MA et al. Efficacy of retrograde coronary sinus cardioplegia in patients undergoing myocardial revascularization: A prospective randomized trial. Ann Thorac Surg 1988; 45:595-602.
9. Bhayana JN, Kalmbach T, Booth FV et al. Combined antegrade/retrograde cardioplegia for myocardial protection: A clinical trial. J Thorac Cardiovasc Surg 1989; 98:956-60.
10. Solorzano J, Taitelbaum G, Chu-Jeng Chiu R. Retrograde coronary sinus perfusion for myocardial protection during cardiopulmonary bypass. Ann Thorac Surg 1978; 25:201-8.
11. Lolley DM, Hewitt RL. Myocardial distribution of asanguineous solutions retroperfused under low pressure through the coronary sinus. J Cardiovasc Surg 1980; 21:286-94.
12. Cohen MV, Matsuki T, Downey JM. Pressure-flow characteristics and nutritional capacity of coronary veins in dogs. Am J Physiol 1988; 255:H834-H846.
13. Partington MT, Ascar C, Buckberg GD et al. Studies of retrograde cardioplegia. J Thorac Cardiovasc Surg 1989; 97:605-12.
14. Stirling MC, McClanahan TB, Schott RJ et al. Distribution of cardioplegic solution infused antegradely and retrogradely in normal canine hearts. J Thorac Cardiovasc Surg 1989; 98:1066-76.
15. Utley J, Carlson El, Hoffman JE et al. Total and regional myocardial blood flow measurements with 25u, 15u, 9u and filtered 1-10u diameter microspheres and antipyrine on dogs and sheep. Circ Res 1974; 34: 391-405.

16. Hoff RP, Salzmann F, Wyler F. Mapping and intramyocardial distribution of microspheres with different diameters in cat and rabbit hearts in vitro. Basic Res Cardiol 1981; 76:630-8.

17. Beck CS, Stanton E, Batiuchok W et al. Revascularization of the heart by graft of systemic artery into the coronary sinus. JAMA 1948; 137:436-42.

18. Hochberg MS. Hemodynamic evaluation of selective arterialization of the coronary venous system. An experimental study of myocardial perfusion utilizing radioactive microspheres. J Thorac Cardiovasc Surg 1977; 74:774-83.

19. Lust RM, Beggerly CE, Morrison RF et al. Improved protection of chronically inflow-limited myocardium with retrograde coronary sinus cardioplegia. Circulation 1988; 78(suppl II): II:217-23.

20. Goldhaber SZ, Newell JB, Ingwall JS et al. Effects of reduced coronary flow on thallium-201 accumulation and release in an in-vitro rat heart preparation. Am J Cardiol 1983; 51:891-96.

21. Piwnica-Worms D, Kronauge JF, Chiu ML. Uptake and retention of hexakis (2-methoxybutyl isonitrile) technetium (I) in cultured chick cells. Mitochondrial and plasma membrane potential dependence. Circulation 1990; 82:1826-38.

22. Bassingthwaighte JB. A concurrent flow model for extraction during transcapillary passage. Circ Res 1974; 35:483-503.

23. Ratajczyk-Pakalska E, Kolff WJ. Anatomical basis for the coronary venous outflow. In: Mohl W, Wolner E, Glogar D, eds. The Coronary Sinus: Proceedings of the First International Symposium on Myocardial Protection via the Coronary Sinus. Darmstadt: Steinkopff-Verlag, 1984; 40-46.

24. Wearner JT, Mettier SR, Klump TG et al. The nature of the vascular communications between the coronary arteries and the chambers of the heart. Am Heart J 1933; 9:143

25. Hammond GL, Austen WG. Drainage patterns of coronary arterial flow as determined from the isolated heart. Am J Physiol 1967; 212:1435-40.

26. Grayson J, Davidson JW, Fitzgerald-Finch A et al. The functional morphology of the coronary microcirculation in the dog: Microvasc Res 1971; 8:20-43.

27. Spaan JAE. Coronary blood flow. Mechanics, Distribution and Control. Dordrecht, The Netherlands: Kluwer Academic Publishers, 1991: 87-98.

28. Bates RJ, Toscano M, Balderman SC et al. The cardiac veins and retrograde coronary venous perfusion. Ann Thorac Surg 1977; 23:83-90.

29. Gregg ED, Shipley RE. Studies of the venous drainage of the heart. Am J Physiol 1947; 151:13-25.

30. Lechleuthner A, Ludinghausen MV. The functional architecture and clinical significance of the cardiac venous system with special reference to the venous valves and Thebesian veins. In: Mohl W, Faxon D, Wolner E, eds. Clinics of CSI. Proceedings of the 2nd International Symposium on Myocardial Protection via the Coronary Sinus. Darmstadt:Steinkopff-Verlag, 1984: 33-9.

31. Tschabitscher M: Anatomy of coronary veins. In: Mohl W, Wolner E, Glogar D, eds. The Coronary Sinus: Proceedings of the First International Symposium on Myocardial Protection via the Coronary Sinus. Darmstadt: Steinkopff-Verlag, 1984: 8-25.

32. Wearn JT. The role of the Thebesian vessels in the circulation of the heart. J Exp Med 1928; 42:293-318.

33. Scharf SM, Bromberger-Barnea B, Permutt S. Distribution of coronary venous flow. J Appl Physiol 1971; 30:657-62.

34. Rhodin JA. Ultrastructure of mammalian venous capillaries, venules and small collecting veins. J Ultrastruc Res 1968; 25:452-500.

35. Spotnitz WD, Kaul S. Intraoperative assessment of myocardial perfusion by contrast echocardiography. Echocardiography 1990; 7:209-228.

36. Keller MW, Spotnitz WD, Matthew TL et al. Intraoperative assessment of regional myocardial perfusion using quantitative myocardial contrast echocardiography: An experimental evaluation. J Am Coll Cardiol 1990; 16:1267-79.

37. Villanueva FS, Kaul S, Glasheen WP et al. Intraoperative assessment of the distribution of retrograde cardioplegia using myocardial contrast echocardiography. Surg Forum 1990; XII:252-54.

38. Aronson S, Lee BK, Liddicoat JR et al. Assessment of retrograde cardioplegia distribution using contrast echocardiography. Ann Thorac Surg 1992; 52:810-14.

39. Maurer G, Punzengruber C, Haendchen RV et al. Retrograde coronary venous contrast echocardiography: Assessment of shunting and delineation of regional myocardium in the normal and ischemic canine heart. J Am Coll Cardiol 1984; 4:577-86.

40. Meerbaum S. Coronary venous myocardial contrast echocardiography. In: Meerbaum S, Meltzer RS, eds. Myocardial Contrast Two-dimensional Echocardiography. Dordrecht: Kluwer Academic Publishers, 1989:141-50.
41. Punzengruber C, Maurer G, Ong CK et al. Factors affecting penetration of retrograde coronary venous injections into normal and ischemic canine myocardium: assessment by contrast echocardiography and digital angiography. Basic Res Cardiol 1990; 85:21-32.
42. Schaper J, Walter P, Scheld H et al. The effects of retrograde perfusion of cardioplegic solution in cardiac operations. J Thorac Cardiovasc Surg 1985; 90:882-887.
43. Taira Y, Kanaide H, Nakamara M. Coronary venous perfusion of the ischemic myocardium during acute coronary artery occlusion in isolated rat hearts. Circ Res 1985; 56:666-75.
44. Masuda M, Yonenaga K, Shiki K et al. Myocardial protection in coronary occlusion by retrograde cardioplegic perfusion via the coronary sinus in dogs. J Thorac Cardiovasc Surg 1986; 92:255-63.
45. Guiraudon G, Campbell CS, McLellan DG et al. Retrograde coronary sinus versus aortic root perfusion with cold cardioplegia: randomized study of levels of cardiac enzymes in 40 patients. Circulation 1986; 74(suppl III):III: 105-15.

CHAPTER 10

Retrograde Cardioplegia in Infants and Children

Steven R. Gundry

Introduction

The coronary venous connections to the capillary bed of the heart have been described for nearly 100 years,[1] yet it was not until the 1940s that clinical application of this concept to treat heart disease was employed by Beck.[2] Since that time surgeons have intermittently used retrograde perfusion of the coronary veins to provide myocardial protection during periods of aortic cross-clamping.[3-6] However up until 1987, cannulation of the coronary sinus was a cumbersome process requiring bicaval cannulation, caval snares, an atriotomy and insertion of a catheter into the coronary sinus under direct vision. This changed with the introduction of "blind" insertion of the coronary sinus catheter through a pursestring in the right atrium, using a flexible stylet to stiffen the catheter, guiding its entrance into the coronary sinus with a finger on the atrio-ventricular groove.[7] Although immensely facilitating adult retrograde cardioplegic techniques, catheter size was clearly too big to allow retrograde techniques to be applied to the infant and pediatric age range. In recent years, this discrepancy has been corrected with the introduction of 6F and 10F cardioplegia cannulas with an integral flexible stylet (Gundry RSCP Cannula, DLP, Inc, Grand Rapids, Michigan).

The Case for Retrograde Cardioplegia in Infants and Children

There is not only debate as to the proper type of myocardial protection in infants and children, but there is little agreement among surgeons as to whether the immature heart is more or less tolerant than an adult's heart to ischemia.[8] However it is clear that ischemia should be modified in some way if an optimal surgical result is to be realized. Whether this is accomplished via crystalloid or blood cardioplegia in single or multiple dose, with or without substrate enhancement, and with or without warm induction or warm termination is beyond the scope of this discussion. Nevertheless, unless one subscribes to the theory that no cardioplegia is the best form of myocardial protection, retrograde cardioplegia via the coronary sinus may be at least as useful as antegrade cardioplegia in producing the desired results regardless of the type of cardioplegic solution.

There is abundant experimental and clinical evidence that retrograde cardioplegia is as efficacious as antegrade cardioplegia in both valvular and coronary artery operations,[5,7] and compelling evidence that it is superior to antegrade cardioplegia in obstructive coronary artery

Coronary Sinus Interventions in Cardiac Surgery, Second Edition edited by Werner Mohl.
©2000 Eurekah.com.

disease or reoperations.[9] But what advantages it may have in infant and pediatric open heart procedures is much less easy to demonstrate clinically. Apparent advantages are several, including: 1) A majority of infant and pediatric heart operations involve opening of the right atrium. Once open, direct vision cannulation of the coronary sinus is effortless. So effortless in fact that multidose cardioplegia may be administered by simply reinserting the catheter prior to each dose; 2) In operations not done through the right atrium, such as arterial switch operations or tetralogy of Fallot repairs performed via a ventriculotomy, introduction of the catheter through an atrial pursestring, using the flexible stylet, has allowed application of this technique even in newborns; 3) in cases of arterial switches where direct cannulation of the coronary arteries may be otherwise required, retrograde cardioplegia allows complete freedom from coronary artery cannulation and its attendant potential for trauma or dissection; and 4) since most congenital heart operations allow air into the ascending aorta, deairing of the aorta must precede each antegrade cardioplegia dose and final aortic unclamping; retrograde cardioplegia pushes any air out of the aorta with each dose and may be further used to deair the aorta and coronary arteries prior to unclamping. Thus, what may initially seem to be a cumbersome addition to the simplicity of antegrade cardioplegia, when more fully contemplated, may actually simplify the entire process of myocardial protection in infants and children.

Technique

The use of the 6F or 10F retrograde cardioplegia catheter with integrated manually inflated balloon and distal pressure monitoring line with a flexible stylet has simplified the application of retrograde cardioplegia to even the smallest infant. In cases where opening of the right atrium is not anticipated, the catheter is introduced via a separate pursestring in the atrium in exactly the same manner as adults. Usually the surgeon holds the catheter in the left hand, while palpating the A-V groove with the right hand. The catheter is ideally placed midway in the great cardiac vein and its positioning confirmed by palpation and/or visual inspection. Egress of blood from the catheter once the stylet is withdrawn, further ensures proper placement. The integrated distal pressure monitoring port is connected via a six foot pressure tubing to the CVP transducer used by the anesthesiologist. Once the cross clamp is in place, retrograde cardioplegia is given, in our preference, 10-15 ml/kg body weight, monitoring the coronary sinus pressure rise, usually keeping the pressure 60 mm Hg or less. Failure to see a pressure rise usually means that the catheter is not in the coronary sinus or that the balloon is not occlusive. In all but the largest children, 1 ml of air adequately seals the coronary sinus.

Addition of a needle hole or vent in the ascending aorta may be added for those cases where no connection exists between the right and left sides of the heart.

Doses can be repeated at the discretion of the surgeon without concern for deairing the ascending aorta, or interrupting the operation to keep the aortic valve competent while giving cardioplegia. Prior to final unclamping, an additional dose of cardioplegia, warm or cold, with or without potassium, may be used to deair the ventricles and aorta, while keeping an aortic vent to suction or air, or while simply putting a needle in the aorta. This may be particularly useful whenever the aorta has been opened or following coronary artery transfer, when almost certainly some air has entered the coronary arteries.

Whenever the entire operation or a portion of it will be performed through an opened right atrium, it is usually more convenient to wait and insert the catheter under direct vision into the coronary sinus once the right atrium is opened. In this case, the stylet is withdrawn and the catheter flushed with cardioplegia and the pressure monitoring port connected and purged prior to insertion into the coronary sinus. Although the catheter can remain within the coronary sinus for the remainder of the procedure, it is frequently easier to remove the catheter following each dose, and reinsert it for each subsequent dose. Any air within the coronary venous system will be flushed out by way of the thebesian veins.

Future Applications

There remain certain operations that are dependent upon near perfect myocardial protection for successful recovery of the patient, notably the Fontan operation. In these cases, myocardial hypertrophy and dilation may have occurred secondary to chronic volume overload. Less than adequate myocardial protection will result in a ventricle that is incapable of "pulling" blood through the lungs, resulting in high right-sided filling pressures and falling systemic output. Experimentally, it has been shown that retrograde cardioplegia preferentially distributes to the subendocardium in hypertrophied hearts, much more so than with antegrade cardioplegia, and may have distinct benefits in these cases.[10]

Finally, warm continuous retrograde cardioplegia has been shown to eliminate myocardial ischemia in adults,[11] but its application has been limited in infants and children, in part due to the strong reliance on deep hypothermia for organ protection in the latter group. Certainly this is an area that deserves exploration, particularly in cases such as Fontan procedures, where myocardial protection is critical to the success of the operation.

Conclusions

The introduction of the 6F and 10F retrograde coronary sinus cardioplegia catheters with their integral flexible stylet has allowed the routine application of retrograde cardioplegia techniques to the infant and child open heart population. Since there are definite advantages of retrograde cardioplegia in adults, the surgeons familiar with cannulation of the coronary sinus can easily apply the technique to this smaller population.

References

1. Pratt FH. The nutrition of the heart through the vessels of Thebesius and the coronary veins. Am J Physiol 1988; 1:86-103.
2. Beck CS. Revascularization of the heart. Surgery 1949; 26:82-88.
3. Lillehei CW, Deverall RA, Gott VL et al. A direct vision correction of calcific aortic stenosis by means of a pre-op oxygenator and retrograde coronary sinus perfusion. Dis Chest 1956; 30:123-32.
4. Daves AL, Hammond GL, Austen WG. Direct left coronary artery surgery employing retrograde perfusion of the coronary sinus. J Thorac Cardiovasc Surg 1967; 54:848-55.
5. Menasche P, Subayi J-B, Piwnica A. Retrograde coronary sinus cardioplegia for aortic valve operations: A clinical report on 500 patients. Ann Thorac Surg 1990; 49:556-64.
6. Blanco G, Adam A, Fernandez N. A direct experimental approach to the aortic valve, acute reperfusion of the coronary sinus. J Thorac Surg 1955; 32:171-7.
7. Gundry SR, Sequiera A, Razzouk AJ et al. Facile retrograde cardioplegia: Transatrial cannulation of the coronary sinus. Ann Thorac Surg 1990; 50:882-7.
8. Bull C, Cooper J, Stark J. Cardioplegia protection of the child's heart. J Thorac Cardiovasc Surg 1984; 88:287-293.
9. Gundry SR, Kirsh MM. A comparison of retrograde cardioplegia versus antegrade cardioplegia in the presence of coronary artery obstruction. Ann Thorac Surg 1984; 38:124-7.
10. Gundry SR. Modification of myocardial ischemia in normal and hypertrophied hearts utilizing diastolic retroperfusion of the coronary veins. J Thorac Cardiovasc Surg 1982; 83:659-669.
11. Gundry SR, Wang N, Bannon D et al. Retrograde continuous warm blood cardioplegia: Maintenance of myocardial homeostasis in humans. Ann Thorac Surg 1993; 55:358-63.

CHAPTER 11

Coronary Sinus Interventions During Surgical Treatment of Acute Myocardial Infarction

Friedhelm Beyersdorf

Introduction

In many centers, coronary artery bypass grafting is currently considered during or soon after an acute myocardial infarction only after failed angioplasty. Emergency coronary artery bypass grafting (CABG) is associated with a higher mortality (6–12%) and an increased risk for developing perioperative myocardial infarction (21–71%) as compared to elective CABG.[28,57,107] During recent years, new observations have been made on the pathophysiology of ischemic and remote myocardium[15,16,22] that gave the impetus for the development for new operative strategies for patients with acute myocardial infarction and cardiogenic shock. These strategies include treatment of the ischemic myocardium during the initial reperfusion phase in order to reduce the damage that follows after reperfusion with normal blood at systemic pressure.[6,17,22]

This new concept of treating the ischemic tissue during the initial reperfusion phase is currently controversial. The attempt to control various components of the reperfusate and the conditions of reperfusion[6,17,22] is based on the following observations: 1) The myocardial cell has an intact structure and function even after a prolonged period of ischemia (6 hours);[14] 2) immediate return of regional contractility after normal blood reperfusion in the beating working heart can not be achieved even after short ischemic periods;[111] and 3) control of the initial reperfusion phase results in an immediate return of contractility after prolonged periods of acute coronary occlusion.[6]

These experimental studies on the beneficial effects of modifying the initial reperfusion phase have been confirmed by other groups, in terms of controlled reflow,[44,87,96,105,117] controlled reperfusion temperature,[74] reduced calcium reperfusion,[77,90,100,104] addition of diltiazem,[72] substrate enhancement,[34,45,46] ventricular unloading,[64] addition of oxygen free radical scavengers,[32,42,79] electromechanical quiescence and initially reduced reperfusion pressure,[31,40,59,58] and leukocyte depletion.[25] Furthermore, confirmation of the superiority of our concept of controlling the conditions of reperfusion and the composition of the reperfusate is reported as well.[26,66,110,112] The results of these experimental studies in the acute model are further supported by a recent report in a chronic dog model where it has been shown that after acute occlusion of the anterior descending coronary artery for 2 hours, controlled surgical reperfusion resulted in a significantly better systolic shortening and less myocardial necrosis immediately and after one week as compared to normal blood reperfusion or no reperfusion at all.[26]

These encouraging experimental data have prompted us as well as others[21] to employ these techniques in patients with acute coronary occlusions.[6,17,18] Most recently, we have evaluated the concept of controlled reperfusion in a multicenter trial, demonstrating the benefits of controlled reperfusion after prolonged ischemia in 156 patients.[7]

This Chapter will concentrate upon the rationale and surgical technique of coronary sinus interventions during surgical treatment of acute myocardial infarction. The aims of this communication are 1) to discuss briefly current understanding of the pathophysiology of acute coronary occlusion on ischemic and nonischemic (remote) myocardium; 2) to summarize the rationale for using retrograde techniques during surgical interventions for acute myocardial infarction; and 3) to describe the technical details of our current surgical strategy for patients with acute myocardial infarction.

Pathophysiology of Acute Myocardial Infarction

Acute coronary occlusion results in immediate systolic bulging (dyskinesia) of the ischemic muscle segment.[15,17,10] Passive bulging occurs because the noncontracting ischemic region is stretched during systole by remote contracting muscle. In order to maintain a sufficient cardiac output to sustain life, remote myocardium not subject to infarction must hypercontract to compensate for dissipation of energy during passive stretching of the ischemic segment.[15] Loss of more than 40% of contracting left ventricular muscle results in cardiogenic shock[84,8] which can occur, e.g., with very proximal coronary occlusions. Survival after an acute coronary occlusion that renders less than 40% of the left ventricle nonfunctional depends upon the compensatory capacity of the remote "nonischemic" myocardium.[15,17,27,77] Left ventricular power failure will develop even if the acute coronary occlusion leads to an ischemic region of the left ventricle less than 40%, if the mass of unaffected myocardium has been reduced by a previous myocardial infarction: reduced contractility (hypokinesis) or even "normal" contractility (normokinesis) in viable remote muscle has grave prognostic implications.[15,50]

Studies of the natural history of acute regional ischemia after coronary occlusion[22] have shown that acute occlusion of a coronary artery not only affects the ischemic myocardium, but causes structural, functional, and metabolic alterations in the remote and adjacent myocardium.[15-17] These changes in the remote myocardium are even more severe if the remote myocardium is supplied by a stenotic artery.[15]

Ischemic Myocardium

The regional wall motion abnormalities after acute coronary occlusion (dyskinesia) are accompanied by progressive ultrastructural[98] and biochemical sequences.[54,52,5] Despite these alterations, the myocardial cell remains intact even after 6 hours of ischemia,[14] as long as the damaged tissue is not exposed to a sudden reperfusion with normal blood. Prolonged ischemia, without reperfusion, causes only mild mitochondrial ultrastructural changes (as demonstrated by the low protein denaturation embedding technique),[14,5,102] a mild decrease in mitochondrial function,[14] and slight calcium accumulation and edema formation.[14]

Studies by Jennings and coworkers[54] suggest that the damage imposed by a 15-minute coronary occlusion can be reversed successfully by normal blood reperfusion. However, after 40 minutes of regional ischemia, massive structural, biochemical, and functional changes (not present before the onset of reflow) occur in the subendocardial muscle after reperfusion of the working heart with normal blood.[51,53] Normal blood reperfusion after longer periods of ischemia (6 hours) produces such extensive transmural necrosis that muscle salvage is unlikely,[53,61] i.e., whether reperfusion injury occurs after normal blood reperfusion depends upon the severity of ischemia.[11] Short ischemic periods or high collateral blood flow[97] during longer ischemic periods might preserve cellular regulatory mechanisms and prevent reperfusion injury.

Based on these pathologic events during ischemia and normal blood reperfusion, our surgical strategy of controlled regional blood cardioplegic reperfusion is intended to prevent cellular overload with calcium, sodium, water, free radicals, etc, in a phase where cellular energy production is still insufficient and normal blood reperfusion might cause persistent and progressive structural damage.

Our current strategy for controlled reperfusion incorporates each of the principles of modification of the conditions of reperfusion and the composition of the reperfusate that evolved from our previous studies.[1-3,16,22,24,55,80,82,83,93,111,113]

Conditions of Reperfusion

The conditions of reperfusion that were modified included 1) *total heart decompression* by vented bypass to prevent the damaged muscle from developing wall tension during reperfusion and thereby increasing its oxygen demands;[1] 2) *gentle reperfusion pressure*, i.e., 50 mm Hg, to limit postischemic edema produced by sudden reperfusion[83] that may also decrease shear stress and minimize endothelial dysfunction[96] and reduce postreperfusion arrhythmias; 3) *regional cardioplegia* to keep energy demands as low as possible during temporarily controlled reperfusion,[80] 4) *normothermia* to optimize the rate of cellular repair;[93] and 5) prolonged reperfusion *duration*, i.e., 20 minutes, to maximize oxygen uptake relative to demands and avoid premature imposition of high-energy demands that divert the limited oxygen utilization capacity to unnecessary electromechanical work.[3]

Composition of the Reperfusate

The reperfusate composition was modified to allow incorporation of the following principles: 1) *oxygenation* with blood to provide substrate (O_2) to generate energy for repair of cellular processes;[3] 2) *cardioplegia* (K^+) to keep the heart from resuming electromechanical activity and raising O_2 demand;[80] 3) *replenishing of amino acid precursors* of Krebs' cycle intermediates, i.e., glutamate aspartate and needed to ensure more effective oxidative metabolism to produce energy for cell repair and subsequent mechanical function[65,95] because it has been shown that both hypoxia[106] and ischemia[14] reduce the tissue concentrations of precursors and some intermediates of the Krebs' cycle, 4) *limitation of calcium influx* by reperfusate hypocalcemia (150 to 250 micromol/L) with citrate-phosphate-dextrose to reduce calcium load and addition of a calcium channel-blocking drug, i.e., diltiazem, that could continue to retard calcium cell entry after normocalcemic reperfusion is started;[2,38] 5) *reversal of acidosis* with a buffer to provide an optimal intracellular milieu for effective resumption of metabolic function;[39] 6) *hyperosmolarity*, i.e., glucose, to minimize postischemic edema and allow cell volume regulation to occur gradually when normothermic blood flow is restored;[82] 7) counteracting of oxygen free radicals with *oxygen free-radical scavenger*, i.e., coenzyme Q_{10}, to limit cytotoxic effects of these compounds;[81] 8) *hyperglycemia* to enhance osmotic effects and perhaps initiate compartmental anaerobic energy production at the start of reperfusion;[82,115] and 9) *leukopenia* to reduce the number of white blood cells that can become activated to generate toxic oxygen species and plug capillaries to contribute to the low-reflow phenomenon.[25,35,63]

Remote Myocardium

The function of remote muscle is the principle determinant of early survival after an otherwise nonlethal coronary occlusion, i.e., 30% of left ventricle at risk.[15] Survival after acute coronary occlusion is determined by a) the infarct size[41,47,108] and b) the capacity of remote, nonischemic myocardium to support the systemic circulation.[15,50,99] Cardiogenic shock or LV power failure occurs if >40% of the LV muscle mass acutely loses its contractile properties[8,84] or if there is insufficient remote myocardium to compensate for the acute loss of <40% of contractile mass. Failure of remote muscle to hypercontract may be caused by one or more of the following factors:

A. A previous myocardial infarction that reduces the available muscle mass in the remote myocardium, i.e., a patient with an acute LAD occlusion and a previous inferior infarction secondary to prior occlusion of the right coronary artery has only a limited capacity to develop hypercontractility in the now "nonischemic myocardium" and might develop cardiogenic shock a short time after acute coronary occlusion.

B. Remote muscle hypercontractility which might be present during the initial few hours after the acute coronary occlusion may decrease progressively to normokinesis and eventually to hypokinesis.[15,116] Our experimental studies have shown that despite maintenance of normal or increased blood flow, i.e., open coronary artery, mild energy and substrate depletion and evidence of anaerobic metabolism in the remote muscle occurs several hours after the acute coronary occlusion:[15] ATP, CP, glycogen and glutamate become depleted in the remote muscle with only LAD occlusion.[15,92] These observations might also serve as an explanation for the development of cardiogenic shock due to acute endocarditis, acute failure of biological valves or mechanical defects, in that the entire left ventricle is now energy depleted and hypercontractility cannot be sustained. Transoesophageal echocardiography reveals global left ventricular hypocontractility in these patients.

C. Remote myocardium may become relatively ischemic if it is supplied by stenotic coronary arteries when called upon to increase contractile function, and compensatory hypercontractility may not either occur or be sustained and lead to cardiogenic shock and/or intractable ventricular fibrillation. We found remote muscle to become progressively hypocontractile with resultant reduction in stroke work index when it was supplied by a noncritically stenotic coronary artery.[15] The functional deterioration was accompanied by moderate substrate- and energy-depletion and more pronounced evidence of anaerobic metabolism despite normal blood flow. Functional impairment despite normal blood flow to remote muscle suggests either autoregulatory failure or substrate-depletion as the cause of hypocontractility.

The critical importance of remote muscle in determining the natural history of patients having acute myocardial infarction is reinforced by a report by Jaarsma and associates[50] showing a 69% mortality rate (usually from left ventricular power failure) in such patients who did not have remote hypercontractility. Schuster and Buckley[99] report a 72% late mortality rate in patients with "ischemia at a distance" and suggest that prognosis appears related more to ischemic events in remote muscle than to the quantity of myocardium lost during the acute infarction.

These data indicate that unimpaired blood flow to remote muscle should be provided by revascularization in patients with multivessel disease and that active resuscitation of the remote muscle is necessary during revascularization.

These observations form the basis for our strategy directed at maximizing myocardial protection of ischemic and remote myocardium during operations for acute coronary occlusion and cardiogenic shock.

Importance for Using Retrograde Techniques
During Surgical Treatment for Acute Myocardial Infarction

Optimal myocardial protection requires adequate distribution of cardioplegic solution to all myocardial regions.[23,43] In the setting of acute coronary occlusion, antegrade delivery of cardioplegia causes maldistribution of the cardioplegic solution and results in inadequate protection of vulnerable cardiac muscle.[48] This disadvantage of antegrade cardioplegia can be circumvented by retrograde cardioplegic administration via either the coronary venous system or right atrium.[73,36] We prefer the direct transatrial cannulation of the coronary sinus, because it can be performed much easier and faster than other retrograde techniques.

In the presence of an occluded left anterior descending coronary artery, antegrade cardioplegia delays cooling and arrest of the anterolateral left ventricle and is associated with delay of early recovery of segmental shortening that impairs complete global recovery after only one hour of ischemia.[86] Retrograde cardioplegia leads to excellent hypothermia of the anterolateral left ventricle and septum, complete return of contractile function in the anterior ventricle, but results in inconsistent right ventricular cooling and recovery (60–100% recovery of function) in canine experiments.[86] However, some recent studies suggest, that there are differences in the canine anatomy as compared to man with predominant venous drainage by Thebesian veins rather than the coronary sinus.[33,9] Furthermore, several clinical studies have suggested superb right ventricular protection by only retrograde cardioplegia.[33,9,37,67]

The importance of including retrograde techniques during surgical interventions for acute coronary occlusions is further strengthened by data showing that the myocardial segment supplied by the obstructed left anterior descending coronary artery receives <10% of flow distributed to the region supplied by the patent circumflex coronary artery, when all cardioplegia is delivered antegrade, and there is selective underperfusion of the subendocardium.[85] In contrast, retrograde cardioplegia delivers to the anterolateral ventricle approximately 60% of the flow of the circumflex distribution and there is selective subendocardial hyperperfusion.[85]

Several reports document the capacity of retrograde cardioplegia to protect myocardium in jeopardy of having intraoperative damage because of the presence of coronary occlusion.[20,71,43] Masuda and colleagues[71] have shown adequate myocardial protection in coronary occlusion by retrograde cardioplegic perfusion via the coronary sinus by the preservation of high energy phosphates, good regional myocardial cooling, and restoration of adequate function of muscle reliant on retrograde cardioplegic protection.

The advantage of retrograde administration of cardioplegia in hearts with coronary occlusions are not only shown in the setting of acute coronary occlusion (Fig. 11.1),[85] but also in patients with chronic coronary occlusions. We have found additional oxygen uptake during retrograde delivery of cardioplegia, after the antegrade dose has been already given, which suggests poor antegrade cardioplegic distribution in patients with occluded coronary arteries (Fig. 11.2).

A prerequisite for the successful myocardial protection by retrograde techniques in the setting of acute coronary occlusions is the correct placement of the coronary sinus catheter. We perform retrograde cannulation either before or after venous cannulation. A 3/0 prolene mattress suture is placed in the low right atrium. A small puncture is made, enlarged, and the cannula is introduced into the right atrium. Advancement into the coronary sinus can usually be accomplished easily, if the tip of the catheter directs towards the patient's left atrium. The correct position of the coronary sinus cannula can be verified by (a) palpation of the tip of the cannula, (b) having dark, desaturated coronary sinus blood coming out of the cannula, and (c) pressure monitoring. A high coronary sinus pressure, i.e., > 20 mm Hg, indicates that the catheter is introduced too far into the coronary sinus; the catheter should be withdrawn approximately 1–2 cm.

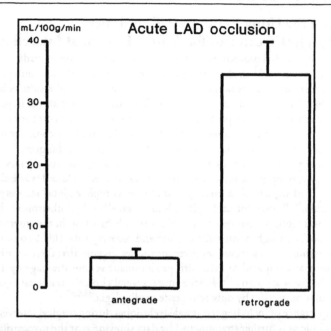

Fig. 11.1. Nutritive flow to the myocardial region supplied by an acutely occluded LAD. Note: Superior flow with retrograde delivery of cardioplegia.[85] With permission Partington MT, Acar C, Buckberg GD et al. Studies of retrograde cardioplegia. 1. Capillary blood flow distribution to myocardium supplied by open and occluded arteries. J Thorac Cardiovasc Surg 1989; 97:605-612. © Mosby-Year Book, 1993.

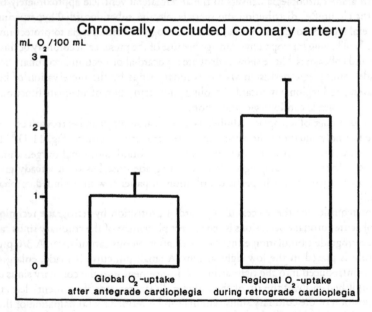

Fig. 11.2. Oxygen uptake in the human heart during antegrade/retrograde delivery of cardioplegia. Note: 1) Reduced global oxygen uptake at the end of antegrade cardioplegia during the first reinfusion (left bar). 2) Increased regional O_2-uptake during the subsequent retrograde delivery of cardioplegia in areas supplied by chronically occluded coronary arteries.

Some patients with acute coronary occlusions are very vulnerable and do not tolerate the placement of the coronary sinus catheter off bypass. In those patients we start extracorporeal circulation first and introduce the coronary sinus catheter on partial bypass.

During retrograde delivery of cardioplegia, the correct position of the cannula is evident from (a) an increase in coronary sinus pressure usually between 30–50 mm Hg, (b) red distended veins on the right and left side of the heart, and (c) cardioplegic outflow from the aortic root.

Coronary sinus pressures >50 mm Hg indicate that the catheter is lodged too far into the coronary sinus or it is in the posterior descending coronary vein; pressures <20 mm Hg during infusions indicate that the self-inflating balloon is not occluding the coronary sinus. Manual compression of the coronary sinus around the catheter is necessary in order to increase the pressure. If retrograde cardioplegia is delivered at 200–250 mL/min, the coronary sinus pressure ranges usually from 30–50 mm Hg.

The coronary sinus pressure may rise occasionally during antegrade cardioplegic delivery suggesting the coronary sinus effluent from the antegrade dose is entering the tip of the retrograde cannula and inflating the balloon. The coronary sinus pressure rarely exceeds 50 mm Hg under these circumstances. Retrograde balloon inflation during antegrade infusion may improve the distribution of antegrade cardioplegia, as either intermittent or fixed coronary sinus occlusion during antegrade cardioplegic administration has been reported to improve protection to areas supplied by occluded vessels.[75,104]

Surgical Technique

The surgical strategy for acute myocardial infarction (Fig. 11.3) can be separated into the phases of 1) total vented bypass, 2) aortic cross-clamping, 3) regional controlled reperfusion, and 4) prolonged beating empty state.

Total Vented Cardiopulmonary Bypass

Extracorporeal circulation is established as quickly as possible by means of single venous and aortic cannulation and connecting them to a membrane oxygenator, primed with lactated Ringer's. The left ventricle is vented routinely by a catheter passed through the right pulmonary vein. For patients who need preoperative cardiopulmonary resuscitation, peripheral cannulation is used for extracorporeal bypass, i.e., the femoral vein is cannulated with a catheter passed into the right atrium (femoro-atrial cannula), and the femoral artery is cannulated in the usual fashion. For antegrade delivery of blood cardioplegia, a cardioplegic needle is inserted into the ascending aorta.

Transatrial Cannulation of the Coronary Sinus

Combined antegrade/retrograde delivery of blood cardioplegia is used for all patients in order to ensure optimal distribution.[6,17,69] A pursestring suture is placed at the lower edge of the right atrium near the inferior caval vein. In hemodynamically unstable patients, cannulation of the coronary sinus is always done on bypass, whereas in stable patients cannulation can also be done before cannulation of the right atrium. The tip of the self-inflating coronary sinus cannula (Retroplegia R, Research Medical Inc.; Salt Lake City, Utah, USA) is directed towards the patient's left atrium and cannulation is usually done very easily. The correct position of the cannula in the coronary sinus is tested by (a) palpating the tip of the cannula in the coronary sinus, (b) measuring the coronary sinus pressure (5–10 mm Hg), and (c) having dark blood coming out of the coronary sinus catheter.

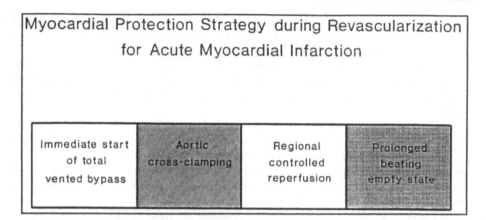

Fig. 11.3. Surgical strategy for acute myocardial infarction.

Choice of Bypass Conduits

For bypass conduits we use only vein grafts into the segment undergoing infarction because the controlled reperfusate has to be administered through these conduits. Internal thoracic artery grafts are feasible only when they are placed in conjunction with vein grafts into the ischemic region, or the remote segment is not large, since (unlike vein grafts) they can not immediate accomodate the high flows that may be needed to supply remote segment containing a large volume muscle mass.

Period of Aortic Cross-Clamping

The strategies for myocardial protection with blood cardioplegia in patients with acute coronary occlusion during the period of aortic cross-clamping may be separated into the phases of (a) induction, (b) maintenance and distribution, and (c) global reperfusion.

The total blood cardioplegic dose is divided equally between antegrade and retrograde delivery for induction, maintenance and reperfusion. The doses are never given simultaneously by the two roots. Furthermore, the duration and volume of cardioplegic delivery should not be increased above that stated in this Chapter because this may lead to markedly excessive volumes of cardioplegia that may cause postoperative myocardial depression.[63]

Induction

Cardioplegia may be induced immediately after extracorporeal circulation has begun and the pulmonary artery is collapsed. Starting the antegrade perfusion before aortic clamping ensures aortic valve competence. The blood cardioplegic solution may be given cold or warm.

Cold blood cardioplegic induction. Patients who are hemodynamically stable receive cold blood cardioplegic induction with the 4 to 8°C blood cardioplegic solution infused at 300 mL/min with the high-potassium solution until arrest and is reduced to a flow of 200–250 mL/min with the low-potassium solution thereafter (Table 11.2). The four-minute period for cold cardioplegic induction is divided into 2 minutes given antegrade and 2 minutes given retrograde.

At the beginning of the retrograde delivery of cardioplegia, the correct position of the cannula inside the coronary sinus has to be tested because the cannula might be 1) too far in the coronary sinus, thus not perfusing the veins of the right side of the heart; 2) the balloon of the cannula may not occlude the lumen of the coronary sinus completely, thus having significant backflow of cardioplegia into the right atrium and a decrease in the amount of nutritive flow effectively delivered to the myocardium; and 3) the cannula might not be in the coronary sinus at all.

The correct position of the coronary sinus cannula (Table 11.1) has to be tested by (a) an increase in coronary sinus pressure up to 20 or 35 mm Hg (however, it should not exceed 50 mm Hg); (b) visualization of red, distended veins on the right and left side of the heart and dark arteries (most important sign); (c) desaturated blood in the aortic root; and (d) if myocardial temperature is measured, decrease in myocardial temperature. Failure to have a significant increase in coronary sinus pressure might indicate significant backflow of cardioplegia into the right atrium and manual compression of the coronary sinus around the self-inflating balloon is necessary. If this also does not increase the coronary sinus pressure, the cannula might not be in the coronary sinus at all. If only the veins of the left ventricle are red and distended and those of the right side of the heart are not, the cannula is usually too far into the coronary sinus and has to be pulled back.

Warm blood cardioplegic induction. Patients in cardiogenic shock or with otherwise depleted energy stores are placed on normothermic bypass and receive warm cardioplegic induction over five minutes (2.5 minutes antegrade and 2.5 minutes retrograde) with a 37°C substrate-enriched (glutamate/aspartate) cardioplegic solution containing 20–25 mEq/mL KCl[94] (Table 7.3). Normothermic blood cardioplegic infusion is started at 250–350 mL/min and causes arrest within 1 to 2 minutes. The infusion rate is then reduced to 150 mL/min to prevent excessive cardioplegic volume, and the warm infusion is continued for a total of 5 minutes (maximum volume 1000 mL). Immediately after the 5 minutes of warm induction, the perfusionist starts systemic cooling to 28°C and the cardioplegic bag is changed to a low-potassium, nonsubstrate-enriched blood cardioplegic solution (Table 7.1). The heater-cooler is switched to the maximum cooling mode and 4–8°C water is circulated through the disposable heat exchanger. The flow rate is increased to 250 mL/min for 3 additional minutes. The cardioplegic solution can be changed at 4 minutes, as the dead space in the cardioplegic line is approximately 175 mL/min, thereby ensuring a full substrate-enriched dose.

During this prolonged cardioplegic induction interval, target coronary arteries on the anterior surface are being prepared for distal anastomosis.

Order of Grafting

The first vein graft is always placed into the vessel involved in the acute coronary occlusion. During vein harvesting, a side branch of the vein is cannulated so that the proximal anastomosis can later be performed while the controlled regional blood cardioplegic reperfusate is delivered (Fig. 11.4).

Table 11.1. Correct position of the coronary sinus cannula during delivery of blood cardioplegia

- Increase in coronary sinus pressure (up to 30–40 mm Hg)

- Bright red, distended veins on the inferior aspect of the right ventricle (e.g., v. interventricularis posterior)

- Desaturated blood in the aortic root

Table 11.2. Cold induction (60 mEq) and maintenance (20 mEq)

Cardioplegic additive	Volume added	Component modified	Concentration delivered
THAM (0.3 mol/L)*	200 mL	pH	7.7–7.8
CPD†	50 mL	Ca++	0.5–0.6 mmol/L
D5 ¼ NS‡	550 mL	Osmol	340–360 mosmol/L
KCl (2 mEq/mL)§			
Induction	30 mL	K+	18–20 mEq/L
Maintenance	10 mL		8–10 mEq/L

* THAM Tromethamine; † CPDcitrate-phosphate-dextrose; ‡ D5 ¼ NS5% dextrose in 0.2 N normal sodium; § KCl potassium chloride

Complete Revascularization

The importance of complete revascularization of all coronary arteries (ischemic and remote myocardium) is based upon the abovementioned experimental and clinical observations and is reinforced by a recent study by Mooney and coworkers.[76] Failure to completely revascularize the myocardium, e.g., coronary arteries less than 1.0 mm unsuitable for grafting, LAD dissections after PTCA failure with occlusion of larger septal branches, peripheral occlusions, etc., might result in persistent hypo- or akinetic areas and will be the cause for inadequate reversal of cardiogenic shock.

Maintenance of Cardioplegia

Reinfusions of cardioplegia are delivered at approximately 20-minute intervals. Re-infusions are delivered at 200–250 mL/min for 2 minutes, with 1 minute antegrade and 1 minute retrograde. Again, the surgeon must be sure, that the retrograde pressure is >25 mm Hg during reinfusions to ensure proper distribution into the coronary venous system.

The solution for multidose cardioplegia is comparable to the standard solution and differs only in the use of low potassium to reduce systemic hyperkalemia.

Global Reperfusion

After completion of the last distal anastomosis, warm (37°C) diltiazem containing, substrate-enriched blood cardioplegia is given into the aorta and all grafts for 2 minutes at 150 mL/min (Table 11.4). Thereafter the aortic clamp is removed.

Controlled Regional Reperfusion

After removal of the aortic clamp controlled regional blood cardioplegic solution (Table 11.4) is given at a flow rate of 50 mL/min only into the graft supplying the region revascularized for acute coronary occlusion for additional 18 minutes. In patients with acute occlusion of the left main coronary artery or with acute occlusion of two coronary arteries, flow is increased to

Table 11.3. Warm induction

Cardioplegic additive	Volume added	Component modified	Concentration delivered
THAM (0.3 mol/L)*	225 mL	pH	7.5–7.6
CPD**	225 mL	Ca^{++}	0.15 mmol/L
D50W***	40 mL	Osmol	380–400 mosmol/L
Glutamate/Aspartate	250 mL	Substrate	13 mmol/L each
KCl (2 mEq/mL)†	40 mL	K^+	20–25 mEq/L
D5W§	220 mL		

* THAM Tromethamine; ** CPDcitrate-phosphate-dextrose; *** D50W 50% dextrose in water; † KCl potassium chloride; § D5W 5% dextrose in water

Table 7.4. Regional controlled blood cardioplegic reperfusate

Cardioplegic additive	Volume added	Component delivered	Concentration modified
THAM (0.3 mol/L)*	225 mL	pH	7.5–7.6
CPD	225 mL	Ca^{++}	0.15–0.25 mmol/L
D50W	40 mL	Glucose	> 400 mg/dL
D5W	200 mL	Osmol	350-400 mosmol
Glutamate/Aspartate	250 mL	Substrate	13 mmol/L each
KCl (2 mEq/mL)**	15 mL	K^+	8–10 mEq/L
Diltiazem			300 µg/kg bw

* THAM Tromethamine; ** CPDcitrate-phosphate-dextrose

100 mL/min and given into both vein grafts. Normal blood is delivered into the remainder of the heart via the aortic segment not included in the tangential clamp (Fig. 11. 4). Cannulation of a side branch of the vein graft allows delivery of the controlled blood cardioplegic reperfusate while the proximal anastomosis is performed so that no additional ischemic time is imposed on the previously ischemic region (Fig. 11.4). The proximal anastomosis of the vein graft supplying the ischemic region is always constructed first.

Beating Empty State

The heart is kept in the beating empty state for 30 minutes more after completion of the controlled regional cardioplegic reperfusion. Recovery of jeopardized myocardium is best achieved by lowering oxygen demands and increasing oxygen delivery. The oxygen requirements of nonischemic muscle can be reduced to 50% by converting a beating working heart (9 mL/100g/min) into the beating empty state (4.5 mL/100g/min).[1] Whereas the oxygen requirements of dyskinetic muscle are almost 55% of beating working needs,[2,114] decompression by total vented bypass abolished systolic bulging immediately and produced an immediate fall in regional oxygen uptake to 1 mL/100g/min. The importance of lowering oxygen demands by ventricular decompression during ischemia is established further by reports of Pennock, Pierce, and Waldhausen,[88] who showed that 95% cardiopulmonary bypass reduced left ventricular oxygen consumption 30% and that total bypass lowered oxygen demands to 50% of the nonischemic, contracting muscle.

A large right atrial drainage cannula or double cannulation with caval tapes will not ensure continuous left heart decompression, which is also known from clinical experience during elective operations. Some coronary sinus return and/or bronchial flow will enter the left ventricle, distend it, allow wall tension to develop, and result in occasional ejection despite apparent right heart decompression. Therefore, effective left heart decompression requires a ventricular vent, usually placed through the right pulmonary veins.

Extracorporeal circulation is discontinued after 30 minutes of beating empty state; bypass is resumed if cardiac output is not satisfactory.

Conclusions

Recent experimental and clinical studies suggest that myocardial salvage with early recovery of contractile function after acute coronary occlusion is possible beyond the generally accepted 2 hours, provided that the initial reperfusion is controlled carefully. Overall hospital survival depends upon the function of the remote, nonischemic myocardium, since failure of remote muscle compensation may cause cardiogenic shock. Surgical revascularization has to restore and maintain significant hypercontractility in the remote area in order to allow the generation of sufficient cardiac output in patients with left ventricular power failure. Myocardial protection techniques, e.g., antegrade/retrograde blood cardioplegia, controlled reperfusion, prolonged beating empty state, has been described for improving salvage and restoring contractile function in the ischemic area, and for restoring hypercontractility in the remote myocardium. It is to be hoped that subsequent clinical studies will test these approaches, and if confirmatory, will reduce the mortality rate of patients with acute coronary occlusions.

References

1. Allen BS, Rosenkranz ER, Buckberg GD et al. Studies of controlled reperfusion after ischemia. VII. High oxygen requirements of dyskinetic cardiac muscle. J Thorac Cardiovasc Surg 1986; 92:543-552.
2. Allen BS, Okamoto F, Buckberg GD et al. Studies of controlled reperfusion after ischemia. IX. Reperfusate composition: Benefits of marked hypocalcemia and diltiazem on regional recovery. J Thorac Cardiovasc Surg 1986; 92:564-572.

3. Allen BS, Okamoto F, Buckberg GD et al. Studies of controlled reperfusion after ischemia. XII. Effects of "duration" of reperfusate administration versus reperfusate "dose" on regional functional, biochemical, and histochemical recovery. J Thorac Cardiovasc Surg 1986; 92:594-604.

4. Allen BS, Okamoto F, Buckberg GD et al. Studies of controlled reperfusion after ischemia. XIII. Reperfusion conditions. Critical importance of total ventricular decompression during regional reperfusion. J Thorac Cardiovasc Surg 1986; 92:605-612.

5. Allen BS, Okamoto F, Buckberg GD et al. Studies of controlled reperfusion after ischemia. XV. Immediate functional recovery after 6 hours of regional ischemia by careful control of conditions of reperfusion and composition of reperfusate. J Thorac Cardiovasc Surg 1986; 92 (suppl):621-635.

6. Allen BS, Buckberg GD, Schwaiger M et al. Studies of controlled reperfusion after ischemia. XVI. Consistent early recovery of regional wall motion following surgical revascularization after eight hours of acute coronary occlusion. J Thorac Cardiovasc Surg 1986; 92 (suppl): 636-648.

7. Allen BS, Buckberg GD, Fontan F et al. Superiority of controlled surgical reperfusion versus PTCA in acute coronary occlusion. J Thorac Cardiovasc Surg 1993; 105:864-884.

8. Alonso DR, Scheldt S, Post M et al. Pathophysiology of cardiogenic shock: Quantification of myocardial necrosis, clinical, pathologic and electrocardiographic correlations. Circulation 1973; 48:588-596.

9. Arom KV, Emery RW. Coronary sinus cardioplegia: Clinical trial with only retrograde approach. Ann Thorac Surg 1992; 53:965-971.

10. Banka VS, Helfant RH. Temporal sequence of dynamic contractile characteristics in ischemic and nonischemic myocardium after acute coronary ligation. Am J Cardiol 1974; 34:158-163.

11. Becker LC, Schaper J, Jeremy R, Schaper W. Severity of ischemia determines the occurrence of myocardial reperfusion injury. Circulation 1991; 84 (Suppl II):II-254.

12. Beggerly CE, Austin EH, Chitwood WR Jr. Current coronary artery surgery practices: a national survey. J Am Coll Cardiol 1987; 9:123A.

13. Berg RJ, Selinger SL, Leonard JL, Grunwald RP, O'Grady WP. Immediate coronary artery bypass for acute evolving myocardial infarction. J Thorac Cardiovasc Surg 1981; 81:493-497.

14. Beyersdorf F, Allen BS, Buckberg GD et al. Studies on prolonged acute regional ischemia. I. Evidence for preserved cellular viability after six hours of coronary occlusion. J Thorac Cardiovasc Surg 1989; 98:112-126.

15. Beyersdorf F, Acar C, Buckberg GD et al. Studies of prolonged acute regional ischemia. III. Early natural history of simulated single and multivessel disease with emphasis on remote myocardium. J Thorac Cardiovasc Surg 1989; 98:368-380.

16. Beyersdorf F, Acar C, Buckberg GD et al. Studies on prolonged acute regional ischemia. IV. Aggressive surgical treatment for intractable ventricular fibrillation after acute myocardial infarction. J Thorac Cardiovasc Surg 1989; 98:557-566.

17. Beyersdorf F, Sarai K, Maul FD et al. Immediate functional benefits after controlled reperfusion during surgical revascularization for acute coronary occlusion. J Thorac Cardiovasc Surg 1991; 102:856-866.

18. Beyersdorf F. Acute myocardial infarction and cardiogenic shock. In: Seminars of Thoracic and Cardiovascular Surgery. Loop FL, ed. Saunders Company 1993; 5:125-133.

19. Beyersdorf F, Mitrev Z, Sarai K et al. Changing patterns of patients undergoing emergency surgical revascularization for acute coronary occlusion. Importance of myocardial protection techniques. J Thorac Cardiovasc Surg 1993; 106:137-148.

20. Bolling SF, Flaherty JT, Bulkley BH et al. Improved myocardial preservation during global ischemia by continuous retrograde coronary sinus perfusion. J Thorac Cardiovasc Surg 1983; 86:659-666.

21. Bottner RK, Wallace RB, Visner MS et al. Reduction of myocardial infarction after emergency coronary artery bypass grafting for failed coronary angioplasty with use of normothermic reperfusion cardioplegia protocol. J Thorac Cardiovasc Surg 1991; 101:1069-1075.

22. Buckberg GD. Studies of Controlled Reperfusion after Ischemia. J Thorac Cardiovasc Surg 1986; 92:483-648.

23. Buckberg GD. Antegrade/retrograde blood cardioplegia to ensure cardioplegic distribution: Operative techniques and objectives. J Cardiac Surg 1989; 4:216-238.

24. Buckberg GD, Allen B, Okamoto F et al. Immediate functional recovery after 6 hours coronary occlusion using regional blood cardioplegic reperfusion and total vented bypass without thoracotomy. A new concept (abstr). Circulation 1984; Suppl 2:172.

25. Byrne JG, Appleyard RF, Chin Lee C et al. Controlled reperfusion of the regionally ischemic myocardium with leukocyte-depleted blood reduces stunning, the no-reflow phenomenon, and infarct size. J Thorac Cardiovasc Surg 1992; 103:66-72.

26. Cheung EH, Arcidi JM, Dorsey LMA et al. Reperfusion of infarcting myocardium: Benefit of surgical reperfusion in a chronic model. Ann Thorac Surg 1989; 48:331-338.
27. Corday E, Kaplan L, Meerbaum S et al. Consequences of coronary arterial occlusion on remote myocardium: Effects of occlusion and reperfusion. Am J Cardiol 1975; 36:385-394.
28. Cowley MJ, Dorros G, Kelsey SF et al. Emergency coronary bypass surgery after coronary angioplasty: The national heart, lung, and blood institute's percutaneous transluminal coronary registry experience. Am J Cardiol 1984; 53:22C–26C.
29. Diehl JT, Eichhorn, EJ, Konstam MA et al. Efficacy of retrograde coronary sinus cardioplegia in patients undergoing myocardial revascularization: A prospective randomized trial. Ann Thorac Surg 1988; 45:595-602.
30. DeWood MA, Spores J, Notske R et al. Medical and surgical management of myocardial infarction. Am J Cardiol 1979; 44:1356-1364 .
31. Digerness SB, Kirklin JW, Naftel DC et al. Coronary and systemic vascular resistance during reperfusion after global myocardial ischemia. Ann Thorac Surg 1988; 46:447-454.
32. Ding M, Dyke CM, Abd-Elfattah AS et al. Efficacy of a hydroxyl radical scavenger (VF 233) in preventing reperfusion injury in the isolated rabbit heart. Ann Thorac Surg 1992; 53:1091-1095.
33. Douville EC, Kratz JM, Spinale FG et al. Retrograde versus antegrade cardioplegia: Impact on right ventricular function. Ann Thorac Surg 1992; 54:56-61.
34. Engelman RM, Rousou JA, Flack JE III et al. Reduction of infarct size by systemic amino acid supplementation during reperfusion. J Thorac Cardiovasc Surg 1991; 101:855-859.
35. Engler RL, Schmid-Schönbein GW, Pevelec RS. Leukocyte capillary plugging in myocardial ischemia and reperfusion in the dog. Am J Physiol 1986; 84:815-822.
36. Fabiani JN, Swanson J, Deloche A et al. Right atrial cardioplegia. In: Roberts AJ, ed. Myocardial Protection in Cardiac Surgery. New York: Marcel-Dekker, 1986:505.
37. Fiore AC, Naunheim, KS, Kaiser GC et al. Coronary sinus versus aortic root perfusion with blood cardioplegia in elective myocardial revascularization. Ann Thorac Surg 1989; 47:684-688.
38. Follette D, Fey K, Livesay J et al. The beneficial effects of citrate reperfusion of ischemic heart on cardiopulmonary bypass. Surg Forum 1976; 26:244-246.
39. Follette DM, Fey K, Buckberg GD et al. Reducing postischemic damage by temporary modification of reperfusate calcium, potassium, pH and osmolarity. J Thorac Cardiovasc Surg 1981; 82:221-238.
40. Fujiwara T, Kurtts T, Silvera M et al. Physical and Pharmacological Manipulation of Reperfusion Conditions in Neonatal Myocardial Preservation. Circulation 1988; 78 (Suppl II):II-444.
41. Geltman EM, Ehsani AA, Campbell MK et al. The influence of location and extent of myocardial infarction on long-term ventricular dysrhythmia and mortality. Circulation 1979; 60:805-814.
42. Gharagozloo F, Melendez FJ, Hein RA et al. The effect of oxygen free radical scavengers on the recovery of regional myocardial function after acute coronary occlusion and surgical reperfusion. J Thorac Cardiovasc Surg 1988; 95:631-636.
43. Gundry SR, Kirsh MM. A comparison of retrograde cardioplegia in the presence of coronary artery obstruction. Ann Thorac Surg 1984; 38:124-127.
44. Gundry SR, de Begona JA, Kawauchi M et a l. Successful transplantation of hearts harvested 30 minutes after death from exsanguination. Ann Thorac Surg 1992; 53:772-775.
45. Haas GS, DeBoer LWV, O'Keefe DD et al. Reduction of postischemic myocardial dysfunction by substrate repletion during reperfusion. Circulation 1984; 70 (Suppl I):I-65–I-74.
46. Haan C, Lazar H, Yang X et al. Reduction of infarct size with substrate enhanced coronary venous retroperfusion. Circulation 1991; 84 (Suppl II):II-716.
47. Herlitz J, Hjalmarson A, Waldenstrom J. Relationship between enzymatically estimated infarct size and short- and long-term survival after acute myocardial infarction. Acta Med Scand 1984; 216: 261-267.
48. Hilton CJ, Teubl W, Acker M, McEnany MT. Inadequate cardioplegic protection with obstructed coronary arteries. Ann Thorac Surg 1979; 28:323-334.
49. Hochberg MS, Austen WG. Selective retrograde coronary venous perfusion. Ann Thorac Surg 1980; 29:578-588.
50. Jaarsma W, Visser CA, Van Einige JM et al. Prognostic implication of regional hyperkinesia and remote asynergy of noninfarcted myocardium. Am J Cardiol 1986; 58:394-398.
51. Jennings RB, Ganote CE. Structural changes in myocardium during acute ischemia. Circ Res 1974; 34/35(Suppl III):156-168.
52. Jennings RB, Reimer KA. Lethal myocardial ischemic injury. Am J Pathol 1981; 102:241-255.
53. Jennings RB, Reimer KA. Factors involved in salvaging ischemic myocardium: effect of reperfusion of arterial blood. Circulation 1983; 68:Suppl I:25-36.

54. Jennings RB, Schaper J, Hill ML et al. Effect of reperfusion late in the phase of reversible ischemic injury. Circ Res 1985; 56:252-278.
55. Julia P, Young HH, Buckberg GD et al. Studies of myocardial protection in the immature heart. IV. Improved tolerance of immature myocardium to hypoxia and ischemia by intravenous metabolic support. J Thorac Cardiovasc Surg 1991; 101:23-32.
56. Kalmbach T, Bhayana JN. Cardioplegia delivery by combined aortic root and coronary sinus perfusion. Ann Thorac Surg 1989; 47:316-317.
57. Killen DA, Hamaker WR, Reed WA. Coronary artery bypass following percutaneous transluminal coronary . Ann Thorac Surg 1985; 40:133-138.
58. Kirklin JK. The science of cardiac surgery. Eur J Cardio-thorac Surg 1990; 4:63-71.
59. Kirklin JK, Neves J, Naftel DC, Digerness SB, Kirklin JW, Blackstone EH. Controlled initial hyperkalemic reperfusion after cardiac transplantation: Coronary vascular resistance and blood flow. Ann Thorac Surg 1990; 49:625-631.
60. Kirklin JW, Frye RL, Blackstone EH, Naftel DC. Some comments on the indications for the coronary artery bypass graft operation. Int J Cardiol 1991; 31:23-30.
61. Kloner RA, Ellis SG, Carlson NV, Braunwald E. Coronary reperfusion for the treatment of acute myocardial infarction: postischemic ventricular dysfunction. Cardiology 1983; 70:233-246.
62. Kloner RA, Ellis SG, Lange R, Braunwald E. Studies of experimental coronary artery reperfusion. Effects on infarct size, myocardial function, biochemistry, ultrastructure and microvascular damage. Circulation 1983; 68(Suppl I):8-15.
63. Kofsky ER, Julia PL, Buckberg GD et al. Overdose reperfusion of blood cardioplegic solution: a preventable cause of postischemic myocardial depression. J Thorac Cardiovasc Surg 1991; 101:275-283.
64. Laschinger JC, Grossi EA, Cunningham JN et al. Adjunctive left ventricular unloading during myocardial reperfusion plays a major role in minimizing myocardial infarct size. J Thorac Cardiovasc Surg 1985; 90:80-85.
65. Lazar HL, Buckberg GD, Manganaro AJ et al. Reversal of ischemic damage with amino acid substrate enhancement during reperfusion. Surgery 1980; 80:702-709.
66. Lazar HL, Wei J, Dirbas FM et al. Controlled reperfusion following regional ischemia. Ann Thorac Surg 1987; 44:350-355.
67. Lichtenstein SV, Abel JG, Slutsky AS. Warm retrograde cardioplegia. J Thorac Cardiovasc Surg 1992; 104:374-380.
68. Lillehei CW, DeWall RA, Gott VL et al. The direct vision correction of calcified aortic stenosis by means of pump-oxygenator and retrograde coronary sinus perfusion. Dis Chest 1956; 30:123-132.
69. Loop FD, Higgins TL, Panda R et al. Myocardial protection during cardiac operations. Decreased morbidity and lower cost with blood cardioplegia and coronary sinus perfusion. J Thorac Cardiovasc Surg 1992; 104:608-618.
70. Lüdinghausen MV. Nomenclature and distribution pattern of cardiac veins in man. In: Mohl W, Faxon D, Wolner E, eds. Clinics of CSI. New York: Springer-Verlag, 1986:13-32.
71. Masuda M, Yonenaga K, Shiki K et al. Myocardial protection in coronary occlusion by retrograde cardioplegic perfusion via the coronary sinus in dogs. J Thorac Cardiovasc Surg 1986; 92:255-263.
72. Melendez FJ, Gharagozloo F, Sun SC et al. Effects of diltiazem cardioplegia on global function, segmental contractility, and the area of necrosis after acute coronary artery occlusion and surgical reperfusion. J Thorac Cardiovasc Surg 1988; 95:613-617.
73. Menasche P, Subayi JB, Veyssie L et al. Efficacy of coronary sinus cardioplegia in patients with complete coronary artery occlusions. Ann Thorac Surg 1991; 51:418-423.
74. Metzdorff MT, Grunkemeier GL, Starr A. Effect of initial reperfusion temperature on myocardial preservation. J Thorac Cardiovasc Surg 1986; 91:545-550.
75. Mohl W. Coronary sinus interventions: From concept to clinics. J Card Surg 1987; 2:467.
76. Mooney MR, Arom KV, Joyce LD, Mooney JF, Goldenberg IF, Von Rueden TJ, Emery RW. Emergency cardiopulmonary bypass support in patients with cardiac arrest. J Thorac Cardiovasc Surg 1991; 101:450-454.
77. Naccarella FF, Weintraub WS, Agarwal JB, Helfant RH. Evaluation of "ischemia of a distance": Effects of coronary occlusion on a remote area of the left ventricle. AM J Cardiol 1984; 54:869-874.
78. Nayler WG. The role of calcium in the ischemic myocardium. Am J Pathol 1981; 102:262-270.
79. Ohara H, Kanaide H, Yoshimura R, Okada M, Nadamura M. A protective effect of coenzyme Q_{10} on ischemia and reperfusion of the isolated perfused rat heart. Gen Mol Cell Cardiol 1981; 13:65-74.
80. Okamoto F, Allen BS, Buckberg GD et al. Studies of controlled reperfusion after ischemia. VIII. Regional blood cardioplegic reperfusion during total vented bypass without thoracotomy. A new concept. J Thorac Cardiovasc Surg 1986; 92:553-563.

81. Okamoto F, Allen BS, Buckberg GD et al. Studies of controlled reperfusion after ischemia. X. Reperfusate composition: supplemental role of intravenous and intracoronary coenzyme Q_{10} in avoiding reperfusion damage. J Thorac Cardiovasc Surg 1986; 92:573-582.

82. Okamoto F, Allen BS, Buckberg GD et al. Studies of controlled reperfusion after ischemia. XI. Reperfusate composition. Interaction of marked hyperglycemia and marked hyperosmolarity in allowng immediate contractile recovery after four hours of regional ischemia. J Thorac Cardiovasc Surg 1986; 92:583-593.

83. Okamoto F, Allen BS, Buckberg GD et al. Studies of controlled reperfusion after ischemia. XIV. Reperfusion conditions. Importance of ensuring gentle versus sudden reperfusion during relief of coronary occlusion. J Thorac Cardovasc Surg 1986; 92:613-620.

84. Page DL, Caulfield JB, Kastor JA et al. Myocardial changes associated with cardiogenic shock. N Engl J Med 1971; 285:133-137.

85. Partington MT, Acar C, Buckberg GD et al. Studies on retrograde cardioplegia. I. Capillary blood flow distribution to myocardium supplied by open and occluded arteries. J Thorac Cardiovasc Surg 1989; 97:605-612.

86. Partington MT, Acar C, Buckberg GD et al. Studies on retrograde cardioplegia. II. Advantages of antegrade/retrograde cardioplegia to optimize distribution in jeopardized myocardium. J Thorac Cardiovasc Surg 1989; 97:613-622.

87. Peng CF, Murphy ML, Colwell K et al. Controlled vs. hyperemic flow during reperfusion of jeopardized ischemic myocardium. Am Heart J 1989; 117:515-522.

88. Pennock JL, Pierce WF, Waldausen JA. Quantitative evaluation of left ventricular bypass in reducing myocardial ischemia. Surgery 1976; 79:523-533.

89. Phillips SJ, Kongtahworn C, Skinner JR et al. Emergency coronary artery reperfusion: A choice therapy for evolving myocardial infarction. Results in 339 patients. J Thorac Cardiovasc Surg 1983; 86:679-688.

90. Pich S, Klein HH, Lindert S et al. Therapie des Reperfusionsschadens mit Calcium Antagonisten und verminderter freier coronarer Calcium Konzentration beim experimentellen Myokardinfarkt. Z Kardiol 1989; 78 (Suppl 1):137.

91. Pratt FH. The nutritition of the heart through vessels of the Thebesius and the coronary veins. Am J Physiol 1898; 1: 86-93.

92. Puri PS. Contractile and biochemical effects of coronary reperfusion after extended periods of coronary occlusion. Am J Cardiol 1975; 36:244-251.

93. Rosenkranz ER, Vinten-Johansen J, Buckberg Gd et al. Benefits of normothermic induction of blood cardioplegia in energy-depleted hearts with maintenance of arrest by multidose cold blood cardioplegic infusions. J Thorac Cardiovasc Surg 1982; 84:667-676.

94. Rosenkranz ER, Buckberg GD, Laks H et al. Warm induction of cardioplegia with glutamate-enriched blood in coronary patients with cardiogenic shock who are dependent on inotropic drugs and intraaortic balloon support: Initial experience and operative strategy. J Thorac Cardiovasc Surg 1983; 86:507-518.

95. Rosenkranz ER, Okamoto F, Buckberg GD et al. Safety of prolonged aortic clamping with blood cardioplegia. III. Aspartate enrichment of glutamate-blood cardioplegia in energy-depleted hearts after ischemic and reperfusion injury. J Thorac Cardiovasc Surg 1986; 91:428-435.

96. Sawatari K, Kadoba K, Bergner KA et al. Influence of initial reperfusion pressure after hypothermic cardioplegic ischemia on endothelial modulation of coronary tone in neonatal lambs. J Thorac Cardiovasc Surg 1991; 101:777-782.

97. Schaper W, Pasyk S. Influence of collateral flow on the ischemic tolerance of the heart following acute and subacute coronary occlusion. Circulation 1976; 53 (Suppl I):I-57-I62.

98. Schaper J. Ultrastructure of the myocardium in acute ischemia. In: Schaper W, ed. The Pathophysiology of Myocardial Perfusion. Elsevier/North-Holland Biomedical Press, 1979:581-673.

99. Schuster EH, Bulkley BH. Early postinfarction angina: Ischemia at a distance and ischemia in the infarct zone. N Engl J Med 1981; 305:1102-1105.

100. Shine KI, Douglas AM, Ricchiuti NV. Calcium, strontium, and barium movements during ischemia and reperfusion in rabbit ventricle. Circ Res 1978; 43:712-720.

101. Shine KI, Douglas AM. Low calcium reperfusion of ischemic myocardium. J Mol Cell Cardiol 1983; 15:251-260.

102. Sjöstrand F, Allen BS, Buckberg GD et al. Studies of controlled reperfusion after ischemia. IV. Electron microscopic studies. Importance of embedding techniques in quantitative evaluation of cardiac mitochondrial structure during regional ischemia and reperfusion. J Thorac Cardiovasc Surg 1986; 92 (suppl): 512-524.

103. Solorzano J, Taitelbaum G, Chiu RCJ. Retrograde coronary sinus perfusion for myocardial protection during cardiopulmonary bypass. Ann Thorac Surg 1978; 25:201-208.
104. Sun SC, Raza ST, Tam SKC et al. Effects of antegrade cardioplegic infusion with simultaneously controlled coronary sinus occlusion on preservation of regional ischemic myocardium after acute coronary artery occlusion and reperfusion. J Thorac Cardiovasc Surg 1988; 96:626.
105. Swanson DK, Myerowitz PD. Effect of reperfusion temperature and pressure on the functional and metabolic recovery of preserved hearts. J Thorac Cardiovasc Surg 1983; 86:242-251.
106. Taegtmeyer H. Metabolic responses to cardiac hypoxia. Circ Res 1978; 43:808-815.
107. Tebbe U, Ruschewski W, Knake W et al. Will Emergency Coronary Bypass Grafting After Failed Elective Percutaneous Transluminal Coronary Angioplasty Prevent Myocardial Infarction? Thorac cardiovasc Surgeon 1989; 37:308-312.
108. Thanavaro S, Kleiger RE, Province MA et al. Effect of infarct location on the in-hospital prognosis of patients with first transmural myocardial infarction. Circulation 1982; 66:742-747.
109. Tschabitscher M. Anatomy of coronary veins. In: Mohl W, Wolner E, Glogar D, eds. The coronary sinus. New York: Springer-Verlag, 1984:8-22.
110. Vinten-Johansen J, Edgerton TA, Howe HR et al. Immediate functional recovery and avoidance of reperfusion injury with surgical revascularization and short-term coronary occlusion. Circulation 1985; 72:431-439.
111. Vinten-Johansen J, Buckberg GD, Okamoto F et al. Studies of controlled reperfusion after ischemia. V. Superiority of surgical versus medical reperfusion after regional ischemia. J Thorac Cardiovasc Surg 1986; 92:525-534.
112. Vinten-Johansen J, Faust KB, Mills SA et al. Surgical revascularization of acute evolving infarction without blood cardioplegia fails to restore postischemic function in the involved segment. Ann Thorac Surg 1987; 44:66-72.
113. Vinten-Johansen J, Rosenkranz ER, Buckberg GD et al. Studies of controlled reperfusion after ischemia. IV. Metabolic and histochemical benefits of regional blood cardioplegic reperfusion without cardiopulmonary bypass. J Thorac Cardiovasc Surg 1986; 92:535-542.
114. Weiss HR. Effect of coronary artery occlusion on regional arterial and venous O_2 saturation, O_2 extraction, blood flow, and O_2 consumption in the dog heart. Circ Res 1980; 47:400-407.
115. Weiss J, Hilbrand B. Functional compartmentalization of glycolytic vs oxidative metabolism in isolated rabbit heart. J Clin Invest 1985; 55:436-447.
116. Wyatt HL, Forrester JS, da Luz PL et al. Functional abnormalities in nonoccluded regions of myocardium after experimental coronary occlusion. Am J Cardiol 1976; 37:366-372.
117. Yamazaki S, Fujibayashi Y, Rajagopalan RE et al. Effects of staged versus sudden reperfusion after acute coronary occlusion in the dog. J Am Coll Cardiol 1986; 7:564-572.

CHAPTER 12

Coronary Venous Interventions
(Experimental Clinical Studies)

Samuel Meerbaum

Introduction

The thrust of advances in interventional cardiology has been aimed at treatment of myocardial jeopardy associated with coronary insufficiency. With surgical coronary artery bypass firmly established, the clinical armamentarium was more recently enriched by thrombolytic reperfusion to combat acute myocardial infarction and various modes of angioplasty to reverse the consequences of significant coronary artery obstructions.

With an ever increasing number of antegrade coronary interventions, including thrombolysis and percutaneous transluminal coronary (PTCA), being applied in high risk settings, serious consideration had to be given to protective support in case of marginal effectiveness, intolerable transient ischemia, or intervention failure leading to persistent coronary occlusion. In the latter situations, it may be essential to at least temporarily maintain the viability of jeopardized myocardium, pending revascularization.

Among antegrade support techniques, perfusion through special PTCA balloon catheters was shown to improve myocardial oxygen supply and to permit extended balloon inflations. This effective approach has a few disadvantages, e.g., a larger profile limiting catheter maneuvering and balloon positioning in small or torturous vessels and potential interference with perfusion at coronary branches. A systemic support, e.g., intraaortic balloon counterpulsation, newer hemopumps or percutaneous cardiopulmonary bypass may be applied during interventions in high risk settings, which could otherwise lead to hemodynamic decompensation, cardiogenic shock, refractory arrhythmias and even cardiac arrest.

Retroperfusion constitutes an alternate support delivered via the coronary veins. Clinically oriented methods usually feature transient obstruction of a coronary vein along with retrograde resupply of regionally jeopardized myocardium. Two primary systems have been developed and validated, largely for treatment of left anterior descending coronary artery (LAD) occlusions: 1) intermittent coronary sinus occlusion (ICSO or its advanced pressure controlled variety PICSO) without extracorporeal retroinfusate pumping, and 2) an ECG-synchronized retroperfusion (SRP) with pump controlled diastolic coronary vein occlusion and arterial blood retroinfusion, phased to facilitate physiologic systolic coronary venous drainage. It will be the objective of this Chapter to describe the evolution, state of the art and limitations of these and related retrograde support modalities.

Largely promising experimental results have recently led to clinical evaluations of SRP and ICSO. In particular, a series of SRP support studies during PTCA balloon inflations examined safety, logistics and effectiveness, while several trials of ICSO investigated its benefits during thrombolytic treatment. Due, in part, to diverse protocols, technical limitations and inadequate measurements in the various studies which will be reviewed here, it will not be possible to provide a meta-analysis or firm conclusions as to the effectiveness of the retrograde support techniques. Nonetheless, the clinical studies established that both SRP and ICSO can be safely applied and help to ameliorate the high risk derangements associated with acute myocardial ischemia.

It is recognized that detailed understanding is as yet lacking of the complex intramyocardial processes during retrograde interventions. Great variability and species-related differences in the profuse anastomotic coronary venous anatomy and drainage patterns make it difficult to prescribe standardized and optimal coronary venous intervention strategies. There is also a paucity of data on the range of coronary venous pressures and retrograde flows, which are safe as well as effective when applied during specific periods of retrograde intervention. Therefore, further clarification will be sought of pertinent mechanism and safety-effectiveness criteria.

A historical or detailed description of the many past research endeavors will not be presented, in view of the numerous surveys available in the literature.[1-9] The expanding retrograde cardioplegic procedures will also not be covered here. Rather, emphasis will be placed on recent evaluations of SRP and ICSO. An attempt will also be made to describe newer directions, including proposed modifications of current retrograde methods, and retroinfusion of pharmacologic agents or myocardial echo contrasts.

SRP Evolution and Experimental Studies

The need for reassessment of retroperfusion techniques was evident to the pioneering investigators led by Dr. Claude Beck,[10] who developed in the 40s the surgical aorta-to-coronary sinus bypass procedure. Their studies revealed that persisting coronary sinus obstruction plus arterial blood retroinfusion yielded excessive flow rates and/or coronary venous pressures, creating an unphysiologic impediment to coronary venous drainage which—if protracted—produced damaging vascular injury, hemorrhages, myocardial edema and fibrosis. It was clear to them that a diastolic retroinfusion would be preferable in view of normal coronary venous drainage occurring primarily in systole.

Credit for potentiating clinically oriented efforts should be given to Dr. Goffredo Gensini,[11] who in the early 1960s conjectured about a retrograde coronary venous method with "pulsating occlusion and phasic distal injection of arterial blood...". His group actually wedged catheters into the posterior interventricular, left marginal or the anterior interventricular vein, retroinjecting normal saline, 5% glucose, renografin 76 and venous or arterial blood. Dr. Gensini discussed a nonsurgical emergency temporary retrograde treatment of ischemic myocardium, and proposed experiments with LAD and left circumflex coronary artery occlusions with a view to eventual application in patients with myocardial infarction. A suitable retroperfusion balloon catheter was being developed, the coronary venous anatomy was studied, and implications for regional retroperfusion were investigated using coronary arteriography and venography.[12]

Inception of SRP

My colleagues and I began in the early 70s investigations of a system featuring ECG synchronized retroperfusion (SRP): diastolic retroinfusion into an obstructed coronary vein alternating with facilitated drainage by ceasing both the obstruction and retroinfusion in systole. We presented a preliminary report in 1975,[13] and followed by a more detailed paper in 1976.[14] The general concept also appealed to Markov et al,[15] who commented on problems they encountered with edema, hemorrhages and petechiae in dogs with nonphased retroperfusion.

In the open-chest dog experiments reported by Meerbaum et al,[14] the LAD was acutely occluded for 75 min. Thirty min after the LAD occlusion, synchronized pumping delivered arterial blood from the brachial artery into the anterior interventricular coronary vein via a nonwedging catheter. Compared to untreated controls, diastolic retroperfusion resulted in significant enhancement in the ischemic zone: regional dysfunction and ECG signs of ischemia were partly reversed (Fig. 12.1) while improved myocardial perfusion was inferred from changes in coronary outflow from and pO_2 in the distal LAD region. Diastolic phasing minimized the hemorrhages and edema encountered with nonphased retroperfusion.

Continuing development of SRP was described in 1978 by Farcot et al.[16] A special autoinflatable balloon catheter was positioned within the great cardiac vein (GCV), and coronary vein balloon occlusion as well as arterial blood retroinfusion were timed to occur in diastole (Fig. 12.2). Systolic release of the balloon, along with simultaneous interruption of the

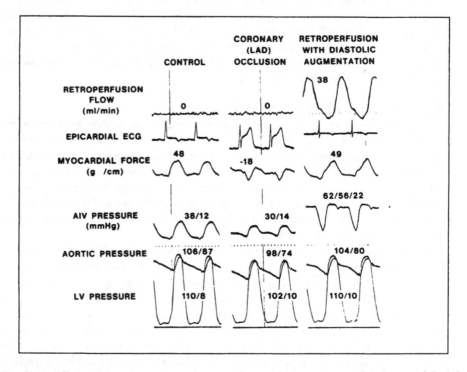

Fig. 12.1. Effects of diastolic augmented retroperfusion after 30 minutes of occlusion of the left anterior descending coronary artery (LAD) in one of the experiments in which retroperfusion effectively improved the ischemic zone contractile dysfunction. The diastolic anterior interventricular venous (AIV) pressure was increased by the synchronized pumping to 56 mm Hg, thus providing augmented retroperfusion in diastole. Programmed phasing of the coronary venous pressure also facilitated systolic drainage from the regional coronary vein around the nonocclusive catheter into the coronary sinus. After coronary occlusion, ischemic zone myocardial force measurements indicated pronounced segmental dyskinesia coupled with epicardial S-T segment elevations. Retroperfusion caused a return to preocclusion regional mechanics and reversal of S-T elevation in the ischemic zone. Small changes in aortic and left ventricular (LV) pressure were observed during the coronary occlusion and subsequent reperfusion periods. ECG = electrocardiogram. Reprinted with permission from Meerbaum et al. Diastolic retroperfusion in myocardial ischemia. Am J Cardiol 1976; 37:595.

retroinfusion resulted in normal coronary venous drainage to the right atrium. In closed-chest dog experiments, the LAD was balloon occluded for 4 hrs, and the dogs were randomized after the first hour of acute LAD occlusion to either untreated controls or 3 hr SRP treatment. The following mean effects were observed: SRP significantly decreased mean left ventricular end-diastolic pressure (LVEDP) from 11 to 5 mm Hg; peak systolic blood pressure and systemic vascular resistance dropped by 20 and 25%, respectively; ischemic region ECG-ST segment elevation decreased 40%, and its potassium loss was reduced by 92%; LAD pO_2 distal to the occlusion decreased 36%, suggesting oxygen delivery to and extraction by the jeopardized myocardium; ventriculography revealed an increase in LV ejection fraction, and reversal of ischemic segment dyskinesia by SRP. Limited infarct size study indicated significant reduction in the amount of necrosis. There was evidence that SRP minimized ischemic arrhythmias. Based on these two studies, SRP was envisioned as a prompt temporary emergency treatment of otherwise not readily accessible, profoundly ischemic myocardium.

Berdeaux et al[17] examined with microspheres the effects of SRP on regional myocardial blood flow during experimental ischemia in open-chest dogs. In both treated and untreated dogs, hemodynamics, ECG-ST segments and regional myocardial blood flow deteriorated similarly up to 1 hr of LAD occlusion, at which time SRP was instituted. As early as 15 min after the start of SRP, ST elevations had significantly decreased, versus no change in the control series. After 1 hr of SRP, mean regional transmural flow increased in the nonischemic zone from .84 to 1.05 ml/min/g. In the ischemic zone, transmural flow increased 59.3% from .3 ml/min/g (collateral supply) to .5 ml/min/g, with favorably greater enhancement of endocardial flow. Such improvement in myocardial perfusion could be significant in maintaining viability of ischemic myocardium.

Corroborative SRP Studies

Smith et al[18] performed SRP in baboons during 4 hrs of proximal LAD occlusion, following which antegrade perfusion was restored. SRP was initiated 15 min post LAD occlusion,

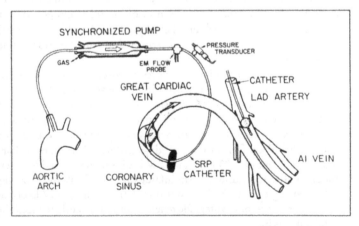

Fig. 12.2A. Schematic diagram of synchronized retroperfusion experimental system. Arterial blood is shunted from the brachial artery into the great cardiac vein and the regional anterior interventricular (AI) coronary vein that adjoins the left anterior descending (LAD) coronary artery. The latter is occluded by means of an intracoronary balloon catheter to create a zone of acute ischemia to be treated by retroperfusion. Arterial blood is pumped by means of an electrocardiograph-synchronized gas-actuated bladder pump that propels blood in a retrograde manner during diastole through a special auto-inflatable balloon catheter into the coronary vein. The retroperfusion flow rate and blood pressure are monitored by means of an electromagnetic flowmeter (EM FLOW) probe and a pressure transducer. SRP = synchronized retroperfusion. Reprinted with permission from Farcot et al. Synchronized retroperfusion of coronary veins. Am J Cardiol 1978; 41;1192.

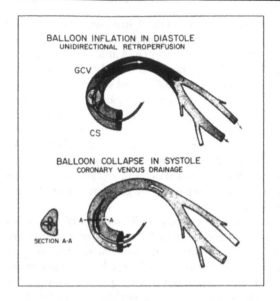

Fig. 12.2B. Phasic operation of synchronized retroperfusion. During cardiac diastole, arterial blood is pumped through the catheter placed within a regional coronary vein such as the great cardiac vein (GCV). This also inflates the catheter balloon, ensuring unidirectionality of the retrograde flow. During systole, the electrocardiographic synchronized pump stops forward flow, causing a sharp decrease in pressure within the catheter. This leads to rapid balloon collapse, which facilitates coronary venous drainage. Note the characteristic mode of balloon folding in the form of a star around the body of the catheter (SECTION A-A). CS = coronary sinus. Reprinted with permission from Farcot et al. Synchronized retroperfusion of coronary veins. Am J Cardiol 1978; 41:1192.

and another series of baboons served as LAD occlusion-reperfusion controls. Epicardial ECG measured at sites overlying the ischemic region showed that SRP significantly reduced ischemic injury. Mean infarct size at 24 hrs was 4.8% (percent of LV mass) in the SRP series, compared to 30.6% in controls. In an associated baboon study, Geary et al[19] quantitated infarct size when SRP was initiated later, between 1 and 4 hrs after LAD occlusion, followed by reperfusion. At 24 hrs, a mean 94.1% of the regional LAD perfusion bed was infarcted in the untreated group, whereas infarction in the SRP supported series was 57.4%. Gundry et al[20] reported on diastolic retroperfusion of myocardial ischemia in normal and chronically hypertrophied left ventricles. LV function (sonomicrometry) was severely depressed in all dogs throughout 40 min LAD occlusion. On the other hand, 30 min of diastolic retroperfusion restored 37% of systolic shortening and normalized all other physiological and hemodynamic parameters. Following reperfusion, 10 of 13 treated dogs recovered normal function, while only 2 of 13 untreated dogs survived.

Most recently, Hatori et al[21] addressed specifically the SRP effects on the often observed reperfusion derangements. The LAD in dogs was occluded for 2 hrs and SRP applied during the last 30 min of the occlusion prior to 5.5 hr of antegrade reperfusion. During untreated LAD occlusion, there was severe regional myocardial underperfusion (colored microspheres). Ischemic zone measurements after 3.5 hrs reperfusion indicated a significantly higher subendocardial blood flow in the SRP dogs (mean .51 ml/min/g) than in untreated occlusion-reperfusion controls (.29 ml/min/g). While both control and SRP series exhibited similar dysfunction after reperfusion, mean infarct size (% of risk area) was significantly smaller in the SRP treated group (17.2%) vs. controls (36.0%). Thus, in LAD occluded dogs, relatively short SRP treatment prior to antegrade reperfusion significantly reduced the eventual extent of myocardial necrosis.

Preclinical SRP Validation

As the time approached for clinical SRP validation, Yamazaki et al[22] performed detailed two-dimensional echo (2DE) measurements in closed-chest anesthetized dogs with 6 hr proximal LAD occlusion, with SRP initiated 30 min postocclusion. Mean LV ejection fraction dropped from 50.7% to 28.1% in untreated control dogs, but decreased significantly less (from

55.9% to 41.8%) in the SRP series. Ischemic segment function was markedly depressed at 30 min LAD occlusion; major dysfunction persisted throughout the untreated LAD occlusion, but was largely reversed with 5.5 hr SRP. 5 min interruptions of SRP at 1 hr postocclusion reduced ischemic zone function (2 DE fractional change) from 33.0% to 12.2%, and this depression was promptly reversed (to 33.6%) when SRP was resumed. In contrast with untreated sudden antegrade reperfusion, there was no increase in ischemic zone diastolic wall thickness and no arrhythmias in the SRP series, perhaps because of a more gradual retrograde resupply.

A similar protocol was used in a second preclinical study of SRP safety and efficacy by Drury et al.[23] Mean infarct size (percent risk area) was significantly lower with SRP (19%) than 6 hr untreated occlusion controls (58%). Morphological examination of the coronary sinus and regional cardiac veins showed no damage from SRP, and no excess myocardial edema was noted. The treatment caused no significant red cell hemolysis or platelet destruction. It therefore appeared that SRP is a safe and effective treatment of experimental acute myocardial ischemia.

SRP During Very Short LAD Occlusions

Smalling[24] reviewed his experience with SRP support of brief periods of acute myocardial ischemia, analogous to coronary angioplasty balloon inflations. Lightly anesthetized dogs were chronically instrumented with LAD cuff occluders, and regional function was measured in several LV regions (sonomicrometry). After baseline measurements, data were obtained during a 5 min untreated LAD occlusion, throughout recovery (with mobilization of SRP) and during two SRP treated 5 min LAD occlusions. Hemodynamics were not significantly changed. Percent LAD zone segmental shortening during the brief acute LAD occlusions changed from dyskinetic (-2.8%) to hypokinetic (+2.2%), a significant yet modest improvement. Smalling cautioned that SRP effects seemed variable. He stated that a high diastolic coronary sinus pressure (up to 140 mm Hg) was needed to achieve normalization of regional function with SRP, and thought such a high pressure would be safe for up to 1-5 min of LAD and left circumflex occlusion.

Berk et al[25] reported negative results in anesthetized pigs, with SRP throughout a 20 min LAD occlusion. Regional systolic wall thickening was completely abolished in untreated animals during the 20 min occlusion, and this dysfunction was not altered by SRP. Recovery during a subsequent 2 hr reperfusion also did not differ between the two groups. The SRP flow rate was relatively low (30-50 ml/min), and when this rate was increased in a few cases to 150 ml/min (producing coronary sinus pressures of 80-120 mm Hg), a marked and reproducible improvement in myocardial thickening by SRP was noted. However, extended periods of such high coronary sinus pressures can cause progressive myocardial edema.

SRP Limitations

While evidently safe, SRP involves a sophisticated pumping device as well as arterial and venous access. The method's invasiveness and required operator skill suggest that SRP justification depends on substantial demonstrated benefits. So far, SRP with GCV diastolic augmentation of 30-40 mm Hg (during LAD occlusions) seemed capable of partly enhancing regional dysfunction toward normal levels. As already discussed, complete reversal of ischemic dysfunction by SRP may be achieved when coronary vein pressures are augmented to around 100 mm Hg, but such pressures might be tolerated only over as yet uncertain very short time periods.

The evidence for SRP effects during left circumflex coronary artery occlusions is still extremely meager. Little indication exists that a right coronary occlusion could be selectively treated with SRP. The significant though partial improvement in LAD territory function was not always consistent, despite efforts to properly position the SRP catheter within the GCV and augmenting the SRP flow rate. To assure adequate retrograde pressure levels, e.g., for brief SRP support during PTCA balloon occlusions, diastolic retroinfusion could be combined with nonsynchronized intermittent coronary vein occlusions (see below).

SRP Mechanisms

The enhancement of myocardial washout by SRP (as well as retrograde blood delivery) during acute myocardial ischemia was examined in dogs by Chang et al.[26] Renografin was sequentially injected into the LAD via the center lumen of an occlusive intracoronary balloon catheter, and videodensitometric contrast washout rate was determined in the myocardial region subserved by the LAD (Fig. 12.3). Prior to LAD occlusion, the mean washout rate was 22.4 min^{-1}. Five min after occlusion, the washout rate dropped sharply to 2.0 min^{-1}. With 50 ml/min SRP treatment during the LAD occlusion, the washout rate was promptly and significantly enhanced to 5.0 min^{-1}. The washout rate was higher at elevated SRP flows. Indirect evidence of retrograde SRP delivery to ischemic myocardium (in spite of the small diastolic retrograde stroke volume) was noted in sequential digital angiographic images (Fig. 12.4). More directly, monastral blue dye was retroinfused through the SRP pump into the GCV before the dog was sacrificed, and transverse heart slices were then studied by detailed microscopy. Scoring the regional intramicrovascular dye content between 0 (no dye) and 3 (maximal dye), SRP delivery during LAD occlusion yielded a mean myocardial capillary blue dye content of 2.3 in the ischemic anterior vs. 1.7 in the nonischemic posterior aspects of the LV. Conversely, antegrade dye injections during untreated LAD occlusion resulted in greater concentrations in the nonischemic posterior myocardium. Thus, when antegrade access is limited, SRP via the GCV appears to both selectively deliver substrates to the acutely ischemic myocardium, and significantly enhance washout from this underperfused region.

The ability of SRP to support the circulation and metabolism of ischemic myocardium was investigated with positron emission tomography (PET) by O'Byrne et al.[27] The PET study was performed in open-chest dogs with LAD occlusion and during SRP treatment begun 20 min postocclusion. Retrogradely delivered flow tracer uptake was observed in the risk zone in the intervention dogs. Fluorine-18 deoxyglucose uptake in the risk zone was increased in 5 of 6 SRP treated dogs, but was reduced in 5 of 6 untreated control occlusion dogs. The risk zone to normal myocardial F18 count ratio was higher in the SRP treated than in the control occlusion group (mean 1.13 vs .59). Infarction (percent of risk zone) was 70% lower in the treated group as compared to controls. PET revealed that SRP did retrogradely deliver the arterial blood to and maintained metabolism in the risk zone myocardium beyond the LAD occlusion. The PET methodology appears particularly well suited to investigate myocardial blood flow, metabolism and tissue viability.

ICSO-PICSO Evolution and Experimental Studies

The concept of intermittent coronary sinus occlusion (ICSO) was first reported by Arealis et al in 1977.[28] These investigators inserted a balloon catheter from the jugular vein into the coronary sinus and intermittently inflated the balloon to cause cyclic coronary sinus occlusions at a rate of 60/min. It appears that, during each cycle, the balloon was inflated 70% and deflated 30% of the time, the latter period permitting coronary venous drainage. Experiments were performed in thoracotomized dogs and sheep with branches of the left coronary artery ligated. Coronary artery occlusion resulted in arrhythmias and deterioration of hemodynamics as well as myocardial function, but when ICSO was repeatedly instituted, improvements were noted in most of the animals. Another similar ICSO procedure, described in 1979 by Tzigorlou et al,[29] modified the timing such that 2–3 beats had coronary sinus occlusion followed by balloon release to facilitate coronary venous drainage.

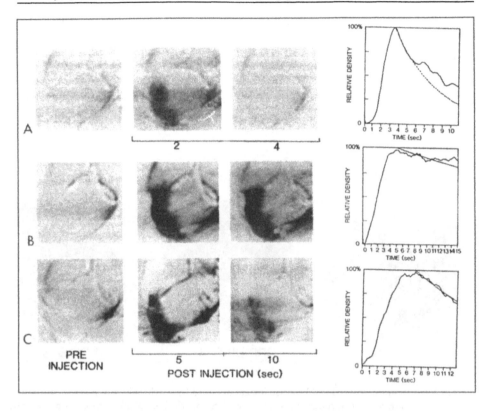

Fig. 12.3A. Injection of Renografin-76 into the left anterior descending coronary artery before occlusion resulted in complete opacification of the anterior left ventricular myocardium (2), followed by a rapid return to preinjection intensity levels within 4 seconds (4). The washout rate (right) was 16 min-1. B. Myocardial opacification was obtained after injection of 1 ml Renografin-76 into the left anterior descending artery distal to the balloon occlusion before synchronized retroperfusion. Contrast injection resulted in myocardial opacification of the ischemic zone, with persistence of contrast 10 seconds after injection. The washout rate was 1.2 min^{-1}. C. Application of synchronized retroperfusion (50 ml/min) demonstrates a significant increase in ischemic zone washout rate at 10 seconds despite maintained coronary occlusion. The washout rate (k) was 3.8 min^{-1}. Reprinted with permission from the American College of Cardiology (J Amer Coll Cardiol) Chang et al. Synchronized retroperfusion in ischemic myocardium. 1987; 9:1093.

Conceptualization of PICSO

In the early 80s, Mohl et al conceived a coronary sinus pressure feedback controlled ICSO system (PICSO) (Fig. 12.5), and commenced a series of investigations of ICSO and PICSO effects on myocardial function and infarct salvage in animals with LAD coronary artery occlusion. A balloon catheter was inserted into the coronary sinus, and balloon occlusions alternated with periods of coronary sinus release (washout). As the coronary sinus systolic pressure rapidly rose to a plateau following the balloon occlusion (Fig. 12.6), this pressure was not allowed to exceed the safe limit of 60 mm Hg. In the most frequently used ICSO, coronary sinus occlusion duration was usually fixed at 90% of the observed plateau pressure, with a release phase of 2–4 sec, whereas in the more sophisticated PICSO controls continuously adjusted the coronary sinus occlusion release timing based upon the varying intracoronary vein pressure.

In their first open-chest dog study, myocardial function was assessed with ultrasound transit devices and found to be improved in the ischemic zone (beyond severe stenosis or occlusion of the

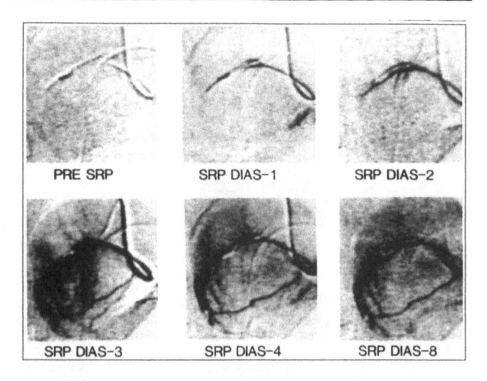

Fig. 12.4. Six end-diastolic (DIAS) cardiac images obtained by synchronized retrograde infusion of 2.5 ml of Renografin-76 through the synchronized retroperfusion (SRP) catheter into the great cardiac vein during left anterior descending coronary artery occlusion. Myocardial opacification noted as early as the third diastole (SRP DIAS 3) suggests an early cumulative effect of the retroinfusate with retroperfusion. The contrast intensity gradually decreased after completion of the Renografin injection. Reprinted with permission from the American College of Cardiology (J Amer Coll Cardiol) Chang et al. Synchronized retroperfusion in ischemic myocardium. 1987; 9:1095.

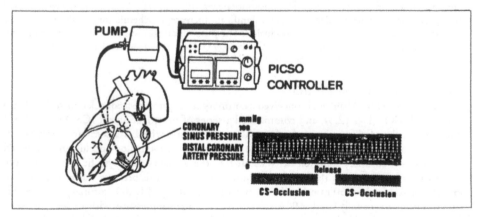

Fig. 12.5. Scheme of PICSO system. A 7F balloon catheter is advanced into the coronary sinus. Balloon blockade is achieved by a coronary sinus pressure controlled pneumatic pump device. Coronary sinus pressure and distal coronary artery pressure are shown during obstruction and release of the coronary venous drainage.

LAD) during ICSO treatment.[30] The systolic pressure in the LAD distal to the obstruction increased significantly during ICSO. In another study by Mohl et al[31] the emphasis was on evaluating infarct size without or with ICSO in dogs with LAD occlusion. ICSO was begun 15 min after LAD occlusion and continued until termination of the experiment 6 hrs later. Compared to untreated control LAD occlusions, ICSO resulted in an average 45% reduction in myocardial infarct size. A further ICSO study in closed-chest dogs[32] featured standardized 2DE measurements of LV function during ICSO treated LAD occlusions. A moderate functional improvement was noted in severely ischemic segments (from dyskinesis to hypokinesis), whereas a further deterioration was noted in the untreated LAD occlusions.

A large number of ICSO presentations were included at the First International Symposium on Myocardial Protection via the Coronary Sinus (Vienna, 1984). In one of these, Mohl et al[33] reported on ICSO-induced enhancement of washout of myocardial edema in dogs. Continuous blood density change measurements in the aorta and coronary sinus were performed in open-chest animals, using a mechanical oscillator device. The arterial-venous blood density difference increased dramatically during LAD occlusion, reflecting edema formation. ICSO resulted in reduced ischemic region edema (Fig. 12.7). Utilizing the density measurements to establish ICSO's optimal coronary occlusion/release timing, Moser et al[34] observed an optimum when the coronary sinus occlusion extended to 90% of the maximal developed systolic pressure. A 2 sec release phase was evidently deemed adequate for washout. The other ICSO mechanism responsible for benefits is believed to be redistribution of retrograde coronary venous flow into the infarcted area during coronary sinus balloon occlusion.

Seitelberger et al[35] reported on ICSO effects on both regional metabolism (lactate and glucose) and function in normal and underperfused canine myocardium, with or without a 30 min ICSO treatment. With normal coronary artery flow, ICSO (inflation/deflation ratio 25/ 2.5 sec) caused a 35% reduction in systolic shortening and a 16% increase in heart rate, while myocardial lactate and glucose uptake were transiently decreased. An untreated 50% reduction in left circumflex coronary artery flow caused an 80% decrease in ischemic region systolic shortening. In this setting of moderate underperfusion, ICSO caused systolic bulging, increased heart rate and further diminished left circumflex flow, while substrate balances remained unchanged. A greater reduction of the left circumflex flow (by 65%) induced systolic bulging, and under these more severe ischemic conditions, ICSO slightly improved function and metabolism in the underperfused area (hemodynamics unchanged). The authors conjectured that a more optimal inflation/deflation timing might improve the ICSO effectiveness. An ICSO

Fig. 12.6. Coronary sinus pressure (CSP) and coronary flow in the CX artery during PICSO. Note how the cyclic pressure variation is reflected in arterial inflow. T96 = 95% rise time of systolic coronary sinus occluded pressure.

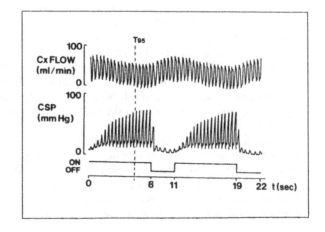

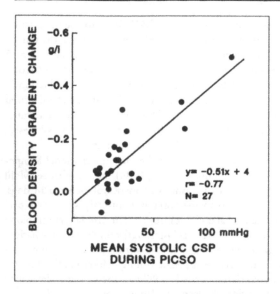

Fig. 12.7. Relationship between washout, measured as the arteriovenous density gradient change, and coronary sinus pressure. With permission from Mohl W. Coronary sinus interventions from concept to clinic. J Cardiac Surg 1987; 2:467-493.

study by Glogar et al[36] concentrated on measurement of myocardial perfusion (microspheres). During 6 hr of ICSO supported LAD occlusion in dogs, there was no significant change in the antegrade underperfusion, yet ICSO did result in significant salvage of ischemic myocardium. It was thought that ICSO leads to an increased border zone perfusion via capillaries or post capillary routes.

Corroborative ICSO Studies

An investigation of ICSO by Ciuffo et al[37] in dogs with 3 hr LAD occlusion indicated that this retrograde intervention (begun 30 min post occlusion) reduced infarction, as compared to untreated controls. Antegrade coronary blood flow measurements (microspheres) indicated no significant change throughout the LAD occlusion. However, circulation in the risk region measured with 133 Xenon (washout) rose significantly from a mean .15-.31 ml/min/g as a result of ICSO. Guerci et al[38] extended this study to include 8–12 days of reperfusion following the 3 hr LAD occlusion. Treatment was begun 30 min post LAD occlusion and lasted for 2.5 hrs. There was no effect on heart rate, blood pressure or mortality when compared to untreated LAD occlusion-reperfusion controls. With risk regions equivalent, percent infarction was about 75% in controls vs only 30% in ICSO treated animals, confirming the ICSO capability to significantly reduce acute ischemic injury and salvage jeopardized myocardium. However, coronary sinus thrombosis was observed in all the survivors of the ICSO treated group vs. none in the untreated controls.

Jacobs et al[39] studied ICSO in open-chest dogs with 3 hr LAD occlusion and 3 hr reperfusion. ICSO treatment of the LAD occlusion from 30 min on was compared with untreated occlusion-reperfusion controls. Mean infarct size (percent of risk area) in controls (32.7%) significantly exceeded infarction in the ICSO treated animals (16.7%). Simon and Jacobs[40] recapitulated the effects of ICSO on LV function observed during reperfusion. When ICSO was started early after coronary occlusion, 34% (vs. 4% in controls) of ischemic segments showed some improvement in systolic wall thickening, measured just prior to reperfusion; following reperfusion, regional improvements were noted in 79% vs. 51% of segments, although ICSO did not enhance regional LV function in the earliest stunning-prone reperfusion. Even when ICSO treatment was initiated just prior to reperfusion, the eventual infarct size (percent of risk area) was still significantly reduced (29% vs 45% in controls).

Contrary to prior investigators, Diltz et al[41] found in an occlusion-reperfusion dog model that their ICSO failed to reduce infarct size or ischemic dysfunction. Relatively long ischemic periods (36 sec proximal coronary sinus occlusions and 30 sec release periods) were applied. The LAD was occluded for 4 hr, followed by 6 hr reperfusion. Compared with untreated LAD occlusion, this ICSO treatment up to reflow yielded a similar infarct size. Ischemic function (segment length shortening) was also not significantly improved by ICSO. Mayr et al[42] investigated in open-chest dogs the effects of ICSO treatment on arrhythmias early after LAD occlusion. ICSO began 15 min after LAD occlusion which continued for 6 hrs. Compared to untreated occlusion controls, ICSO significantly reduced arrhythmias.

ICSO Effects During Brief Ischemia

Jacobs et al[43] examined ICSO's ability to limit ischemia during brief coronary artery occlusions in open-chest dogs. Intermittent coronary sinus occlusions were timed to achieve a pressure plateau (10 sec), followed by rapid balloon deflation (2 sec) to facilitate the coronary venous drainage/washout. Measurements were obtained at baseline, during a 3 min untreated LAD occlusion and subsequent 30 min reflow, a second baseline, and then during ICSO treatment in a second 3 min LAD occlusion, with 30 min reperfusion. ECG-ST segment elevations and LV dysfunction remained unaffected by ICSO, nor was the reperfusion recovery altered by ICSO. ICSO did, however, blunt the hyperemic response in coronary blood flow following release of the LAD occlusion.

ICSO in Pigs

To examine the ICSO effects in the absence of arterial coronary collaterals, Toggart et al[44] studied a swine preparation with controlled perfusion. ICSO (15 sec coronary sinus occlusion, 5 sec release) was started after LAD occlusion control measurements. ICSO caused the mean coronary sinus pressure to rise significantly (from 11.2 to 66.2 mm Hg), and—with a slight delay—mean distal LAD pressure increased from 14.2 to 26.8 mm Hg. Myocardial oxygen consumption was similar in both treated and untreated LAD occluded animals. LVEDP rose early after coronary artery ligation and then gradually decreased in both ICSO treated and control dogs. An apparent increase of LV dp/dt during ICSO was not statistically significant, and the loss of systolic wall thickening in the ischemic myocardium was not modified by ICSO. Both end-diastolic and end-systolic wall thickness increased in the ICSO versus control animals. PostLAD occlusion coronary sinus oxygen saturation was lower in the ICSO dogs. While distal LAD oxygen saturation fell in both groups after LAD ligation, it was lower in the ICSO series. These authors concluded that ICSO facilitated some retrograde delivery to the ischemic bed, however failed to preserve regional or global function in the setting of no collateral flow.

Fedele et al[45] examined in closed-chest swine the effects of ICSO during myocardial ischemia caused by increased demands (maintained pacing at 145 beats/min) in the presence of substantial yet incomplete LAD obstruction (luminal diameter reduced by 80%). A balloon tipped ICSO catheter was positioned in the GCV. After placement of the artificial 80% LAD stenosis, endocardial and transmural blood flow (microspheres) distal to the stenosis declined significantly, and superimposed ICSO did not increase this residual inflow. Myocardial aerobic metabolism changed from lactate, inosine and hypoxanthine consumption before stenosis to production after stenosis. Comparing the ICSO treated and untreated series, the patterns of regional myocardial oxygen and metabolic changes, as well as hemodynamics, showed no significant difference at comparable times. While ICSO treatment in this model did not alter the degree of myocardial ischemia, it did accelerate the rate of resolution of ischemic lactate metabolism.

ICSO Modeling and Mechanisms

Sun reported on a closed loop system for PICSO.[46] In one of a series of mathematical ICSO modeling studies[47] diagnostic quantities, e.g., coronary sinus pressures derived during ICSO in dogs were analyzed in the hope of providing a basis for optimized coronary sinus occlusion-release timing in future human applications. The relationship between coronary artery inflow and coronary venous pressures during ICSO was studied by Neuman et al[48] in the presence of normal antegrade perfusion, LAD occlusion and reperfusion. Systematically varying the ICSO timing, a Fourier analysis was applied to predict the arterial flow curve, based on coronary venous pressure measurements.

Jacobs et al[49] reexamined the ICSO washout hypothesis in open-chest dogs with Xenon injected into the distal LAD 30 min following LAD occlusion. As previously reported, ICSO significantly reduced myocardial edema by increasing ischemic zone circulation. Simon et al[50] raised the question whether supplemental arterial blood retroinfusion would benefit infarct size reduction by ICSO. In a study of open-chest dogs with LAD occlusion, ICSO with or without diastolic arterial blood retroinfusion was instituted 30 min postocclusion and compared with untreated controls. Compared to the control group, both ICSO and ICSO + retroinfusion were found to similarly significantly reduce infarct size, without evidence of synergism.

In a 1991 paper, Jacobs et al[51] tried to rationalize the previously observed limited effects of ICSO on ischemic dysfunction during brief LAD occlusions. An open-chest dog study was refined to meet PICSO objectives through continuous adjustment of the coronary sinus balloon inflation time, thus accounting for differing pressure rise and time to plateau during LAD occlusion and reperfusion. Measurements were obtained at baseline, during a 3 min LAD occlusion, and for 10 min of reperfusion, with or without adenosine infusion to abolish reactive hyperemia. PICSO support during the brief LAD occlusion and reperfusion, did not prevent, reduce or shorten the ischemic zone dysfunction (sonomicrometry). PICSO uniformly blunted reactive hyperemia during reperfusion, but also reduced coronary blood flow (LAD flow probe) during adenosine-induced maximal vasodilatation. The latter was attributed to the coronary vein engorgement. Although it provides substantial salvage in acute myocardial infarction, PICSO appeared ineffective during brief periods of ischemia. In the authors' words, PICSO may be sufficient to maintain cell viability but not cell function.

A recent examination of ICSO effects on coronary sinus pressure dynamics and coronary arterial flow was carried out in open-chest dogs by Matsuhashi et al.[52] In particular, hyperemic response correlated positively with the coronary sinus occlusion duration. Inadequately short release durations significantly lowered the net volume of coronary arterial inflow. Hyperemia was augmented by supplemental coronary sinus retroinfusion, reduced by coronary arterial ischemia, or else abolished by maximally vasodilating the coronary arteries with intravenous adenosine. The authors point to compensatory regulating mechanisms of the coronary circulation as a factor in the retrograde ICSO treatment effectiveness, and urge consideration of both coronary arterial flow as well as coronary sinus pressure dynamics, when selecting optimal ICSO occlusion-release intervals.

Commentary

The bulk of experimental evidence indicates that both SRP and ICSO/PICSO are capable of significant myocardial salvage when applied during LAD coronary occlusions. Both techniques were also shown to ameliorate derangements of reperfusion, whether the retrograde intervention was commenced early during the acute ischemia or even when initiated shortly prior to antegrade reflow. These results would point to a common feature, e.g., washout of ischemic metabolites. Measurements with Xenon and digital angiography indicated that ICSO and SRP produce significant washout, depending on the ICSO occlusion-release timing and on SRP's retroinfusion flow rate. Considering past physiologic investigations of myocardial anoxia vs. ischemia,[53] the question remains whether washout alone can achieve more than a partial extension of myocardial viability, and whether effective treatment does not also mandate adequate retroinfusion. SRP differs significantly from the simpler ICSO system because it retroinfuses arterial blood in diastole, and 2) it occludes the coronary veins only diastole. Reviewing the experimental evidence, one would have to conclude that ICSO treatment during acute coronary occlusions exhibited much less of an effect on functional recovery than was the case with SRP, particularly during very short periods, e.g., 1-5 min. The need of oxidative metabolism for contractile function has been previously emphasized.[54] Jacobs et al argued on the basis of recent experiments that ICSO could maintain myocardial cell viability but not cell function.[51] The significant functional improvements with SRP are often of a partial and variable character, possible reasons including:

1. delimited or vitiated retroinfusion effectiveness because of coronary veno-venous and Thebessian shunting;
2. insufficient retrograde delivery with low stroke volume diastolic infusions;
3. inadequacies of SRP pumping and/or catheter balloon positioning. Such limitations motivated concepts such as hypothermic SRP, combining SRP with ICSO features, or other modifications.

An important (and contested) study by Zalewski et al[55] compared a number of retrograde interventions during a 6 hr LAD occlusion in dogs, including diastolic GCV occlusions with continuous 60 cc/min arterial blood retroinfusion, and an ICSO of the GCV with a 15:4 balloon inflation: release timing. Occluded GCV systolic pressures ranged from 54 mm Hg at 15 min and 46 mm Hg at 6 hrs post LAD occlusion. The diastolic retroperfusion resulted in significant myocardial salvage, infarct size (percent of risk area) being 54% vs. 100% in untreated 6 hr occlusions, while ICSO failed to provide significant salvage (84%). The latter seems at odds with other ICSO studies and still needs to be rationalized. It could be associated with somewhat lower developed pressures in the GCV-based ICSO versus the usual coronary sinus ICSO, more pronounced coronary veno-venous back shunting, or absence of an antegrade collateral supply to the ischemic zone from the left circumflex territory, whose pressures may be augmented by a coronary sinus ICSO.

Taking the sum total of SRP and ICSO experimental experience, one could argue that reversal of ischemia with its associated dysfunction was less likely without than with a certain amount of arterial coronary collateral flow, e.g., in pigs or dogs. Retrograde supplementation by SRP or ICSO may be simply insufficient to overcome the severely compromised myocardial viability and function when there is no collateral supply. Modifications are needed to significantly increase retrodelivery effectiveness. Conversely, a high antegrade perfusion, e.g., approaching normal coronary flow, would compete with the retroinfusion, minimizing retrograde treatment effectiveness and tending to generate edema and other undesirable effects. With ICSO, it is apparently essential that coronary sinus occlusion not be less or exceed the time needed to reach a pressure plateau (of the order of 10 sec), whereas the subsequent balloon release period should be limited to merely assure adequate washout, e.g., 2 sec. Yet, the criticality of continually adjusted precise timing (PICSO) for optimal ICSO effectiveness has not been clearly demonstrated in various settings. ICSO-induced "redistribution" of myocardial blood flow is often referred to, but its extent achieved is uncertain. When the balloon is placed at a very proximal site of the coronary sinus (apart from potential problems with catheter stability), ICSO could conceivably enhance the arterial collateral blood flow toward the LAD obstructed ischemic region (see above), but antegrade blood flow (in the left circumflex) may also be reduced. Based on experimental observations and inferences from early clinical results, reversal of the ischemic zone flow stagnation and washout of its edema and toxic substances appears the most likely favorable mechanism of ICSO. Retroinfusion in conjunction with ICSO is a definitive option, should be developed, and might include oxygenated blood.

Finally, there remains the challenge of providing an effective retrograde treatment of not only LAD occlusions, but also of circumflex and perhaps even right coronary ischemia. The latter is as yet somewhat difficult to envision, but further advances in balloon catheter design and catheterization procedures may well overcome the present limitations. It is also hoped that new diagnostic tools will facilitate individualized definition of available coronary venous pathways and prevailing residual regional myocardial viability, so that catheters can be properly positioned and retrograde treatment adjusted for optimal effectiveness.

Clinical Safety, Logistics and Effectiveness of SRP and ICSO

The SRP and ICSO systems and procedures applied in different clinical settings were arrived at through extensive animal research and preclinical experimental studies. SRP evaluations were largely performed during PTCA balloon inflations in the LAD, while ICSO was initially assessed during surgical revascularization and as a support of thrombolysis. Before describing the clinical results to date, it may be useful to first address the common issue of catheter placement in the appropriate coronary vein.

Percutaneous catheterization must first of all achieve reliable insertion into the coronary sinus. For effective retroinfusion support during LAD coronary artery occlusions, the special balloon catheter is then usually advanced into the GCV. When the coronary sinus is approached from either the right internal jugular vein or the left subclavian vein, the catheterization can be successfully achieved within minutes in 85–90% of cases, with little hindrance by the residual Thebesian and Vieussens valves. The size and location of regional coronary veins are of a great variety and often feature pronounced coronary veno-venous anastomoses.

Utilizing an improved retroperfusion balloon catheter and controlled pumping system, a first limited clinical study reported by Gore et al in 1986[56] involved SRP in five patients with unstable angina refractory to maximal medical therapy. Beneficial SRP support—occasionally for periods beyond the 24 hrs investigated in limited animal experiments—significantly lowered the frequency of anginal episodes, reduced the need for antianginal drugs, and satisfactorily stabilized the patients. Commenting on logistics, the authors remarked on the ease with which SRP could be instituted in these patients. The SRP procedure was not only safe but did not interfere with scheduled patient care. Of the five patients, three underwent successful emergency coronary artery bypass surgery. The two remaining patients had diffuse disease and were not considered candidates for bypass; after SRP support was discontinued, they were treated with intraaortic balloon pumping (IABP), and died 48 and 72 hrs after IABP was terminated.

PTCA Support by SRP

One of the logical settings for SRP evaluation is a PTCA balloon inflation in the LAD (see Fig. 12.8), yet only few experimental efforts were devoted to SRP or ICSO treatment of very brief coronary artery occlusions. Use of coronary angioplasty has, of course, greatly expanded and is now being increasingly applied in high risk unstable ischemic syndromes, occasionally in patents with severe left ventricular dysfunction, and even in acute myocardial infarction or cardiogenic shock. Thus, even brief PTCA occlusions of a coronary artery may not be tolerated without support. Apart from methods aimed primarily at unloading of the heart and reducing oxygen demands, selective myocardial perfusion support is provided by currently proposed antegrade as well as retrograde methods, each of which has distinct advantages as well as limitations.

In a first 1986 report, Weiner et al[57] described three cases of elective LAD angioplasty supported by SRP. A special 8F balloon catheter was placed in the coronary sinus, and SRP treatment during PTCA inflations was compared with unsupported inflations. SRP significantly delayed the onset of chest pain (from about 28-100 sec), and time to equivalent ECG-ST elevations (from 60-137 sec). It was anticipated that SRP support of the ischemia would allow use of longer PTCA balloon inflations in the LAD. No complications were reported, but SRP did not prevent the PTCA-induced ischemic changes. The question remained whether these particular PTCA-SRP results were perhaps due to insufficient retroperfusion flow rates, or inadequate coronary venous diastolic pressure augmentation.

A more systematic evaluation of SRP supported PTCA was detailed by Berland et al in 1990.[59] In 16 patients, after successful therapeutic PTCA balloon dilation of the LAD, an SRP supported PTCA inflation was compared with an equivalent untreated control. Following successful coronary sinus catheterization (within less that 2½ min), the SRP catheter balloon was most often positioned in the GCV. There were no complications, SRP interfered minimally with the PTCA procedure, and significant though modest benefits were reported. Thus, only 31% of the SRP treated PTCA inflations led to pain or discomfort, compared with 72% during controls. SRP supported balloon inflations significantly lowered and delayed ECG-ST segment elevations and ameliorated regional as well and global LV function. Substantial variability in effectiveness was attributed to the variable human coronary venous anatomy, nonoptimal SRP catheter positioning, and apparently insufficient GCV diastolic pressure augmentation and/or retroinfusion rate.

A recent paper by Kar et al[60] reported on 30 patients with significant LAD stenosis, undergoing elective PTCA, some balloon inflations being treated by an SRP system capable of higher retroinfusion rates. SRP support resulted in delayed and lower angina severity with lesser ST segment changes, when compared to untreated PTCA balloon inflations. The latter

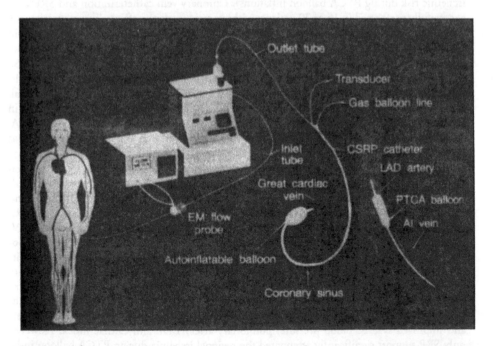

Fig. 12.8. Schematic drawing of the synchronized retroperfusion system. CSRP coronary sinus retroperfusion, A1 vein-anterior interventricular vein. With permission from Jacobs AK, Faxon DP. Retroperfusion and PTCA. In: Topol EI, ed. Textbook of Interventional Cardiology. New York: WB Saunders Co., 1990:477-495.

were characterized by dyskinetic regional wall motion, while SRP support caused a significant, albeit partial, functional improvement in hypokinesis. There were no differences in hemodynamics. The report cites a low SRP-induced coronary venous pressure augmentation (mean 13 mm Hg vs. 8 mm Hg in control), possibly due to occasionally inappropriate catheter positioning or simply because of major coronary veno-venous shunting. Cases of minor transient adverse effects reported in this study included atrial fibrillation, and hematomas or atrial wall staining at the jugular catheter insertion site. Three patients who suffered PTCA complications were successfully treated with extended SRP (2-7 hrs), pending emergency bypass surgery, suggesting that SRP could be particularly effective during failed or complicated angioplasty. Direct inspection indicated no significant coronary vein injury.

Kar also summarized a multicenter SRP-PTCA investigation[61] involving 164 LAD angioplasty patients. Safety and logistics of SRP support during PTCA balloon inflations were demonstrated. On average, observations in this somewhat diverse study indicated the following: angina occurred later (47 sec) and in fewer (44%) SRP-treated than in untreated PTCA balloon inflations (58% at 38 sec); ST segment elevations were significantly reduced by SRP support, 2.4 vs. 3.3 mm in control inflations; mean LV ejection fraction was 35.7% in untreated PTCA inflations vs. 43.6% during SRP support; extent as well as severity of the regional wall motion abnormality were significantly reduced by SRP support. Abrupt LAD closure during PTCA occurred in five patients, and these were successfully supported by SRP over a mean period of 4 hr. PTCA was repeated in one patient, and four had emergency bypass surgery with a satisfactory postoperative course.

Costantini et al[62] examined patients with unstable angina SRP support during high risk PTCA (baseline LV ejection fraction less than 40%, or else more than 40% of the LV at severe ischemic risk during PTCA balloon inflations). Coronary vein catheterization and SRP were successfully performed in 15 of 20 patients without serious adverse effects. Target vessels were: left main coronary artery in two, LAD in ten, left circumflex in one, right coronary artery in two. Unsupported PTCA balloon inflations (mean duration 44 sec) led to significant reduction in cardiac index from a mean baseline level of 2.5-1.7 l/min m², and stroke work from 52 to 27 g/m², whereas these indices decreased less (to 2.1 1/min/m² and 37 g/m²) during SRP-treated inflations (mean duration 144 sec). Similarly, LV ejection fraction and regional wall function dropped from a baseline mean of 55-27% and from 49% to 11%, respectively, in control inflations, but were improved (to 39% and 27%, resp.) during SRP supported PTCA. Judging from this study, SRP during high risk angioplasty appeared to provide global as well as regional benefits.

In an abstract[63] Nishida et al reported on 30 patients undergoing 120 sec PTCA balloon dilatations (SRP treated vs. unsupported) of proximal LAD lesions. Unsupported PTCA balloon inflations resulted in angina in 13 of 30 patients, mean ECG-ST segments of 2.0 mm and mean pulmonary artery end-diastolic pressure (EDP) of 13.4 mm Hg. With a mean SRP retroperfusion flow rate of 198 ml/min, treated balloon inflations led to angina in 8 of the 30 patients, a moderately yet significantly lower mean ECG-ST of 1.6 mm, and a mean pulmonary artery EDP of 11.3 mm Hg. A second recent abstract by these investigators[64] merits attention since it alludes to SRP supported PTCA in eight patients with left main coronary artery disease. In this high risk setting, SRP treatment of PTCA balloon inflations was compared with cardiopulmonary bypass assisted and unsupported inflations. Both support techniques equally extended the tolerable mean PTCA balloon inflation time from 38.6-57.5 sec, and improved systolic blood pressure, pulmonary artery EDP and cardiac index. However, only SRP support significantly attenuated the regional ischemia during PTCA balloon inflations, judged from reduced ECG segment elevations. This unique but insufficiently described study suggests that SRP is capable of providing both myocardial and systemic support in high risk PTCA.

Nienaber et al[65] raised the question whether SRP support is really needed during elective PTCA with duration of 60–300 sec. Fifteen patents with proximal LAD stenosis were studied during PTCA in a setting presumably not considered high risk. Comparing SRP support (200–250 cc/min) vs. untreated PTCA balloon inflations in the LAD, chest pain incidence and score were not altered, but ECG-ST elevations were significantly reduced, while echocardiographic regional wall motions improved. The obvious comment was that SRP support may not be needed whenever elective PTCA is devoid of complications, while SRP support might be quite desirable in instances of failed PTCA.

Other as yet unreported SRP-PTCA studies are believed to corroborate the above observations. In high risk situations, SRP may well permit extending the duration of PTCA balloon inflations without causing severe hemodynamic or symptomatic deterioration. The few transient complications reported with SRP are considered minor. In addition to the jugular route, a femoral vein approach to the coronary sinus may also be used. There is some uncertainty about the reliability of SRP balloon catheter positioning within the GCV and the variable amount of coronary veno-venous and drainage. A serious limitation is that, so far, protection of right coronary artery occlusion has not been demonstrated, and even left circumflex coronary artery occlusion may not now be effectively treated with SRP.

In the single reported application of ICSO during PTCA, Komamura et al[66] applied this intervention in ten patients with severe LAD stenosis during brief PTCA balloon inflations. The ICSO used had a constant coronary vein occlusion and release timing (10 and 5 sec). It was initiated 3 min prior to the PTCA balloon inflations and was maintained throughout the LAD dilatation as well as up to 3 min postinflation. Although detailed comparisons with untreated controls are not reported, the patient's hemodynamics were said to have been stabilized during the ICSO treatment.

ICSO Supported Reperfusion

In a 1985/1986 trial by Mohl et al,[67] 30 consecutive patients undergoing bypass surgery were evaluated. The more sophisticated PICSO was applied in 15 patients for 1 hr during the early reperfusion period, using average coronary sinus occlusion and release periods of 6.7 and 4.3 sec, respectively. Analyzing regional wall motion with 2DE, moderately hypokinetic myocardial segments were found to be significantly better preserved in the PICSO treated patients as compared to the 15 unsupported patients. Differences in global function and in severely hypokinetic segments were not statistically significant. A positive relationship was established between cumulative CK release and coronary sinus occluded pressure levels, suggesting metabolite washout by PICSO. Three months after the operation, function was similar in both groups. PICSO was shown to be a safe procedure with short term potential benefits. The importance of continuous coronary sinus pressure monitoring became evident in this study.

Details on feasibility, safety and effectiveness of ICSO in acute myocardial infarction were provided by Komamura and Kodama.[68] Twelve ICSO treated patients with primary transmural acute myocardial infarction (9 anterior, one lateral and 2 inferior AMI) as well as 22 unsupported anterior AMI patients had successful intracoronary thrombolysis with urokinase. A 7F balloon catheter was inserted into the coronary sinus (for right or left circumflex occlusions) of the GCV (for LAD occlusions), and a 1 hr ICSO treatment (10 sec coronary sinus occlusions, 5 sec release periods) was initiated just before the lytic treatment. With ICSO occlusions, mean coronary sinus pressure rose from 8.3 to 38.1 mm Hg. There were no adverse effects on hemodynamics, no serious ventricular arrhythmias, no hemolysis or fall in platelet counts. There was no difference in LV function, but the ICSO group exhibited fewer abnormally contracting segments than the control group. In the whole ICSO group, no significant differences were found in peak CK activity, total amount of CK release and time from onset to peak CK activity. However, in four patients in whom cardiac enzyme release into the coronary sinus was determined serially, peak CK, total amount of CK release and peak transcardiac difference of CK were greater, and peak time to transcardiac CK difference shorter in the ICSO group than in controls. This study does not provide firm conclusions regarding ICSO-generated washout effects.

In yet another study, Komamura et al[69] applied ICSO in patients with acute anteroseptal myocardial infarction treated successfully with tissue plasminogen activator. There were no adverse effects on hemodynamics, no serious ventricular arrhythmias, no hemolysis or fall in platelet count during ICSO. In this ICSO application, the mean CK activity, total CK release, peak time of CK, as well as mean lactate extraction ratios, were not significantly different from those in the unsupported control group. ICSO did not result in any differences in abnormally contracting segments or in ejection fractions. The investigators concluded that, while ICSO support during thrombolytic treatment of AMI was feasible and had no adverse effects, it offered few benefits.

The implications of these limited studies are unclear. A case can apparently still be made for ICSO myocardial support during thrombolytic reperfusion; the latter may be associated with reperfusion injury, and ischemic yet viable myocardium might benefit from a more gradual retrograde flow distribution. To provide clarification, ICSO support of lytic treatment was examined by Nakazawa et al[70] in a controlled dog study. The authors tested the effectiveness of ICSO (coronary vein occlusion time 12 sec, release period 5 sec) during low dose intravenous urokinase administration, comparing it to unsupported high and low dose intravenous administration, as well as to low dose intracoronary urokinase infusions. Lytic therapy and ICSO was started 1 hr after angiographic confirmation of complete thrombotic coronary occlusion of the LAD. The reperfusion success rate in the ICSO supported group was significantly higher (6 of 8 dogs) than in the unsupported high dose intravenous group (1 of 10) and almost as high as with intracoronary infusions (7 of 8). The incidence of ventricular premature contractions was significantly lower in the ICSO group (4/min) than with intracoronary infusion (38/min), but similar to the non-ICSO high dose (3/min) and low dose intravenous urokinase administration (6/min). It remains to be shown how these animal study data are relevant to clinical ICSO, and whether the method can be optimized as a support during thrombolytic treatment of AMI patients.

Commentary

Relating the general experience of the 1940s "Beck era" to the currently proposed SRP and ICSO/PICSO techniques, one is reminded to be realistic and cautious. Thus, based on currently available evidence, safety demands that intracoronary vein pressures during SRP or ICSO be limited, i.e., to 60 mm Hg peak, 40 mm Hg mean. Further data might indeed reveal the safety of higher coronary vein pressures when applied during very short periods of LAD occlusion, but it would be unreasonable to base any protocols upon less than rigorous data on potential damage in a particular setting.

Conversely, achievement of optimal effectiveness with coronary venous interventions usually requires approaching the highest permissible coronary vein pressures and flows. Evidence from human trials is that—due to a significantly different vascular anatomy—the coronary venous pressures developed during the retrograde interventions were frequently lower than those observed in the encouraging animal studies. Upgrading of retrograde methods will be aimed, in part, at higher pressure differentials between the coronary vein and the regional occluded coronary artery. The inevitable trade-off between safe limits and maximal effectiveness will always have to be considered against the background of a specific human coronary venous anatomy. Given newer pumping devices, advanced catheter technology and experience with coronary vein catheterization, as well as new diagnostic tools such as PET or retrograde echo contrast, optimal effectiveness in a particular SRP or ICSO application may be approached by appropriate catheter tip positioning relative to the treated zone and tailoring of retrograde pressures and flows, possibly even curtailing undesirable coronary veno-venous shunting.

PTCA is increasingly used to treat complex coronary disease patients with unstable ischemic syndromes and occasionally severe global dysfunction. In such high risk subsets, coronary artery occlusion during unsupported PTCA balloon inflations can become intolerable, jeopardize the regional myocardium, and potentially lead to life threatening hemodynamic collapse. Retrograde interventions during high risk PTCA, and arterial blood SRP in particular, appear to effectively provide a partial myocardial support, along with possible (but as yet uncertain) systemic benefits. The multicenter SRP-PTCA evaluation corroborates the potential benefits without any serious complications, and suggests that SRP may permit longer PTCA procedures. Retrograde myocardial perfusion does not interfere with antegrade catheter maneuvers in the presence of complexities of coronary arteries.

Even when assisted, established interventions may fail in some high risk cases, leading to abrupt vessel closure; in these difficult circumstances, occasionally exacerbated by inevitable delays before emergency revascularization, temporary maintenance of myocardial viability and function is of highest priority. The retrograde methodologies could certainly be envisioned as a complement, or temporary emergency bridge to the more permanent revascularization procedures. It appears that further development and optimization of the coronary venous interventions will now focus on treatment in high risk settings, where the retrograde approach could help resupply regional acutely ischemic tissue while also washing out accumulated toxic metabolites which exacerbate injury.

Modified SRP or Alternate Retrograde Interventions

Hypothermic SRP

The concept of hypothermic synchronized retroperfusion (HSRP) treatment of myocardial ischemia was described by Meerbaum et al in 1982.[71] In initial closed-chest dog experiments, SRP was combined with an arterial blood supply cooled to 20°C, the LAD was occluded for 3 or 6 hr, while HSRP was started 30 min post LAD occlusion. Hemodynamic measurements, contrast cineangiography and 2DE were used sequentially. The ischemic area at risk and the extent of necrosis were measured in transverse slices of the LV. While untreated control dogs deteriorated further during LAD occlusion, 2.5-5.5 hrs of HSRP significantly reduced the rate-pressure product, mean LVEDP decreased (by 39.5 or 51.4%), and LV ejection fraction increased (by 28 or 33%). HSRP caused no arrhythmias and led to much less necrosis of ischemic risk myocardium after 6 hrs LAD occlusion (28.9%), vs. 72.3% in untreated controls. Thus, moderately hypothermic retroperfusion in closed-chest dogs protected reversibly injured myocardium and improved cardiac function. Improved effectiveness over and above SRP alone was apparently achieved, with regional myocardial temperatures reduced by about 3°C.

Haendchen et al[72] extended the above HSRP study to include 7 days reperfusion. HSRP was applied from 30 min up to 3 hr proximal LAD occlusion. Compared with untreated LAD occlusion-reperfusion controls, HSRP significantly reduced heart rate and rate-pressure product, decreased LV volumes and improved ejection fraction during the occlusion period. HSRP significantly improved ischemic zone function (systolic wall thickening). During the reperfusion period, untreated control dogs exhibited more severe derangements in hemodynamics and wall motion, while HSRP minimized the complications of reperfusion. Mortality in the control group was 30.7% vs. 16.7% with HSRP treatment. Mean infarct size on the 7th day (% of LV) was 12.0% in controls and 4.2% in the HSRP treated dogs. In a separate limited group, it also appeared that HSRP was more effective than SRP alone.

Recently, Wakida et al[73] reexamined the regional myocardial temperature distribution and infarct size in open-chest dogs with 3.5 hr of LAD occlusion, treated with HSRP. The dogs were randomized after 30 min occlusion to either untreated controls, normothermic SRP (pump infusion temperature 32°C) or HSRP (infusion temperature 15°C).

Regional myocardial temperatures were measured with needle-tipped thermistors at various sites of the heart, including the anterior wall distal to the LAD occlusion. Rectal and pulmonary temperatures were also monitored. In the HSRP group, the anterior LV wall temperature decreased rapidly by 5°C (15 min of HSRP), whereas all other temperatures, decreased linearly over time. Myocardial temperatures in the ischemic area were generally lower than at the other sites, but the highest intra-site temperature difference was only 3.6°C (at 15 min SRP). Mean infarct size (percent of risk area) was significantly smaller in the HSRP group (6.2%) than in controls (64.9%) or in the normothermic SRP dogs (24.1%). These results corroborated that HSRP provides better ischemic myocardial protection than normothermic SRP, through rapid moderate regional cooling of acutely ischemic myocardium, with only small spatial temperature gradients. As to clinical applications, the authors thought that the small temperature changes in the closed-chest would perhaps minimize a shivering response, and suggested metocurine as a possible pharmacologic control, if needed.

Suction-Enhanced SRP

A recently proposed modification involving selective ECG synchronized suction-enhanced retroinfusion of oxygenated blood (SSR) was described by Boekstegers et al.[74] A study was carried out in 15 open-chest dogs subjected to 5 hrs LAD occlusion. The suction period preceding the retrograde pumping period was timed to allow the coronary veins to empty upstream of the retroinfusion catheter tip, thus facilitating the refilling of the veins by the retrogradely pumped oxygenated fluid. SSR with oxygenated Ringers lactate solution was applied between 30 min and 5 hr LAD occlusion. Mean subepicardial pO_2 in the ischemic myocardium of SSR treated dogs increased by 7–12 mm Hg. Mean infarct size was reduced to 5.6% in the treated dogs, compared to 27% in controls. In a most recent abstract, Boekstegers et al[75] presented results in pigs with a 10 min LAD occlusion. During the brief LAD occlusions, 57-79% of regional myocardial function (sonomicrometry) was maintained by the suction-enhanced treatment, in contrast to 1-19% with SRP alone. Reduction of measured surface and intramyocardial pO_2 was also significantly less pronounced in SSR treated pigs. Obviously, this interesting new technique will have to be further validated and corroborated.

Combination of SRP and ICSO

In clinical applications, it appeared difficult to achieve an adequate diastolic coronary vein pressure augmentation. Conversely, retroperfusate redistribution toward the jeopardized ischemic zone is enhanced by maximizing the retrograde arterial infusion and/or the retrograde pressure potentials, subject to safe limits. The suggestion was made to enhance SRP effectiveness in some applications by inclusion of certain ICSO features, in particular to supplement diastolic retroinfusion with extended periods of coronary vein occlusion (vs. occlusion only in diastole during SRP). Some mathematical modeling of this combined treatment was reported by Schreiner et al,[75a] indicating that the combined SRP-ICSO approach could increase the retrograde intramyocardial delivery even with relatively low retroperfusate flow rates. Conversely, delivery could also be markedly enhanced by increasing the SRP flow rates. It must be kept in mind that protracted inhibition of systolic coronary venous drainage and excessive coronary sinus pressures or reperfusion flow rates can be damaging.

Jacobs et al reported in an abstract[76] that the SRP-ICSO combination produced greater myocardial salvage than either SRP or ICSO alone in dogs with 6 hr LAD occlusion, the retrograde intervention commencing 30 min postocclusion. Although not fully reported, Dr. Jacobs referred to a clinical evaluation of the ICSO-SRP support during PTCA balloon inflations in a state of the art survey ("New Left Ventricular Support Techniques for Cardiac Patients"), presented at the 1990 Annual Scientific Session of the American College of Cardiology. Whereas SRP alone is currently designed to retroinfuse up to 250 cc/min, the peak pressure (diastolic) measured in the coronary vein during the clinical SRP trials was generally only of the order of 30 mm Hg. Combining ICSO with SRP, peak pressures tend to occur in systole and are readily augmented to the permissible limit (60 mm Hg) at substantially lower retrograde flows (approx 100 cc/min). During PTCA, ICSO-SRP was compared with SRP support and with untreated LAD balloon inflations in patients with class 3–4 angina, normal LV ejection fractions, and absence of evident coronary arterial collaterals. Statistical evidence has not been published, but a general impression during the PTCA balloon inflations was apparently that combined SRP-ICSO provided substantial benefits, relative to untreated control inflations, beyond those experienced with SRP support alone, i.e., less angina and increased time to onset, lesser ECG changes, lesser decrease in LV ejection fraction and fewer abnormally functioning segments. It was, however, concluded that further data will have to be gathered to resolve questions about optimal effectiveness.

Other SRP Variants

A diastolic coronary sinus retroperfusion variant was described in 1978 by Feola and Weiner.[77] A double lumen balloon catheter was inserted into the coronary sinus of dogs, with one lumen connected to a roller pump to provide steady retroperfusion of arterial blood, and the other lumen to a helium counterpulsing pump to phase balloon inflation in diastole and assure systolic deflation. With a potential developed coronary sinus pressure between 50 and 75 mm Hg, anesthetized open-chest dogs were subjected first to 15 min proximal LAD occlusion alone, followed by 30 min of diastolic coronary sinus perfusion during continued LAD occlusion. Reduction of measured myocardial tissue oxygen tension with simultaneous elevation of the ECG-ST segments characterized the untreated ischemia. Diastolic coronary sinus retroperfusion significantly improved oxygen tension in the ischemic myocardium, reduced ECG-ST elevation, and tended to restore arterial blood pressure. Histologic examination indicated no intramyocardial hemorrhage.

Another variant involves nonsynchronized retrovenous perfusion and was examined by Feindel et al[78] in open-chest pigs with 4 hr LAD occlusion and 1 hr reperfusion. In the arterial group, the coronary sinus was intermittently occluded (5 sec balloon inflation, 5 sec deflation) and arterial blood was retroinfused during each balloon inflation at a 60 ml/min rate, throughout the LAD occlusion. In the venous group, the protocol was identical except that 60 ml/min venous blood was retroinfused. The ICSO group featured the above coronary sinus occlusion-release timing without active retroinfusion. No intervention was performed in the control occlusion-reperfusion group. Mean infarct size (percent of risk area) in control animals was significantly greater (86.3%) than in either the arterial (44.1%) or venous retroperfusion group (57.7%), but was not statistically different in the ICSO series (78.0%). Arterial blood retroinfusion did not achieve statistically greater salvage compared to venous blood retroinfusion, but both were significantly superior to ICSO. Mean coronary sinus pressure was 56.1 mm Hg in the arterial, 38.8 mm Hg in the venous and 17.1 mm Hg in the ICSO group (a rather low pressure). In an extension of the above study,[79] interventions were started 1 or 2 hr post LAD occlusion vs. immediately post LAD occlusion. It was established that in pigs the nonsynchronized retroperfusion was able to limit infarct size even after substantial amounts of myocardium within the area at risk had already undergone necrosis.

Coronary Venous Retroinfusion

It has always been recognized that, in the absence of adequate collaterals, antegrade delivery to an acutely ischemic myocardial region may prove insufficient. The coronary venous system, free of atherosclerosis, constitutes an alternate approach to conventional pharmacologic treatment. In past experiments, Cibulski et al[80] noted that Krypton-85 and Xenon-133 injected via the coronary venous system resulted in high concentrations and selectively greater tracer uptake in the low pressure ischemic region created by either LAD or circumflex coronary artery occlusions. The ratio of ischemic to nonischemic zone delivery was between 4 and 6, indicating that effective selective retroinfusion into the ischemic risk zone could be anticipated.

Drug Retroinfusion

In 1979, Kordenat[81] described clinically oriented retroinfusions in a series of dogs. Methysergide or dipyridamol or a combination were retroinfused in bolus fashion via the GCV after 30 min LAD occlusion, the latter continuing up to 3 hrs. Compared to 3 hr untreated LAD occlusion, which significantly reduced cardiac output and significantly increased total peripheral resistance, retroinfusion of each drug resulted in hemodynamic improvements, without evidence of synergistic effects.

Povzhitkov et al[82] reported on SRP with prostaglandin E₁ retroinfusion for treatment of acute myocardial ischemia in closed-chest anesthetized dogs. Retroinfusion was administered via the GCV between 30 min and 3 hr proximal LAD occlusion. 2DE measurements of global and regional LV function indicated distinct improvements with drug retroinfusion, particularly compared to progressive deterioration in untreated controls, but also relative to partial benefits by SRP alone. Mean infarct size (percent of risk zone) in untreated control dogs was 47.1%, compared to 19.5% for retroinfusion-supplemented SRP. Similar results were reported with manitol retroinfusion.[83]

Bourdarias and Berdeaux[84] studied retroinfusion of verapamil and nitroglycerin via SRP in open-chest dogs with 180 min proximal LAD occlusion. SRP with (controls) or without drug treatment started 10 min postocclusion and was maintained for 170 min. SRP alone significantly increased ischemic zone blood flow, with redistribution toward the endocardium, and improved regional function. Supplemental verapamil and nitroglycerin further enhanced the myocardial perfusion, primarily in the subepicardial layer, thus decreasing the endocardial/epicardial ratio. Functional recovery deteriorated in the ischemic zone, particularly with verapamil. Thus, coronary vasodilator retroinfusion was not beneficial for treatment of myocardial ischemia.

Markov et al[85] described GCV retroinfusion of fructose 1-6 diphosphate in anesthetized dogs. Arterial blood retroperfusion was started 2 hr after LAD occlusion, after which reperfusion was instituted. After an initial retrograde bolus injection, the drug was continuously added to the retroperfusing arterial blood. Compared to untreated LAD occlusions with dextrose infusion, retroinfusion led to decline in LVEDP, and enhancement of cardiac output, blood pressure and LV dp/dt. Since there were no differences in coronary blood flow between retroinfused and control dogs, the drug benefits were attributed to augmented anaerobic carbohydrate utilization and inhibition of oxygen free radical generation by the neutrophils.

Ryden et al[86] investigated metoprolol retroinfusion (GCV) in open-chest pigs with 90 min LAD occlusion. Drug administration commenced 30 min post LAD occlusion and lasted for 5 min, with no effects on heart rate or blood pressure, whether retroinfused or administered intravenously. Plasma metoprolol concentration did not differ significantly in the two groups of pigs, yet myocardial tissue concentration in the ischemic zone was much higher with retroinfusion than with intravenous drug administration. There was also a significant transmyocardial concentration gradient, with highest drug levels in the subepicardial and lowest in the subendocardial layer. Depending on the coronary venous pressures developed during the retroinfusion, regional myocardial concentrations could be as high as those with antegrade coronary artery administration.

Lytic Retroinfusion

In 1983, Meerbaum et al[87] reported another potential application of retroinfusion: lysis of a coronary artery thrombus by low dose coronary venous streptokinase retroinfusion. Both repeated brief periods of retrograde administration into an occluded coronary vein, or else streptokinase retroinfusion along with arterial blood SRP, proved similarly effective. In closed-chest dogs with an intra-LAD thrombus, full retrolysis and consequent reperfusion occurred within about 50 min, whereas lysis by intravenous streptokinase took substantially longer (about 130 min) and was highly variable. A recent follow-up study with rt-PA was described by Miyazaki et al.[88] The rt-PA retroinfusion began 60 min after LAD occlusion and was continued for 30 min. Similar to trends established in the prior study, mean time to full thrombolysis in the retroinfusion group was shorter (13.4 min) than in vena cava rt-PA administration controls (27.8 min). Sixty min after reperfusion, 2D echo revealed functional recovery in the retroinfusion group, whereas reperfusion after systemic thrombolysis was associated with apparent myocardial stunning. Mean infarct size (percent of risk area) after 3 hr was 34.9% in the retroinfused dogs vs. 54.5% for the intravenous group. No myocardial hemorrhages or damage to the coronary venous system were observed. These studies showed that lytic agent retroinfusion can provide rapid LAD clot lysis, improved functional recovery and greater infarct size reduction, as compared to equivalent dose systemic intravenous administration.

Antiarrhythmic Retroinfusion

Otsu et al[89] reported on retroinfusion of lidocaine into a briefly (1 min) obstructed coronary sinus, following a 24 hr LAD occlusion in dogs. Compared to intravenous drug administration, retroinfusion was most effective in interrupting ventricular tachycardia, attributed to significantly higher concentrations of lidocaine achieved at the border of the infarcted myocardium. Simon et al[90] delivered lidocaine via the coronary sinus in ischemic dogs (between 30 and 60 min LAD occlusion) in conjunction with ICSO. Retroinfusion provided regionally elevated myocardial drug levels, with low systemic concentrations. Davy et al[91] described lidocaine, esmolol, adenosine or deferoxamine retroinfusions in sheep with LAD occlusion. There was a general trend toward lower myocardial necrosis and minimal ventricular fibrillation in the retroinfusion survivors.

Karagueuzian et al[92] investigated in conscious dogs procainamide retroinfusion (vs. intravenous administration) for management ventricular tachycardia during permanent LAD occlusion. The selective retroinfusion via the GCV was a significantly more effective treatment of both spontaneous (24 hr post LAD occlusion) and electrically induced (3–12 days postocclusion) ventricular tachycardia. Compared to systemic administration, significantly lower doses of procainamide could be used with retroinfusion. With retroinfusion, myocardial tissue drug concentration reached much higher levels in the infarcted and ischemic zones, and this probably explains the greater antiarrhythmic drug efficacy.

Retroinfusion Treatment of Reperfusion

Recent investigations pursued a variety of drug retroinfusions, for amelioration of myocardial ischemia as well as reperfusion derangements. The simplest procedure might involve retrograde coronary venous infusion, e.g., with a pump, during a 2–3 min balloon inflation within the appropriate coronary vein, e.g., GCV for LAD occlusions.

Ikeoka et al[93] described effects of diltiazem retroinfusion (SRP balloon catheter in GCV) on myocardial infarction and reperfusion in anesthetized dogs with 4 hr treated coronary occlusion followed by 1 hr reperfusion. There were no significant differences in hemodynamics, compared with untreated control occlusions. Diltiazem retroinfusion benefited the ischemic myocardium directly, without systemic hemodynamic changes. Reperfusion hemorrhage was significantly less than in either controls or in an alternate intravenous diltiazem treatment.

Diltiazem retroinfusion was also studied in pigs by Tadokoro et al.[94] This study compared retrograde vs. antegrade administration in pigs with a 60 min LAD occlusion, followed by 3 hr reperfusion. The drug administration began 10 min prior to reperfusion and lasted 30 min. In addition to drug retroinfusion via the GCV, other pigs had equivalent diltiazem infusion into the right atrium, or saline infusions into either the GCV or the right atrium. Measurements of regional myocardial blood flow indicated no differences among these groups, during either occlusion or reperfusion. However, infarct size was significantly less in the retroinfused pigs, compared to either saline infusions or right atrial diltiazem. Diltiazem seemed to have a direct protective effect on the myocardium, rather than acting through changes in myocardial blood flow.

Tadokoro et al[95] hypothesized that adenosine retroinfusion might reduce reperfusion injury and infarct size. Twenty-four pigs were subjected to 60 min LAD occlusion followed by 3 hr reperfusion, and adenosine was retroinfused for 30 min beginning 15 min prereperfusion. In controls, the same amount of adenosine was infused into the right atrium. Retrograde coronary venous adenosine treatment significantly reduced infarct size, but it did not resolve the functional reperfusion derangements.

Recently, Hatori et al[96] reported on effects of superoxide dismutase and catalase retroinfusion upon reperfusion arrhythmias, myocardial function and infarct size. Anesthetized closed-chest dogs had 90 min LAD occlusion, followed by 3 hr reperfusion. A 30 min continuous or bolus drug infusion, (begun 15 min before reperfusion) was carried out into the right atrium, or else via GCV retroinfusion along with right atrial infusion. Mean infarct size (percent of risk area) was significantly smaller in the retroinfusion group (11.3 %) than in either the right atrial drug infusion group (31.3%) or in untreated control dogs (43.0%). 2DE measurements of ischemic zone function indicated significantly better post-reperfusion recovery and fewer arrhythmias in the retroinfusion group.

Deferoxamine retroinfusion for reduction of infarct size was studied by Kobayashi et al[97] in open-chest pigs with a 60 min LAD occlusion, followed by 3 hr reperfusion. The drug was administered into the anterior interventricular vein over a 5 min period, at 15 min before reperfusion. Mean infarct size (percent of risk area) was 73.9% in a control group with iv saline administration, 70.6% in a systemic deferoxamine series, and 48.5% in the retroinfused pigs. There were no differences in hemodynamics or regional myocardial function between the groups. The lack of hemodynamic effects by the drug, and persisting myocardial dysfunction during "reperfusion stunning", suggested a direct cardioprotective effect.

Clinical Retroinfusion

Berland et al[98] reported a limited retroinfusion attempt in the human. Effects of low dose nifedipine retroinfusion on global and regional LV function were examined in five patients. The coronary sinus was occluded (by a special catheter balloon) and 10 ml saline or else 10 ml saline with 200 µg nifedipine were retroinfused for 1 min under continuous coronary sinus pressure monitoring (mean pressure not to exceed 40 mm Hg). In three of the patients with severe proximal LAD stenosis, there was a significant decrease in LV function during the nifedipine retroinfusion. This contrasted with no effect in one patient with hypertrophic cardiomyopathy without coronary lesion and with saline retroinfusion alone. Reflecting on the regional changes of wall motion, the investigators felt that there was a selective retrodelivery into the ischemic area.

Retrograde Myocardial Contrast 2D Echo

Developments in myocardial contrast echocardiography stimulated an application in which echo contrast agents (with microbubbles of the order of 10 micron) are injected into coronary veins, in conjunction with ultrasonic assessment of the resulting myocardial contrast enhancement. Punzengruber et al[99] reported on factors affecting the retrograde penetration of echo contrast into normal and ischemic canine myocardium. Fifteen closed-chest dogs were studied with coronary venous administration of renografin before and after coronary artery occlusion. Digital subtraction venography was used to assess delivery, drainage and shunting of the retrograde injectate. Mean values of baseline systolic/diastolic blood pressure in the GCV were 7/1 mm Hg, increased to 29/5 mm Hg after coronary sinus occlusion, and further to 55/15 mm Hg during coronary sinus contrast injection. In a 2 DE midpapillary LV short axis cross section, baseline myocardial contrast echo appearance was limited to the anteroseptal region, extending to a mean 28.4% of the sectional circumference after GCV injections vs. 35.3% after coronary sinus injections (nonsignificant difference). After LAD occlusion, GCV contrast injections resulted in opacification of 36.6% of the sectional circumference (nonsignificant vs. preocclusion baseline) and opacified most but not all of the asynergic segments. After occlusion of the circumflex coronary artery, myocardial echo contrast uptake was restricted to the septum and the anterior wall. The ischemic and asynergic posterolateral myocardial segments were not opacified. In spite of coronary sinus balloon occlusion, digital subtraction coronary venography revealed rapid drainage of retrogradely injected contrast to the right atrium via veno-venous anastomoses. It was thought that retrograde coronary venous contrast injections might be of particular help in defining myocardial regions which are accessible with retrograde coronary venous interventions.

Nishida et al[100] applied retrograde coronary venous myocardial contrast echocardiography in eight patients during LAD angioplasty. While long axis cross sectional images of the LV were recorded by 2DE, 10 ml of agitated echo contrast was retroinfused into the temporarily obstructed GCV, generating high mean systolic (81 mm Hg) and augmented diastolic (43 mm Hg) levels of coronary venous pressure. Myocardial perfusion was then evaluated by analysis of enhanced grey levels in various myocardial regions, caused by GCV retroinfusion or antegrade LAD injections. Brief retroinfusion caused no adverse effects and resulted in confluent and transmural regional opacification. A mean baseline grey level of 3 was enhanced to 12 by low GCV pressure and 20 with high pressure GCV contrast retroinfusions, compared to 26 for antegrade echo contrast infusion. It was confirmed that GCV retroinfusion can deliver agents into myocardium distal to an LAD occlusion, but effective retrodelivery into the ischemic region apparently requires a hazardously high coronary venous pressure.

Commentary on Obstacles for Coronary Venous Interventions

Most intensive competitive research efforts give rise to enthusiasm. This has its benefits, but needs to be matched by realistic reevaluation and confirmation, as major clinical applications are contemplated. It is true that both SRP and the simpler ICSO appear safe in the human and logistically satisfactory. However, both support techniques are still plagued by questions about the underlying mechanisms, and only partial effectiveness has been demonstrated in a limited number of settings. Following comprehensive experimental development and a few promising clinical evaluations, there remain several challenging issues:

1. The human coronary venous system differs significantly from that in animals, and it apparently features markedly more coronary veno-venous and Thebesian shunting. This makes it difficult to achieve the levels of coronary venous pressure observed in experiments and presumably required for reliable and effective retrograde myocardial resupply. Balloon catheter technology and procedures for coronary venous interventions need to be refined to provide options, including

     a) stable balloon occlusions very near the coronary sinus entrance;

     b) stable balloon catheter positioning deep in the GCV without wedging;

     c) catheter balloon configurations capable of intermittently occluding not only the target coronary vein, but also major shunts.

2. As a corollary, and perhaps also germane to other investigations, diagnostic tools need to be mobilized to define blood perfusion and myocardial viability, e.g., with PET, and to assess—in individual cases—the retrograde coronary venous pathways available for the retroperfusion intervention, e.g., using retrograde myocardial contrast echocardiography.

3. Retroperfusion balloon catheter technology and catheterization methods should be tailored so as to facilitate retrograde treatment of non LAD territory, i.e., myocardial regions subserved by an occluded left circumflex and possibly right coronary artery.

4. Further studies should provide a firmer definition of the hazards to be anticipated over a range of times, pressures and retrograde flows. This will allow appropriate engineering of retrograde pumps and control systems.

5. Coronary sinus catheterization techniques from the femoral, jugular or other approaches need to be refined.

6. Retroinfusion procedures need to be optimized and standardized through further validations.

7. It is essential to review all available evidence to clarify the effects of coronary venous occlusions with or without arterialization as well as the maximal nutritive microcirculatory delivery that can be achieved with retroinfusion. The role of washout of toxic metabolites from ischemic myocardium needs to be further elucidated, for both SRP and ICSO/PICSO.

References

1. Mohl W, Wolner E, Glogar D, eds. The Coronary Sinus. Darmstadt: Steinkopff Verlag, 1984.

2. Meerbaum S. Coronary venous retroperfusion delivery of treatment to ischemic myocardium. Herz 1986; 11:41-54.

3. Corday E, Meerbaum S, Drury JK. The coronary sinus: An alternate channel for administration of arterial blood and pharmacologic agents for protection and treatment of acute cardiac ischemia. J Am Col Cardiol 1986; 7:711-714.

4. Mohl W, Faxon DP, Wolner E, eds. Clinics of CSI. Darmstadt: Steinkopff Verlag, 1986.

5. Faxon DP, Jacobs AK. Coronary sinus retroperfusion and intermittent occlusion. In: Topol EJ, ed. Acute Coronary Intervention. New York: Alan Liss, 1988:255-269.

6. Meerbaum S, ed. Myocardial Perfusion, Reperfusion, Coronary Venous Retroperfusion. Darmstadt: Steinkopff Verlag, 1990.

7. Jacobs AK, Faxon DP. Retroperfusion and PTCA. In: Topol EJ, ed. Textbook of Interventional Cardiology. New York: WB Saunders Co, 1990:477-495.

8. Haendchen RV, Corday E. Coronary sinus interventions for reduction of myocardial ischemia. In: Kulick DL, Rahmintoola SH, eds. Techniques and Applications in Interventional Cardiology. New York: Mosby Year Book, 1991.

9. Corday E, Haendchen R. Introduction. In: Seminar on Coronary Venous Delivery Systems for Support and Salvage of Jeopardized Ischemic Myocardium. J Am Coll Cardiol, 1991; 18 (No. l):253-256.

10. Beck CS. Revascularization of the heart. Surgery 1949; 26:82-88.

11. Gensini GG, DiGiorgi S, Murad-Nettor S. Coronary venous occluded pressure. Arch Surg, 1963; 86:72-80.

12. Gensini GG, DiGiorgi S, Murad S, Delmonico JE. Percutaneous retrograde venous perfusion of the myocardium (Abstract #22). 1962; 6th Scientific Session of the American College of Cardiology.

13. Meerbaum S, Lang TW, Osher J et al. Coronary venous retroperfusion treatment of jeopardized myocardium. (Abstract P1.67). 1975; 28th Annual Conference on Engineering in Medicine and Biology:425.
14. Meerbaum S, Lang TW, Osher JV et al. Diastolic retroperfusion of acutely ischemic myocardium. Am J Cardiol 1976; 37: 588-598.
15. Markov AK, Lehan PH, Hellems HK. Reversal of acute myocardial ischemia in closed-chest animals by retrograde perfusion of the coronary sinus with arterial blood. Acta Cardiol 1976; 31:185-190.
16. Farcot JC, Meerbaum S, Lang TW et al. Synchronized retroperfusion of coronary veins for circulatory support of jeopardized ischemic myocardium. Am J Cardiol 1978; 41:1191-1201.
17. Berdeaux A, Farcot JC, Boudarias JP et al. Effects of diastolic synchronized retroperfusion on regional coronary blood flow in experimental myocardial ischemia. Am J Cardiol 1981; 417:L033-L040.
18. Smith GT, Geary GG, Blanchard W et al. Reduction in infarct size by synchronized selective coronary venous retroperfusion of arterialized blood. Am J Cardiol 1981; 48:1064-1070.
19. Geary GG, Smith GT, Suebiro GT et al. Quantitative assessment of infarct size reduction by coronary venous retroperfusion in baboons. Am J Cardiol 1982; 50: 1424-1430.
20. Gundry SR. Modification of myocardial ischemia in normal and hypertrophied hearts, utilizing diastolic retroperfusion of the coronary vein. J Thor Cardiovasc Surg 1982; 83:659.
21. Hatori N, Uriuda Y, Isozima K et al. Short term treatment with synchronized coronry venous retroperfusion before full reperfusion significantly reduces myocardial infarct size. Am Heart J 1992; 123:1166-1174.
22. Yamazaki S, Drury JK, Meerbaum S et al. Synchronized coronary venous retroperfusion: Prompt improvement of left ventricular function in experimental myocardial ischemia. J Am Coll Cardiol 1985; 5:655-663.
23. Drury JK, Yamazaki S, Fishbein M et al. Synchronized diastolic coronary venous retroperfusion: Results of a preclinical safety and efficacy study. J Am Coll Cardiol 1985; 6:328-335.
24. Smalling RW, Ekas R, Tiberi M et al. Effects of synchronized coronary sinus retroperfusion on regional left ventricular function during acute regional ischemia. (Abstract 34) 1986; 2nd International Symposium of Myocardial Protection via the Coronary Sinus:51.
25. Berk L, Hartog JM, Rensen RJ et al. On the time course of systolic myocardial wall thickening during coronary artery occlusion and reperfusion in the absence and presence of synchronized retroperfusion in anesthetized pigs. (Abstract 35) 1986; 2nd International Symposium of Myocardial Protection via the Coronary Sinus:51.
26. Chang BL, Drury JK, Meerbaum S et al. Enhanced myocardial washout and retrograde blood delivery with synchronized retroperfusion during acute myocardial ischemia. J Am Coll Cardiol 1987; 9: 1091-1098.
27. O'Byrne GT, Ninaber CA, Miyazaki A et al. Positron emission tomography demonstrates that coronary sinus retroperfusion can restore regional myocardial perfusion and preserve metabolism. J Am Coll Cardiol 1991; 18:257-70.
28. Arealis EG, Moulopoulis SD, Kolff WJ. Attempts to increase blood supply to an acutely ischemic area of the myocardium by intermittent occlusion of the coronary sinus (preliminary results). Medical Research Engineering 1971: 4-7.
29. Tzigorlou AG, Raphael SS, Troulinis AE. Attempt to increase the blood supply to an acutely ischemic area of myocardium by intermittent occlusion of the coronary sinus. Proc Eur Soc Artif Organs 1979; 6:49
30. Mohl W, Gueggi M, Haberzerth K et al. Effects of intermittent coronary sinus occlusion (ICSO) on tissue parameters after ligation of LAD. Bibl Anat 1980; 20: 517-121.
31. Mohl W, Glogar DH, Mayr H et al. Reduction of infarct size induced by pressure controlled intermittent coronary sinus occlusion. Am J Cardiol 1984; 53:923-928.
32. Mohl W, Punzengruber C, Moser M et al. Effects of pressure controlled intermittent coronary sinus occlusion on regional ischemic myocardial function. J Am Coll Cardiol 1985; 5:939-947.

33. Mohl W, Moser M, Aigner A et al. Enhancement of washout of myocardial edema by intermittent coronary sinus occlusion. (Abstract 42) lst International Symposium on Myocardial Protection Via the Coronary Sinus 1984:15.
34. Moser M, Mohl W, Kenner T. The arterial venous density gradient as an index of myocardial function. In: Mohl W, Wolner E, Glogar D, eds. The Coronary Sinus. Darmstadt: Steinkopff Verlag 1984:497-507.
35. Seitelberger R, Mohl W, Winkler M et al. Effects of pressure controlled intermittent coronary sinus occlusion (PICSO) on metabolism and regional function in the normal and underperfused canine myocardium. (Abstract 48) lst International Symposium on Myocardial Protection via the Coronary Sinus 1984:18.
36. Glogar DH, Mohl W, Mayr H. Pressure controlled intermittent coronary sinus occlusion affects the myocardium at risk and reduces infarct size. (Abstract 43) lst International Symposium on Myocardial Protection via the Coronary Sinus 1984:15.
37. Ciuffo AA, Guerci AD, Halperin H et al. Intermittent obstruction of the coronary sinus following coronary ligation in dogs reduces ischemic necrosis and increases myocardial perfusion. In: Mohl W, Wolner E, Glogar D, eds. The Coronary Sinus. New York: Springer Verlag 1984:454-464.
38. Guerci AD, Ciuffo AA, DiPaula AF et al. Intermittent coronary sinus occlusion in dogs: Reduction of infarct size 10 days after reperfusion. J Am Coll Cardiol 1987; 9:1075-1081.
39. Jacobs AK, Faxon DP, Minihan A et al. Pressure controlled intermittent coronary sinus occlusion reduces myocardial necrosis during reperfusion. (Abstract 54) 2nd International Symposium on Myocardial Protection via the Coronary Sinus 1986:57.
40. Simon E and Jacobs AK. The effects of PICSO on left ventricular function during reperfusion. International Working Group on Coronary Sinus Interventions. Newsleter Vol. 1 (3) 1987.
41. Diltz EA, Mannes RN, Lee JW et al. Intermittent coronary sinus occlusion does not reduce infarct size or ischemic dysfunction in an occlusion-reperfusion model. (Abstract) Circulation Suppl. III 1985; 72:120.
42. Mayr H, Glogar D, Mohl W et al. Effect of PICSO treatment on arrhythmias during early myocardial ischemia. (Abstract 67) 2nd International Symposium on Myocardial Protection via the Coronary Sinus 1986:60.
43. Jacobs AK, Faxon DP, Coats DW et al. The effect of intermittent coronary sinus occlusion during ischemia. (ABstract 45) lst International Symposium on Myocardial Protection via the Coronary Sinus 1984:17.
44. Toggart EJ, Nellis SH, Liedtke AJ. The efficacy of intermittent coronary sinus occlusion in the absence of coronary artery collaterals. Circulation 1987; 76 (No.3): 667-677.
45. Fedele FA, Capone RJ, Most AS et al. Effect of pressure controlled intermittent coronary sinus occlusion on pacing-induced myocardial ischemia in domestic swine. Circulation 1988; 77:(No.6) 1403-1413.
46. Sun Y. A closed-loop system for pressure controlled intermittent coronary sinus occlusion. Biomedical Instrumentation and Technology 1989; 23:136-143.
47. Schreiner W, Neuman F, Schuster J et al. Computation of derived diagnostic quantities during intermittent coronary sinus occlusion in dogs. Cardiovas Research 1988; 22:265-276.
48. Neuman F, Mohl W, Schreiner W. Coronary sinus pressure and arterial flow during intermittent coronary sinus occlusion. Am J Physiol 1989; 256:H906-H915.
49. Jacobs A, Rothendler J, Faxon D et al. Enhancement of ischemic zone perfusion by intermittent coronary sinus occlusion. (Abstract 31) 3rd International Symposium on Myocardial Protection via the Coronary Sinus 1988:37.
50. Simon P, Jacobs A, Hogfeldt V et al. Infarct size reduction using coronary sinus technique: is arterial blood necesssary? (Abstract 34) 3rd International Symposium on Myocardial Protection via the Coronary Sinus 1988:38.
51. Jacobs AK, Faxon DP, Coats DW. Coronary sinus occlusion: effect on ischemic left ventricular dysfunction and reactive hyperemia. Am Heart J 1991; 121:442-449.
52. Matsuhashi H, Hasele M, Kawamura Y. The effect of intermittent coronary sinus occlusion on coronary sinus pressure dynamics and coronary arterial flow. Jap Circ J 1992; 56:272-285.

53. Rovetto MJ, Whitma JT, Neely JR. Comparison of the effects of anoxia and whole heart ischemia on carbohydrate utilization in isolated working rat hearts. Circ Res 1973; 32:699.
54. Gropler RJ, Geltman EM, Sanpathkumaran K et al. Functional recovery after coronary revascularization for chronic coronary artery disease is dependent on maintenance of oxydative metabolism. J Am Coll CArdiol 1992; 20:569-577.
55. Zalewski A, Goldberg S, Slysh S et al. Myocardial protection via coronary sinus interventions: superior effects of arterialization compared with intermittent occlusion. Circulation 1985; 71:1215-1223.
56. Gore JM, Weiner BH, Benotti JR et al. Preliminary experience with synchronized coronary sinus retroperfusion in humans. Circulation 1986; 74:381-388.
57. Weiner BH, Gore JM, Sloan KM et al. Synchronized coronary sinus retroperfusion (SCSR) during LAD angioplasty. (ABstract) J Am Coll Cardiol 1986; 7:64A.
58. Beatt K, Verdow P, Serruys P. Synchronized coronary sinus retroperfusion. International Working Group on Coronry Sinus Intervention. Newsletter 1987 vol 1 #2.
59. Berland J, Farcot JC, Barrier A et al. Coronary venous synchronized retroperfusion during percutaneous transluminal angioplasty of left anterior descending coronary artery. Circulation 1990; 81:(suppl) 35-42.
60. Kar S, Drury JK, Hajduczki I et al. Synchronized coronary venous retroperfusion for support and salvage of islchemic myocardial during elective and failed angioplasty. J Am Coll Cardiol 1991; 18:271-2822.
61. Kar S for the investigators of the multicenter coronary venous retroperfusion clinical trial group. Reduction of PTCA-induced ischemia by synchronized coronary venous retroperfusion: Results of a multicenter clinical trial. (Abstract) J Am Coll Cardiol 1990; 15:250A.
62. Costantini C, Sampaolin A, Serra CM et al. Coronry venous retroperfusion support during high risk coronary angioplasty in patients with unstable angina. J Am Coll Cardiol 1991; 18:283-292.
63. Nishida K, Nanto S, Hirayama A et al. Reduction of myocardial ischemia during PTCA by synchronized coronary venous retroperfusion. Jap Circ J 1991; 55: (Suppl A).
64. Nishida K, Masai T, Nanto S et al. Beneficial effects of synchronized coronary venous retroperfusion during high risk PTCA compared with those of cardiopulmonary bypass. (Abstract) J Am Coll CArdiol 1991; 17:(No.2) 904.
65. Nienaber CA, Abend M, Rehders T, Chen CH. Synchronized coronary venous retroperfusion: Support or superfluous with coronary angioplasty. Circulation Suppl.II 1991; 84:(No.4) 156.
66. Komamura K, Nanto S, Yamamoto K, Kodama K. Time controlled intermittent coronary sinus occlusion during LAD coronary angioplasty in man. (Abstract 50) 3rd International Symposium on Myocardial Protection via the Coronary Sinus 1988:43.
67. Mohl W, Simon P, Neuman F et al. Clinical evaluation of pressure-controlled intermittent coronary sinus occlusion: Randomized trial during coronary artery surgery. Ann Thorac Surg 1988; 46:192-201.
68. Komamura K, Kodama K. Human experience with intermittent coronary sinus occlusion in acute myocardial infarction. (Abstract 32) 3rd International Symposium on Myocardial Protection via the Coronary Sinus 1988:37.
69. Komamura K, Mishima M, Kodama K. Preliminary clinical experience with intermittent coronary sinus occlusion in combination with thrombolytic therapy in acute myocardial infarction. Jap Circ J 1989; 53:(No.9) 1152-1163.
70. Nakazawa K, Ikeoha K, Tateishi J et al. The effect of coronary thrombolysis by intermittent coronary sinus occlusion (ICSO) in combination with intravenous administration of urokinase (UK). (Abstract 39) 3rd International Symposium on Myocardial Protection via the Coronary Sinus 1988:40.
71. Meerbaum S, Haendchen RV, Corday E et al. Hypothermic coronary venous phased retroperfusion: A closed-chest treatment of acute regional myocardial ischemia. Circulation 1982; 65:(No. 7) 1435-1445.
72. Haendchen RV, Corday E, Meerbaum S et al. Prevention of ischemic injury and early reperfusion derangements by hypothermic retroperfusion. J Am Coll Cardiol 1983; 1 (4):1067-1080.

73. Wakida Y, Haendchen RV, Kobayashi S et al. Percutaneous cooling of ischemic myocardium by hypothermic retroperfusion of autologous arterial blood: Effects on regional myocardial temperature distribution and infarct size. J Am Coll Cardiol 1991; 18:(No.1) 293-302.

74. Boekstegers P, Diebold J, Weiss CH. Selective ECG synchronized suction and retroinfusion of coronary veins: First results of studies in acute myocardial ischemia in dogs. Cardiovasc Res 1990; 24:(No. 6) 456-464.

75. Boekstegers P, v Diegenfeld G, Peter W et al. Protection of regional myocardial function during acute ischemia in pigs. Comparison of ECG synchronized suction and retroinfusion of coronary veins (SSR) to synchronized retroperfusion (SRP). (Abstract P2479) European Cardiology Congress 1992:435.

75a. Schreiner W, Simon P, Nanninga C, Meerbaum S et al. Synchronized retroperfusion combined with coronary sinus occlusion: experimental measurements compared with simulation results and model predictions. Cybernet Sys: Inter J 1990; 21:389-421.

76. Jacobs AK, Simon P, Hogfeld V et al. Increase in myocardial salvage by combining coronary sinus occlusion and retroperfusion. (Abstract) JACC 1989; 13:(No.2) 53 A.

77. Feola M, Weiner L. A method of coronary retroperfusion for the treatment of acute myocardial ischemia. Cardiovasc Diseases Bulletin of Texas Heart Institute 1978; 5 (No.3).

78. Feindel CM, Cruz J, Sandhu R et al. The effectiveness of various modes of nonsynchronized retrovenous perfusion in salvage of ischemic myocardium in the pig. Can J Cardiol 1991; 7(8):357-365.

79. Feindel CM, Sandhu R, Cruz J et al. The effects of delay in retroperfusion therapy on infarct size reduction. (Abstract 0158) Circulation Suppl III 1990; 82:(4).

80. Cibulski AA, Markov A, Lehan PH et al. Retrograde radioisotope myocardial perfusion patterns in dogs. Circulation 1974; 50:159-66.

81. Kordenat RK. Retroperfusion of the ischemic myocardium with methysergide and dipyridamole. (ABstract) 7th Internation Congress of Thromb Haem 1979: 6-100.

82. Povzhitkov M, Haendchen RV, Meerbaum S et al. Protective effect of coronary venous prostaglandin El retroperfusion during acute myocardial ischemia. J Am Coll Cardiol 1984; 3:(4) 939-947.

83. Povzhitkov M, Haendchen RV, Meerbaum S. Manitol coronary venous retroperfusion; improvement in ischemic left ventricular function in acute occlusion. (Abstract) Clin Res 1982; 30:17.

84. Berdeaux A, Farcot JC, Giudicelli JF et al. Failure of regional vasodilator drug to potentiate the retroperfusion beneficial effect in ischemic myocardium in dogs. In: Mohl W, Wolner E, Glogar D, eds. The Coronary Sinus. Darmstadt: Steinkopff Verlag 1984:354-359.

85. Markov AK. Myocardial function improvement and reduction of infarct size by delivering fructose 1-6 diphosphate (FDP) via the coronary sinus (CS). (Abstract 51) 3rd International Symposium on Myocardial Protection via the Coronary Sinus 1988:43.

86. Ryden L, Tadokoro H, Sjoquist PO et al. Pronounced accumulation of metropolol in ischemic myocardium after coronary venous retroinfusion. J Cardiovasc Pharm 1990; 15:22-28.

87. Meerbaum S, Lang TW, Povzhitkov M et al. Retrograde lysis of coronary artery thrombus by coronary venous streptokinase administration. J Am Coll Cardiol 1983; I:1262-1267.

88. Miyazaki A, Tadokoro H, Drury JK et al. Retrograde coronary venous administration of recombinant tissue-type plasminogen activator: A unique and effective approach to coronary artery thrombolysis. JACC 1991; 18:(2) 613-620.

89. Otsu F, Carew TE, Maroko PR. Myocardial concentration and antiarrhythmic effects of lidocaine administration via coronary veins. Am Coll Cardiol 1985; 5 (2):467 (Abstract).

90. Simon P, Jacobs A, Faxon D et al. Lidocaine delivery via coronary sinus results in high concentrations in ischemic myocardium. (Abstract 43) 3rd International Symposium on Myocardial Protection via the Coronary Sinus 1988:41.

91. Davy T, Ort JL, Peters JL. Effects of retrovenous myocardial drug delivery after coronary artery occlusion in sheep. ASAIO Transactions 1990; 36:M203-M206.

92. Karagueuzian HS, Ohta M, Drury JK et al. Coronary venous retroinfusion of procaine amide: a new approach for the management of spontaneous and inducible ventricular tachyarrhythmia during myocardial infarction. J Am Coll Cardiol 1986; 7:(no.3) 551-63.

93. Ikeoka K, Nakagawa Y, Kawashima S et al. Effects of synchronized retroinfusion of diltiazem on the size of myocardial infarction and reperfusion hemorrhage. (Abstract 40) 3rd International Symposium of Myocardial Protection via the Coronary Sinus 1988:40.

94. Tadokoro H, Miyazaki A, Satomura K et al. Coronary venous retroinfusion of diltiazem reduces infarct size in pigs. (Abstract 41) 3rd International Symposium of Myocardial Protection via the Coronary Sinus 1988:40.

95. Tadokoro H, Kobayashi S, Corday E. Profound infarct size reduction with retrograde coronary venous administration of adenosine (Abstract 1139) Circulation Suppl III 1990; 82:(No. 4).

96. Hatori N, Miyazaki A, Tadokoro H et al. Beneficial effects of coronary venous retroinfusion of superoxide dismutase and catalase on reperfusion arrhythmias, myocardial function and infarct size in dogs. J Cardiovasc Pharmacol 1989; 14:396-404.

97. Kobayashi S, Tadokoro H, Washida Y et al. Coronary venous retroinfusion of deferoxamine reduces infarct size in pigs. J Am Coll Cardiol 1991; 18:(No.2) 621-627.

98. Berland J, Farcot JC, Cribier A et al. Changes in left ventricular function induced by coronary venous retrinfusion of low dose nifedipine: Preliminary results. (Abstract 20) 3rd International Symposium on Myocardial Protection via the Coronary Sinus 1988:34.

99. Punzengruber C, Maurer G, Chang BL et al. Factors affecting penetration of retrograde coronary venous injections into normal and ischemic canine myocardium: Assessment by contrast echocardiography and digital angiography. Basic Res Cardiol 1990; 85:2-32.

100. Nishida K, Kodama K, Mishima M et al. Retrograde coronary venous myocardial contrast echocardiography in human: Can coronary venous retroinfusion deliver pharmacologic agents to the myocardium? (Abstract 195A) J Am Coll Cardiol 1990; 15(No.2).

Addendum

Coronary Venous Interventions: Update of Recent Developments

This Chapter 12 supplement will review developments since the first edition of this book to provide an appropriate perspective, a certain amount of overlap is inevitable. The historical background and description of earlier efforts need not be amended. Rather, recent directions will be assessed, with emphasis on clinical applications.

Whereas this author was intensively involved in the conceptualization and development of the synchronized retroperfusion (SRP) modality since the early 1970s, it was always understood that the field of coronary venous interventions has many facets and contributors. The comprehensive investigations of the so-called Beck era of the 1940s deserve special credit, even though the application objectives were not achieved. The processes underlying coronary venous treatment of jeopardized myocardium are complex and even now insufficiently understood. In fact, unlike progress in the area of surgical cardioplegic retroperfusion, the potentials of clinically oriented types of retroperfusion in the ever growing interventional cardiology armamentarium are yet to be defined.

As will be apparent, the past several years did not feature an impressive growth of clinical uses of retroperfusion. A survey also revealed that, apart from SRP, most of the alternate coronary vein assist methods remained in the experimental stage. These include primarily intermittent coronary sinus occlusion (ICSO) and its pressure controlled variant (PICSO), suction enhanced synchronized retroperfusion (SSR), nonsynchronized modes of retroperfusion, and retrograde drug infusion. Several studies demonstrated again that short duration SRP is capable of providing significant support during percutaneous transluminal coronary (PTCA), even in high risk settings. Regional dysfunction is reversed and other cardiac derangements alleviated during PTCA balloon inflations. The coronary venous approach is considered safe, is readily implemented, and features high success rates in catheterizing the coronary sinus, usually within minutes. A few anecdotal reports of longer duration SRP, alone or in conjunction with intraaortic balloon pumping (IABP), showed that myocardial viability could be extended following abrupt post-PTCA coronary occlusions or during cardiogenic shock. SRP usually provided bridging support pending emergent coronary artery bypass surgery.

Substantial retroperfusion effectiveness variability is attributed to different degrees of coronary veno-venous and Thebesian shunting, varied localization of the balloon catheter-insufficient retrograde flow rates and frequently inadequate pressure augmentation in the coronary veins. It appears feasible to define the individual coronary venous anatomy and to assess the retrograde myocardial penetration. For effective application, it is helpful to develop rational guidelines for positioning the retroperfusion catheter, selecting an optimal retrograde flow rate, and developing maximally safe coronary venous pressures.

SRP Support During PTCA Balloon Inflations

In a 1992 general review, Kar and Norlander[101] state that, as of mid-1987, the randomized multicenter SRP-PTCA study encompassed 164 patients. No major adverse effects were noted in any of the patients. A comprehensive evaluation appeared difficult, in view of the wide spectrum of conditions covered, including relatively mild and high risk settings. Haendchen and Corday[8] pointed out that SRP flows ranged from 50-250 ml/min. Angina occurred in 60% of untreated 38 sec PTCA inflations, with treatment in only 43% of 48 sec inflations. ECG-ST and left ventricular ejection fraction (LVEF) were significantly improved during the inflations, from 36% (vs 52% control) to 44%. With experience, coronary sinus catheterization success rate reached 93%, achieved mostly within less than 5 minutes. The detailed Kar et al report[60] dealt with a Cedars Sinai Medical Center subset of SRP supported elective PTCA of -70% LAD coronary artery obstructions.

A more recent study of Nienaber et al[102] reported on 26 patients with good cardiac function (LVEF =67 ± 14%) and proximal stenosis of the LAD coronary artery (87 ± 12%). SRP flow rate was 200 ± 46 ml/min. Two or more 60 sec PTCA balloon inflations were performed randomly, with or without SRP support. During inflations, SRP improved regional wall motion score significantly from 5.65 ± 2.88 to 3.55 ± 2.80 (control 1.65 ± 81). Anginal pain perception did not differ, but EC G-ST changes were less pronounced during SRP treatment of the PTCA. Nishida et al[63,64] reported initially on SRP-PTCA in 30 patients. Subsequently,[103] the same group indicated it had studied a further 35 SRP - PTCA procedures. Coronary sinus cannulation success rate was 90% (in 6 ± 3 min). Significant SRP support effectiveness was noted during LADPTCA balloon inflations.

With SRP safety and significant though partial benefits demonstrated in lower risk subsets, the question arose as to the SRP potentials in high risk PTCA. More severe consequences of PTCA balloon inflations would be expected in patients exhibiting an LVEF of the order of 35%, and/or a large proportion (say, 40-50%) of the myocardium in jeopardy. Constantini et al[63] examined SRP supported PTCA in a high risk unstable angina setting. SRP support allowed significantly longer PTCA balloon inflation, and greatly benefited regional wall motion. In a more recent study, Incorvati et al[104] examined SRP support of high risk PTCA in 21 patients. Regional LAD wall motion score during untreated PTCA balloon inflations was 2.7 ± 1.6 and significantly better at 1.7 ± 2.1 when treated with SRP. Supported 173 ± 95 sec

PTCA balloon inflation caused no greater ST deviations than 129 ± 87 sec unsupported PTCA. Mean and peak coronary sinus pressures during SRP were 21 ± 6 and 44 ± 13 mm Hg. Hemodynamic or anginal variables did not differ. The site of SRP application varied between great cardiac vein or coronary sinus, depending on primary coronary lesion site.

In 10 patients with left main coronary artery obstructions, Nanto et al[103] supported PTCA with SRP. Clinical characteristics included effort angina, prior myocardial infarctions, unstable angina. Most lesions were in or near the left main trunk and in the LAD. The left circumflex was obstructed in three patients, right coronary in one. Baseline LVEF was $53 \pm 17\%$, but in four patients ranged from 25-48%. SRP flow rate was 218 ± 54 ml/min, peak SRP-induced coronary sinus pressure 31 ± 15 mm Hg. Without SRP, ST rose from 0 to $.28 \pm .04$ mm vs to only $.14 \pm .12$ mm with SRP support. Since SRP support occurred in first of two PTCA inflations, its effectiveness was thought underrated.

In these limited high risk PTCA applications, SRP was again demonstrated to be safe, rapidly instituted and apparently beneficial. Relatively low diastolic pressure augmentation was observed in the human coronary veins, perhaps due to pronounced coronary venous shunting. To achieve higher coronary vein pressure might require modified SRP balloon catheters and extending coronary vein occlusions during the cardiac cycle, which might prove safe for brief PTCA balloon inflations. SRP systems already have the capability to vary and augment the retroflow.

Extended SRP Treatment of Critically Jeopardized Myocardium

Most of the extensive animal investigations of long term SRP and PICSO demonstrated significant preservation of viable but severely jeopardized ischemic myocardium. Among a few recent experimental studies corroborating the earlier findings, Hata et al reported in 1995 on a 60-70 cc/min SRP into the coronary sinus of swine, during coronary artery occlusions and cardiogenic shock refractory to IABP.[105] SRP reduced the infarction area and cardiac function recovered gradually. When SRP was combined with a left heart bypass, the infarct salvage was even more pronounced. The hearts recovered from cardiogenic shock.

As long ago as in 1988, Gore et al[56] reported on long duration SRP treatment in several patients with unstable angina refractory to maximal medical therapy. SRP was envisioned as a bedside procedure to stabilize the patient, pending catheterization and subsequent treatment. Recently, Barnett et al[106] applied SRP for up to 24 hours in 15 patients, and reported full relief of angina and significantly improved cardiac function. It was concluded that SRP can be beneficial in circumflex as well as LAD obstructions, is rapidly and safely instituted, and facilitated maintenance of the patients during transport for further intervention. The above multicenter study included five patients with post-PTCA abrupt coronary artery occlusion. SRP was maintained for 4 ± 2 hours before bypass surgery. The patients did well postoperatively.

SRP in Conjunction with IABP

For difficult scenarios including circulatory collapse, the potentials of a synergistic combination of support techniques was considered. SRP improves circulation in and supply to critically underperfused myocardium, while IABP provides a beneficial cardiac unloading, along with a less certain antegrade coronary flow potentiation. At the Cedars Sinai Medical Center in Los Angeles, the combination SRP + IABP was tested in the 70s (Fig. A12.1). In 8 dogs, treatment was instituted 1 hour after LAD coronary artery occlusion. Measurements showed potentiation of SRP benefits. Similar experiments were carried out in sheep at the Deseret Research Company in Salt Lake City, Utah. Along with a recent positive report by Katirciggli et al,[107] these SRP-IABP studies appear incomplete, and inadequately reported.

Based on clinical SRP experience, combined support treatments were considered for special situations. Freedman et al[108] reported in 1994 on such an application during impending or manifest cardiogenic shock in four patients, age 67, 58, 69 and 83. The cases involved a history of prior heart surgery, myocardial infarctions, and severe derangements culminating in cardiogenic shock. SRP + IABP stabilized the patients and bridged the dire period pending surgical revascularization efforts. Three patients survived the procedures and had a satisfactory postop course. Freedman et al believe that such support can be very useful. Further evidence is required.

Elucidation and Enhancement of SRP Effectiveness

In a 1996 isolated perfused canine heart study, Mitsugi et al[109] compared SRP with coronary sinus occlusion. SRP does not interfere with coronary venous outflow during systole, and its diastolic coronary sinus pressure augmentation did not affect the coronary artery inflow, in contrast with coronary sinus occlusion-induced systolic pressure elevations. Increasing the myocardial blood volume during systole was found to be deleterious. Two closed-chest dog studies, one by Wakida et al[110] and a prior one by Hatory et al,[21] examined relatively short SRP treatment of prolonged ischemia, and its effects on reperfusion. SRP did reduce infarct size significantly, enhanced cardiac function, minimized myocardial hemorrhages and wall swelling, and moderated the no-reflow phenomena. The observed benefits were thought to be due to a more gradual reperfusion and prior washout of accumulated metabolites. Evidence was presented that SRP selectively improved blood flow in the subendocardium.

Presumably with PTCA applications in mind, a 1994 report by Feld et al[111] describes SRP effects on regional function in dogs during 4 min LAD coronary artery occlusions, as measured with sonomicrometry. A modest but significant improvement in regional function was demonstrated. Such SRP benefits could be shown in the presence of a circumflex coronary occlusion. This limitation might perhaps have been overcome by SRP catheter repositioning and increasing retroperfusion flows.

There were a number of additional studies of SRP drug retroinfusion. As reported in 1996 by Tadokoro et al,[112] infarct size reduction following coronary artery occlusion and post-reperfusion

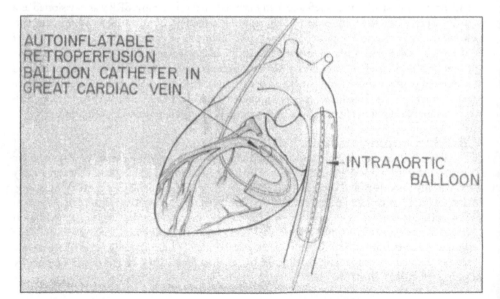

Fig. A12.1. Combined synchronized retroperfusion and counterpulsation

functional recovery were improved through significant diltiazem retrodelivery to the ischemic zone in dogs. Uriuda et al[113] reported on coronary venous felidipine retroinfusion in rats, and Haga et al[114] studied this retroinfusate in the porcine model. Retroinfusion treatment of coronary occlusions prior to reperfusion was found to offer significant protective effects, and will undoubtedly receive further attention.

There was no recent followup of the hypothermic SRP studies of Meerbaum et al,[71] Haendchen et al[72] and Wakida et al.[73] The thrombolytic application of SRP, reported by Meerbaum et al in 1983[87] and later corroborated by Miyazaki et al,[88] was also not pursued. These modalities are thought to warrant further exploration. In the echocardiographic study of Punzengruber et al,[99] great cardiac vein contrast injection opacified most though not all of the asynergic ischemic region during LAD occlusion. Coronary sinus contrast retroinjection during circumflex occlusion failed to opacify the asynergic posterolateral segments. In patients during LAD-PTCA, Nishida et al[100] found that reliable myocardial opacification required high coronary venous pressures. Myocardial contrast echo investigators recently developed agents containing sub-capillary diameter microbubbles. Retrograde injections of such echo contrasts might allow reliably define myocardial regions treatable by coronary venous interventions.

Recent Investigations Involving ICSO or PICSO

Chapter 8 reports on experimental studies applying the relatively simple ICSO-PICSO technique, as well as on limited clinical or intraoperative applications reported in 1988 by Mohl et al[67] and Komamura et al.[66,68] A search of recent literature did not reveal additional clinical PICSO studies, but several experimental investigations have been reported. In dogs with LAD occlusion and reperfusion, Ikeoka et al[115] demonstrated ICSO benefits, attributed to significantly enhanced washout and associated reduction of post-reperfusion derangements. Matsuhashi et al[116] investigated further the ICSO, coronary sinus pressure dynamics and effects on coronary artery inflow. Lazar et al[117] tested in pigs an ICSO-IABP system, applying a protocol of 1.5 hour treated versus untreated coronary occlusion, followed by .5 hour cardioplegic arrest and 3 hours reperfusion. Ischemic damage was significantly reduced by either ICSO or IABP, but the improvements and recovery were most marked when the two support methods were combined. In another study, Lazar et al[118] combined PICSO with L-glutamate coronary venous substrate enhancement. It was found that this approach significantly decreased ischemic damage. Finally, Lazar et al also studied a combination of PICSO with percutaneous bypass,[119] again establishing in open-chest dogs benefits of the combination.

Kanazawa[120] found regional and global function significantly improved with an intermittent coronary sinus occlusion and retroperfusion. Unfortunately, function was not compared to equivalent ICSO treatment. Following up on substantial mathematical modeling, Schreiner et al[121] discussed the features of PICSO and SRP. So far, coronary venous retroinfusions during PICSO received only limited attention, in spite of likely benefits of supplemental arterialization of the ischemic myocardium. To achieve more adequate SRP coronary vein pressures, modification of SRP balloon occlusion timing might be appropriate, safely permitting.

Alternate Coronary Vein Support Concepts

Following a prior report,[74] Boekstegers et al[122] carried out an experimental study in pigs involving their suction-enhanced retroperfusion. Although preservation of regional function and viability after coronary occlusion was said to be better than with SRP, it is fair to say that further verification is needed. A recent exchange between Kar et al and Boekstegers[123] addressed questions of safe coronary venous pressures, catheterization, and clinical application. Debating SSR vs SRP effectiveness is perhaps not useful at this stage, particularly since protocols and measurement techniques are not always comparable. Both approaches have advantages and limitations, and SSR needs to be further developed as a clinically applicable technique.

Retroperfusion without synchronization of coronary vein occlusions was already studied by Feindel et al.[79] More recently, Ropchan et al[124] reported on another experimental investigation. Their intermittent coronary sinus balloon retroperfusion (ICSR) featured a 5 sec coronary vein occlusion followed by 5 sec release. Arterial blood retroinfusion was limited to the coronary sinus occlusion. Open chest experiments were performed in 12 control pigs with 4 hour LAD occlusion followed by 1 hr reperfusion, while in 13 pigs ICSR was applied at the beginning and throughout the coronary occlusion. The retroflow rate was 60 ml/min. Mean coronary sinus pressures for the inflation-deflation cycle was 51 ± 12 mm Hg. Infarct size as percent of myocardium at risk was $41.5 \pm 15.0\%$ with ICSR, compared to $80.5 \pm 6.1\%$ in the control series. Generally, little damage to the coronary veins was encountered with ICSR, except in two dogs exhibiting obvious epicardial hemorrhage. Regional function was not evaluated.

Bearing in mind the techniques proposed earlier by Feola,[77] ICSR is clearly a simpler system than SRP, as is ICSO or PICSO. Actually, the initial SRP development in dogs was largely motivated by observations in early open-chest experiments that nonsynchronized retroperfusions occasionally led to the above type hemorrhages. The current study apparently featured very high coronary sinus pressures during the ICSR balloon inflation. These may have contributed to effective retrodelivery to the ischemic myocardium, but can hardly be justified for safe applications. Because of near absence of coronary collaterals, the pig model is of interest. As pointed out by Chen et al,[125] a factor influencing retroinfusion effectiveness is the pressure gradient from the coronary veins to the coronary artery distal to occlusion. One should also recall that many of the SRP or ICSO experimental investigations featured a delayed start of retroperfusion, say, 1 hour after coronary artery occlusion. Studies aimed at PTCA support require a protocol featuring brief periods of coronary artery occlusion and retroperfusion.

Nonetheless, the authors' discussion serves a useful purpose. It points out again the meager literature data upon which we base criteria of maximal safe coronary venous pressures for brief or long use of intermittent coronary sinus occlusions, with or without supplemental retroinfusion. Equally disconcerting is the poor understanding of myocardial and microcirculatory processes associated with short and extended nonsynchronized or synchronized interventions in the coronary veins. In spite of attempts at modeling, the degree of retrograde delivery, retropenetration or washout, are all only marginally defined for ICSO, SRP, SSR, or ICSR, delimiting rational refinement of the techniques. There is no shortage of catheter or pumping technology, but only when the above limitations will be overcome through further research is it likely that new useful odifications or concepts will be forthcoming.

Concluding Remarks

As already intimated, the past five years may be classified as a hiatus period in the development of retroperfusion, including its clinical application. Having realized and demonstrated definite though partial effectiveness, e.g., in support of PTCA, it is deemed appropriate that the human coronary venous anatomy and retrograde intervention fundamentals be reassessed, to achieve greater reliability and degree of benefits. Supplemental hypothermia, pharmacologic retroinfusions and combined support warrant further examination. The earlier "Commentary on Obstacles for Coronary Venous Interventions" remains largely valid. New dedicated reevaluation may yet lead to another active period of clinical retroperfusion applications.

References

101. Kar S, Nordlander R. Coronary veins: An alternate route to ischemic myocardium. Heart Lung 1992; 21:148-159.
102. Nienaber ChA, Rehders TCh, Abend M et al. Synchronisierte koronarvenoese Retroperfuions: Ischaemie Protektion by Koronaragngioplastie (PTCA). A Kardio 1992; 81:645-655.

103. Nanto S, Nishida K, Hirayama A et al. Supported angioplasty with synchronized retroperfusion in high risk patients with left main trunk or near left main trunk obstruction. Am Heart J 1993; 125:301-309.
104. Incorvati RL, Taubert SG, Pecora MJ et al. Clinical applications of coronary sinus retroperfusion during high risk percutaneous transluminal coronary . JACC 1993; 22(1) 127-134.
105. Hata M. Experimental application of synchronized coronary sinus retroperfusion (SCSR) and left heart bypass (LHB) for severe cardiogenic shock. Nippon Kyobu Geka Gakkai Zasshi 1995; 43(9):1646-1656.
106. Barnett JC, Freedman RJ, Touchon R et al. Coronary venous retroperfusion of arterial blood for the treatment of acute myocardial ischemia. Catheterization and Cardiovascular Diagnosis 1993; 28:206-213.
107. Katircioglu SF, Kucukaksu DS, Gokce P et al. Coronary sinus retroperfusion combined with intra-aortic balloon pumping to perfuse the acutely ischemic myocardium. Thorac Cardiovasc Surg 1994; 42(6):330-332.
108. Freedman RJ, Lasorda DM, O'Neill WW. Combined intra-aortic balloon counterpulsation with synchronized coronary venous retroperfusion: The United States experience. Catheterization and Cardiovascular Diagnosis 1994; 33:362-367.
109. Mitsugi MS, Saito T, Saitoh S et al. Effects of synchronized retroperfusion on the coronary arterial pressure-flow relationship. Cardiovasc Rec 1996; 32(2):335-343.
110. Wakida Y, Nordlander R, Kobayashi S et al. Short-term synchronized retroperfusion before reperfusion reduces infarct size after prolonged ischemia in dogs. Circulation 1993; 88(1):2370-2380.
111. Feld S, Ekas RD, Felli P et al. Differential effects of synchronized coronary sinus retroperfusion on regional myocardial function during brief occlusion of the left anterior descending and circumflex coronary arteries. Catheterization and Cardiovascular Diagnosis 1994; 32;70-78.
112. Tadokoro H, Myazaki A, Satomura K et al. Infarct size reduction with coronary venous retroinfusion of diltiazem in the acute occlusion/reperfusion porcine heart model. J Cardiovasc Pharmacol 1996; 28(1):134-141.
113. Uriuda Y, Wang QD, Lei SX et al. Coronary venous drug infusion in the ischaemic-reperfused isolated rat heart. Cardiovasc Rec 1996; 31(1):82-92.
114. Haga Y, Hatori N, Nordlander M et al. Coronary venous retroinfusion of felodipine reducing infarct size without affecting regional myocardial blood flow. Heur Heart J 1993; 14(10):1386-1393.
115. Ikeoka K, Nakagawa Y, Kawashima S et al. Effects of intermittent coronary sinus occlusion on experimental myocardial infarction and reperfusion hemorrhage. Japanese Circ J 1990; 54:1258-1272.
116. Matsuhashi H, Hasebe N, Hawamura Y. The effect of intermittent coronary sinus occlusion on coronary pressure dynamics and coronary arterial flow. Jpn Circ J 1992; 56:272-285.
117. Lazar HL, Yang XM, Rivers S et al. Retroperfusion and balloon support to improve coronary revascularization. J Cardiovasc Surg (Torino) 199s; 33(5):538-544.
118. Lazar HL, Haan CK, Yang X et al. Reduction of infarct size with coronary venous retroperfusion. Circulation 1992; 86(5):II352-II357.
119. Lazar HL, Treanor P, Rivers S et al. Combining percutaneous bypass with coronary retroperfusion limits myocardial necrosis. Ann Thorac Surg 1995; 59(2):373-378.
120. Kanazawa M. Effects of intermittent coronary sinus retroperfusion on global and regional ventricular function during acute coronary occlusion in dogs. Nippon Kyobu Geka Gakkai Zasshi 1994; 42(7):1007-1015.
121. Schreiner W, Simon P, Nanninga C et al. Synchronized retroperfusion combined with coronary sinus occlusion. Experimental measurements compared with simulation results and model predictions. Cybernetics and Systems: An International Journal 1990; 21:382-421.
122. Boekstegers P, Peter W, von Degenfeld G et al. Preservation of regional myocardial function and myocaridal oxygen tension during acute ischemia in pigs: Comparison of selective synchronized suction and retroinfusion of coronary veins to synchronized coronary venous retroperfusion. JACC 1994; 23(2):459-469.

123. Kar S, Barnett JC, Freedman RJ et al. Synchronized coronary venous retroperfusion (Letter to the Editor) and Boekstegers P, Peter W, Werdan K et al. (Reply). JACC 1994; 24(2):578-582.
124. Ropchan GV, Findel CM, Wilson GJ et al. Salvage of ischemic myocardium by nonsynchronized retroperfusion in the pig. J Thorac Cardiovasc Surg 1992; 104:619-625.
125. Chen S, Chang B, Meerbaum S et al. The pattern of delivery and distribution of coronary venous retroinfusate in canine hearts. Proc Cams & PUMC 1989; 4(1):19-25.

CHAPTER 13

Coronary Sinus Interventions in Experimental Research: A Review

Harold L. Lazar and Richard J. Shemin

Introduction

Despite optimal myocardial protection, ventricular dysfunction may still occur in the postoperative period following the revascularization of acutely ischemic myocardium. As more high risk patients with acute ischemic syndromes and reduced ejection fractions present for surgical revascularization, established techniques of cardioplegic arrest may be inadequate to protect these hearts. As the incidence of patients with unstable angina and evolving myocardial infarction increases, interventions directed at the coronary venous system have emerged as alternative techniques of myocardial protection. There is currently a renewed interest in protecting jeopardized myocardium during regional and global ischemia using coronary sinus retroperfusion techniques.

Pressure-controlled intermittent coronary sinus occlusion (PICSO) has emerged as one of these coronary sinus techniques. The PICSO technique was developed by Mohl and his colleagues at the Second Surgical Clinic at the University of Vienna.[1] PICSO redistributes coronary venous blood by changes in pressure gradients throughout the coronary venous system. In the PICSO technique, a balloon-tipped catheter is positioned in the orifice of the coronary sinus and is connected to a pneumatic pump. The pump automatically increases and decreases the pressure in the coronary venous system according to a preset cycle. Based on earlier experimental work, an inflation cycle of 8-10 seconds with a deflation period of 4 seconds is thought to be the optimal PICSO cycle.[2] During the occlusion phase, there is a slow increase in coronary sinus pressure until a plateau is reached. This results in pressure changes throughout the coronary venous system so that blood flow is redistributed toward underperfused areas. After the period of occlusion, the pneumatic pump automatically deflates the balloon. This results in an abrupt decrease in coronary sinus pressure and allows for drainage of the venous system. When the coronary sinus pressure returns to baseline levels, the balloon is automatically inflated and the PICSO cycle is repeated. The intermittent nature of the inflation and deflation cycle avoids the potential complications of hemorrhage, edema, thrombosis, arrhythmias and conduction disturbances despite peak coronary sinus pressure as high as 50 mm Hg.

Coronary Sinus Interventions in Cardiac Surgery, Second Edition edited by Werner Mohl.
©2000 Eurekah.com.

Experimental studies involving regional ischemia without cardiopulmonary bypass showed that PICSO effectively reduced infarct size, improved regional myocardial function and enhanced the washout of ischemic metabolic by-products.[2-4] These beneficial effects of PICSO prompted us to perform a series of experimental studies to determine whether PICSO would decrease ischemic myocardial damage during surgical revascularization. Surgical revascularization of acutely ischemic myocardium is unique in that there are three potential periods where ischemic damage may occur. First, there is the period of "normothermic ischemia" which follows the onset of coronary insufficiency and is prior to the period of cardioplegic arrest. This would be similar to the period following a coronary occlusion during a failed percutaneous transluminal coronary (PTCA) as the patient is being transported to the operating room. The second period is the period of "cardioplegic arrest" where the presence of coronary occlusions may interfere with the distribution of cardioplegia when given by standard antegrade techniques. And, finally, there is the period of "reperfusion" during which time changes in myocardial metabolism and cellular organelle dysfunction can lead to ventricular dysfunction and further necrosis. Would PICSO be as effective in reducing ischemic damage following surgical revascularization compared to nonsurgical conditions? Would the effects of cardiopulmonary bypass and cardioplegic arrest alter the protective benefits of retrograde perfusion? Would PICSO be as beneficial during reperfusion or should these techniques be instituted as soon as ischemia develops? And, finally, would retrograde perfusion not only limit necrosis but also enhance ventricular function and prevent "stunning"?

This chapter will attempt to answer these questions by reviewing our experimental studies using PICSO and retrograde perfusion techniques to decrease ischemic damage during urgent surgical revascularization. In addition, we will discuss how these interventions can be used clinically to potentially decrease the morbidity and mortality involved in the revascularization of acutely ischemic myocardium.

Experimental Models and Techniques

Although no experimental study can ever completely mimic a clinical situation, we believe that our model of acute coronary occlusion in the pig with subsequent reperfusion closely simulates the events that occur following a failed PTCA leading to CABG surgery. The coronary anatomy of the pig has less collateral flow than in dogs and sheep and more closely mimics human anatomy. Infarct size following a coronary occlusion in the pig is greater than in the dog. Hence, interventions which significantly reduce infarct size in the pig will undoubtedly have an important role in clinical practice. In our studies, the occlusion of the second and third diagonal vessels just distal to the takeoff of the LAD has consistently resulted in an area of risk of approximately 10-11%. While this may seem like a relatively small area, one must remember that in patients with triple vessel disease, the presence of collateral flow probably limits the actual amount of ventricular tissue which is at risk for an infarction. In addition, we have found that this degree of jeopardized myocardium allows for a stable preparation so that measurements of ventricular function can be made under steady state conditions. This model also allows us to define exactly the area of risk and to determine the effects of our interventions on pH, wall motion, and histochemical staining. These variables can be more precisely measured in our experimental model than in clinical studies. The coronary sinus orifice in pigs is patulous and the sinus communicates with the azygous vein. Because of this, the azygous vein has been ligated in all our studies. We have found no detrimental effects of ligation of the azygous vein on left ventricular function. Our initial studies showed that PICSO increased peak coronary sinus pressures from $1 \pm .04$ to 52 ± 1.40 mm Hg and had no effect on left ventricular (LV) pressure-volume relationships, LV stroke work index (LVSWI), or myocardial pH.[5] In addition, PICSO did not result in any sustained atrial or ventricular arrhythmias. In our earlier studies, PICSO was instituted with a 7 F double-lumen catheter (Meditech Labs, Watertown, MA) inserted just beyond the orifice of the coronary sinus via a pursestring suture in the right atrium. The catheter was then connected to a pneumatic pump (Meditech Labs, Watertown, MA) which automatically inflates and deflates the balloon according to its preset cycle. In subsequent studies, we used a 9 F triple-lumen balloon tipped catheter (DLP, Inc., Grand Rapids, MI) identical to the type we use to administer retrograde cardioplegia in our clinical practice. In addition to measuring pressure and inflating and deflating the balloon, the extra lumen allows us to infuse various solutions into the coronary sinus.

To assess changes in metabolism in the area at risk, we measured myocardial tissue pH using a tissue pH probe (Khuri Tissue Ischemia Moniter, Vascular Technology, Inc., No. Chelmsford, MA). Control pH measurements are made after a 30 minute period of equilibration and were standardized according to LV temperature which was measured simultaneously with a temperature probe. Experimental and clinical studies have shown that myocardial tissue pH is a sensitive indicator of ischemic injury, the adequacy of cardioplegic protection, and a predictor of postischemic LV function.[6,7] In analyzing our pH data, we looked at both absolute pH values and the change in tissue pH from the onset of ischemia (Δ pH). This approach overcame the problem of differences in the absolute value of pH at the onset of ischemia. Hence, every animal serves as its own control.

Two-dimensional echocardiograms, obtained with a hand-held 3.5 MH$_z$ ultrasound transducer (ATL, Tempe, AZ), were used to assess regional wall motion changes. Left ventricular end-diastolic volume (LVEDV) was obtained by planimetry of a perpendicular long-axis length and a short-axis area as previously described.[8] The same echocardiographic short-axis sections were also used to assess wall motion changes. The ventricle was arbitrarily divided into eight anatomical areas and wall motion was qualitatively analyzed by a numerical score in which 4 = normal, 3 = mild hypokinesis, 2 = moderate hypokinesis, 1 = severe hypokinesis, 0 = akinesis, and -1 = dyskinesis. Echocardiographic sections for wall motion analysis were obtained as left ventricular end-diastolic pressure was varied using the right heart bypass technique at a constant afterload (mean aortic pressure = 65 mm Hg). Measurements were made in a blinded fashion by an experienced echocardiographer. Only sections with the same LVEDV during the preischemic, coronary occlusion, and reperfusion periods were used for analysis so that preload conditions were similar. Hence, the right heart bypass method allows for preischemic and postischemic wall motion measurements to be made in a working heart with comparable afterloads at a consistent LVEDV. The area of risk and area of necrosis were determined by histochemical staining techniques.[9,10] After the 3 hour reperfusion period, the second and third diagonal branches were reoccluded. The ascending aorta was cross-clamped, and the area of risk was determined by injecting 60 ml of phthalo-blue dye (Harshaw-Filtrol, Cleveland, OH) into the aortic root through a 9 F catheter. The left ventricle was then excised and cut into 5 to 10 mm cross-sectional slices. The infarct area was determined by incubating the slices in triphenyl-tetrazolium chloride (Sigma Chemical Co., St. Louis, MO) for 30 minutes and then placing them in formaldehyde overnight. The next morning the stained slices were placed under a glass plate and traced on clear plastic sheets. With reperfusion of ischemic myocardium, there is washout from the nonviable cells of dehydrogenases necessary to reduce nitro blue tetrazolium, and these areas remain pale. The areas of risk and infarct were then measured by planimeter for each slice to obtain the area of risk compared with the total left ventricular mass and the percent area of infarct in the area of risk.

All animals in our experimental studies received humane care in compliance with the "Principles of Laboratory Animal Care" formulated by the National Society of Medical Research and the "Guide for the Care and Use of Laboratory Animals" prepared by the National Academy of Sciences and published by the National Institute of Health (NIH Publication No. 80-23, revised 1978).

Effects of PICSO During Reperfusion

The beneficial effects of PICSO after regional ischemia prompted us to perform an experimental study to determine whether PICSO could alter reperfusion damage after a period of ischemic arrest with cardiopulmonary bypass in the presence of a coronary occlusion.[5] Previous research had concentrated on decreasing reperfusion damage by modifying the reperfusate to meet the changing needs of the ischemic myocardium. This study was unique in that the venous and not the arterial reperfusate was being manipulated in an attempt to reverse reperfusion damage.

Fourteen pigs were placed on cardiopulmonary bypass and underwent 2 hours of aortic crossclamping during which time the mid-LAD was occluded with a snare. Hearts were protected with cold (4°C) crystalloid, potassium (25 mEq/L) cardioplegia given every 20 minutes (5 ml/kg) through an aortic root catheter supplemented with topical and systemic (28°C) hypothermia. After aortic unclamping, the LAD snare was released. All hearts were immediately defibrillated and kept on cardiopulmonary bypass for 60 minutes at which time postischemic measurements of pH, LVSWI, LVEDP, and LVEDV were made. During the reperfusion period, hearts were treated in one of two ways. In seven pigs, PICSO was instituted and maintained throughout the reperfusion period. In another seven pigs, the balloon-tipped catheter was positioned in the coronary sinus but PICSO was not performed. We chose this model because our earlier studies had shown that 2 hrs of cardioplegic arrest with the LAD occluded resulted in heterogenous delivery of antegrade cardioplegia and the subsequent development of significant reperfusion damage.[11]

The results are summarized in Figures 13.1-13.3. Neither the PICSO nor the non-PICSO hearts showed any significant changes in their pressure-volume curves from control (Fig. 13.1). Hearts treated with PICSO had significantly higher myocardial pH values in the distal LAD following 60 minutes of reperfusion (6.99 ± 0.06 versus 6.67 ± .05; p<0.01: Fig. 13.2). These changes in pH were reflected in the parameters of postischemic ventricular function. PICSO treated hearts had significantly higher LVSWI (0.87 ± 0.07 versus 0.61 ± 0.05 gm-m/kg at LVEDP = 10 mmHg; p<0.01; Fig. 13.3). Ejection fraction returned to control levels in the PICSO treated group and was significantly higher than the nonPICSO hearts (50% ± 2 versus 33 ± 6%; p<0.01). Wall motion scores in the area at risk were higher in the PICSO hearts but did not reach statistical significance (1.8 ± 0.4 versus 1.5 ± 0.4; NS).

From these results, we concluded that PICSO does result in a significant decrease in reperfusion damage following a prolonged period of "heterogenous" cardioplegic arrest. Although regional wall motion remained depressed, global ventricular function was significantly improved and there was less tissue acidosis. This appeared to support earlier studies which showed that PICSO enhanced lactate washout during ischemia.[4]

Effects of PICSO During Cardioplegic Arrest

Having shown that PICSO effectively reverses reperfusion damage following periods of global and regional ischemia on cardiopulmonary bypass, we turned our attention toward the period of cardioplegic arrest. In previous studies, we and others had shown that the presence of a coronary occlusion results in heterogenous distribution of antegrade cardioplegia which leads to further myocardial dysfunction upon reperfusion.[11-14] We hypothesized that since the PICSO technique was able to redistribute blood retrograde throughout the coronary venous system, it might also be able to redistribute antegrade cardioplegic flow toward areas of the myocardium distal to a coronary occlusion. Therefore, we designed an experimental study to determine whether PICSO would improve antegrade cardioplegic distribution in the presence of a

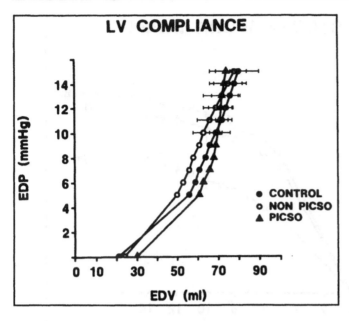

Fig. 13.1. Left Ventricular Compliance. NOTE: a) LVEDP/LVEDV curves are shown during control and postischemic periods. b) LVEDP/LVEDV curves following ischemia are unchanged from control values in both the PICSO and nonPICSO groups. Reprinted with permission from Lazar HL et al. J Thorac Cardiovasc Surg 1988; 95:637-642.

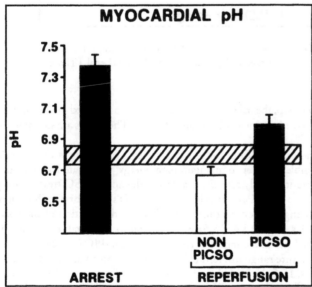

Fig. 13.2. Myocardial pH in the Distal LAD. NOTE: a) The horizontal cross-hatched bar represents the control LAD pH in all hearts. b) pH increases above control during cardioplegic arrest in all hearts. c) Following reperfusion, PICSO treated hearts have a significantly higher tissue pH. Reprinted with permission from Lazar HL et al. J Thorac Cardiovasc Surg 1988; 95:637-642.

coronary occlusion, thereby reducing ischemic injury.[15] We used a protocol similar to our previous reperfusion experiments.

Twenty pigs were placed on CPB and the aorta was crossclamped for 2 hours, during which time the mid-LAD was occluded with a snare. Hearts were protected with hypothermic, crystalloid, antegrade, potassium cardioplegia given every 20 minutes. We intentionally did not use topical hypothermia so that only the effects of cardioplegia delivery could be studied. Following aortic unclamping, the LAD snare was released, and all hearts were reperfused on CPB for 60 minutes. During the period of cardioplegic arrest, hearts were treated with or without PICSO. In the 10 PICSO treated hearts, PICSO was initiated only during each infusion of antegrade

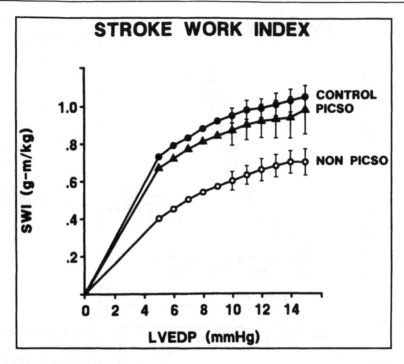

Fig. 13.3. Stroke Work Index. NOTE: Stroke Work Index (SWI) returned to control levels and is significantly higher in PICSO treated hearts. Reprinted with permission from Lazar HL et al. J Thorac Surg 1988;
95: 637-642.

cardioplegia. In the nonPICSO group, the balloon-tipped catheter was positioned in the coronary
sinus but PICSO was not performed during cardioplegic infusions. The results are summarized
in Figures 13.4–13.7.

　　One of the most important prerequisites for any cardioplegia technique is to achieve a
complete arrest as soon as possible in order to maintain high-energy phosphate levels. In this
study, PICSO treated hearts arrested nearly four times as fast as the non-PICSO treated group
(27 ± 5 versus 102 ± 21 seconds, p<.05). Further evidence of PICSO's superior distribution of
cardioplegia was seen in the changes in temperature and pH in the distribution of the distal
LAD and the circumflex arteries (Figs. 13.4, 13.5) Although mean temperature was in the
10°C to 18°C range in both the LAD and circumflex regions in the nonPICSO-treated hearts,
this supposedly optimal temperature range still resulted in significant postischemic changes in
LV compliance and LVSWI (Figs. 13.6, 13.7). Although temperature differences in the circumflex
region were not significantly different between PICSO-treated and nonPICSO-treated hearts,
there was a significant difference in pH between the two groups (Fig. 13.4). In the LAD
region, PICSO-treated hearts achieved lower temperatures (16.8 ± 0.3°C vs 18.6 ± 0.5°C;
p<0.02) and had significantly fewer changes in pH (ΔpH) from control values (Fig. 13.5).
These changes in pH persisted during the reperfusion period. The higher pH in the
PICSO-treated hearts resulted not only from PICSO's ability to better redistribute cold
cardioplegia, which lowers tissue temperature and increases the ph of water, but also from
PICSO's washout of acid metabolites which are known to accumulate during ischemic arrest.
The improved distribution of cardioplegia in the PICSO-treated hearts was reflected in the indices
of postischemic LV function. PICSO hearts generated a higher LVSWI (Fig. 13.7) and had no
change in their postischemic compliance as reflected in pressure-volume curves (Fig. 13.6).

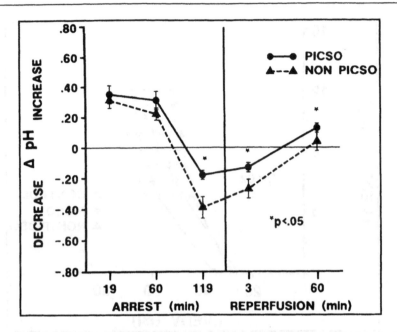

Fig. 13.4. pH Changes in the Distribution of the Circumflex Artery. NOTE: a) An initial rise in pH above control occurred in both groups. b) Subsequently, the decrease in pH was more pronounced in the nonPICSO-treated group at the end of the cross-clamp period. c) Values in both groups returned toward control pH values during the reperfusion period. Reprinted with permission from Ann Thorac Surg 1988; 46:202-207. Cardiovasc Surg 1988; 95:637-642.

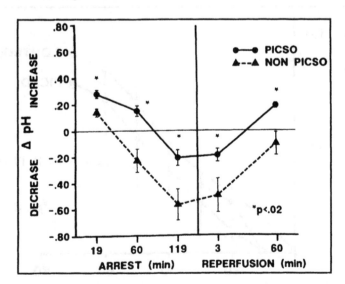

Fig. 13.5. pH Changes in the Distribution of the LAD. NOTE: a) Although there was a steady decrease in pH from control levels in both groups during ischemic arrest, ΔpH was consistently less in the PICSO-treated group. b) During reperfusion, pH returned toward control levels in the PICSO-treated hearts but remained below control in the nonPICSO-treated group. Reprinted with permission from Ann Thorac Surg 1988; 46:202-207.

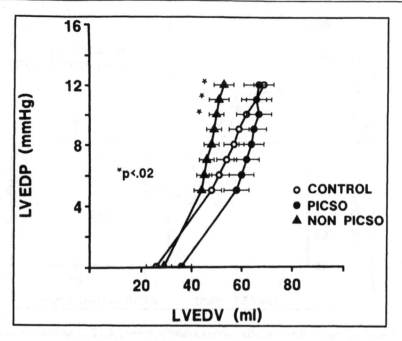

Fig. 13.6. LV Compliance. NOTE: Postischemic pressure-volume curves in nonPICSO hearts was shifted to the left, indicated a stiffer, less compliant heart. Reprinted with permission from Ann Thorac Surg 1988; 46:202-207.

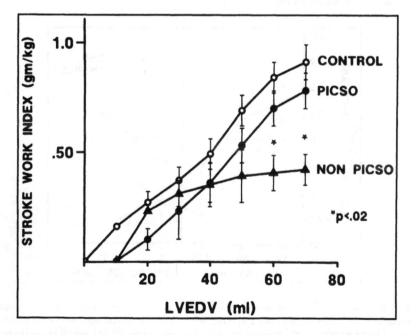

Fig. 13.7. LV Stroke Work Index (SWI). NOTE: Postischemic hearts treated with PICSO generated a significantly higher LVSWI as LVEDV increased. Reprinted with permission from Ann Thorac Surg 1991; 51:408-412.

The superior myocardial protection afforded by PICSO during antegrade cardioplegic arrest in the presence of an occluded coronary artery prompted us to compare the effects of retrograde coronary sinus cardioplegia with standard antegrade techniques. Although experimental studies had shown that in the presence of coronary occlusions, retrograde cardioplegia resulted in more complete recovery of regional and global myocardial function,[16,17] several clinical studies in patients undergoing CABG surgery failed to show any added protection with retrograde techniques.[18,19] In these clinical studies, patients had normal ventricular function and stable angina patterns. A more accurate assessment of the potential advantages of retrograde cardioplegia would be in the setting of acute coronary ischemia such as that which occurs after a failed PTCA. We, therefore, designed an experimental study in a setting analogous to a failed PTCA to determine whether retrograde coronary sinus cardioplegia would result in more optimal myocardial protection than antegrade cardioplegia.[20] In addition to looking at the recovery of wall motion in the jeopardized myocardium at risk, we sought to determine whether retrograde cardioplegia might also decrease the amount of myocardial necrosis.

In 20 pigs, the second and third diagonal vessels just distal to the takeoff of the LAD were occluded with snares for 1.5 hours. Animals were then placed on CPB and underwent 30 minutes of ischemic arrest with multidose, hypothermic potassium crystalloid cardioplegia supplemented with topical and systemic hypothermia. In 10 animals the cardioplegia was given antegrade through the aortic root, whereas in 10 others it was given retrograde through the coronary sinus. After the arrest period, the coronary snares were released and all hearts were reperfused for 3 hours on CPB.

During the period of cardioplegic arrest, there was no difference in temperature between the two cardioplegic techniques in the area beyond the coronary occlusions. However, there appeared to be less acidosis in the retrograde group in the area at risk immediately before aortic unclamping, although this did not reach statistical significance (Fig. 13.8). We suspect that the short aortic crossclamp time combined with the use of topical hypothermia may have masked

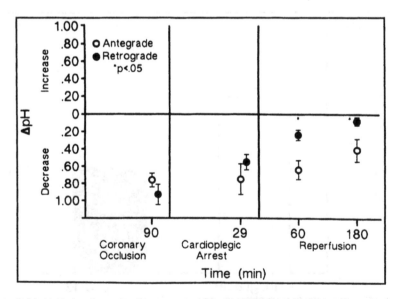

Fig. 13.8. Changes in Myocardial pH. NOTE: a) During cardioplegic arrest, pH values tend to be higher in the retrograde group. b) During reperfusion, pH values are significantly higher in the retrograde cardioplegia protected hearts. Reprinted with permission from Ann Thorac Surg 1991; 51:408-412.

the temperature differences seen in previous studies comparing retrograde and antegrade cardioplegia.[16,17] Nevertheless, there was significantly less tissue acidosis in the area at risk during reperfusion, suggesting that this area received more uniform cardioplegic distribution during arrest. As in our previous studies using PICSO and antegrade cardioplegia, we could find no difference in the degree of protection provided by either technique in areas of myocardium supplied by unobstructed vessels. Hearts protected with retrograde coronary sinus cardioplegia had significantly less infarcted tissue in the area at risk ($43.4\% \pm 3.6$ versus $73.3 \pm 3.5\%$; $p<0.0001$; Fig. 13.9). This occurred despite the absence of significant improvement in wall motion scores in the area of risk between the two cardioplegic techniques. We suspect that this persistent depression in systolic shortening is due to "stunned myocardium" and provides further evidence that depressed wall motion immediately after reperfusion is not a valid index of the degree of myocardial necrosis.[21]

These experimental studies clearly showed that in the presence of a coronary occlusion, techniques employing retrograde perfusion such as PICSO and coronary sinus cardioplegia, resulted in more uniform distribution of cardioplegia, especially to potentially jeopardized areas of myocardium. As a result, there was more complete recovery of ventricular function and less necrosis.

With these experimental studies, we established that the PICSO technique effectively reduced ischemic damage during the reperfusion and cardioplegic arrest period. It had been traditional for surgeons to concentrate their efforts on decreasing ischemic damage during surgical revascularization to the periods of cardioplegic arrest and reperfusion. However, in recent years, an increasing number of patients present for surgical revascularization with ongoing ischemia and necrosis. In a series of patients undergoing CABG surgery after a failed PTCA at the Boston University Medical Center, 64% of patients had some evidence of myocardial necrosis by ECG or enzyme criteria.[22] The presence of new ECG changes immediately after coronary occlusion in the catheterization laboratory in this series was one of the factors that

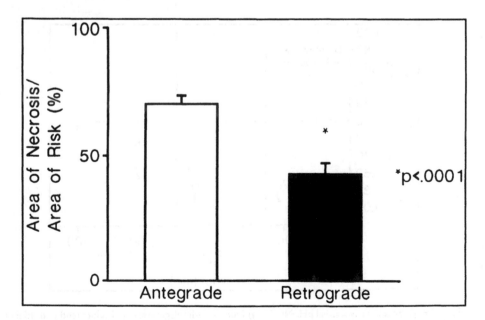

Fig. 13.9. Area of Necrosis/Area of Risk NOTE: Hearts protected with retrograde cardioplegia have significantly less myocardial necrosis. Reprinted with permission from Ann Thorac Surg 1991; 51:408-412.

predisposed to a perioperative myocardial infarction. In a recent series from the same institution, the surgical mortality for CABG surgery after failed PTCA was 11% with 35% of patients having a documented Q-wave myocardial infarction.[23] In this series, the use of antegrade reperfusion catheters failed to result in a decrease in infarct rates. These studies suggest that strategies aimed at reducing myocardial necrosis after acute coronary occlusion must begin immediately in the catheterization laboratory or the coronary care unit once ischemic changes are detected. The period of normothermic ischemia prior to cardioplegic arrest in the operating room became the focus for our next series of experiments to determine whether the initiation of PICSO immediately following coronary occlusion would result in more complete recovery of acutely ischemic myocardium.

Effects of PICSO and Retroperfusion Immediately Following Coronary Occlusion

We used our standard experimental protocol of 1.5 hours of occlusion of the second and third diagonal vessels, 0.5 hour of cardioplegic arrest and 3 hours of reperfusion to simulate the events following a failed PTCA. Ten animals had no interventions. In 10 others, PICSO was instituted immediately following the coronary occlusion and continued throughout the periods of cardioplegic arrest and reperfusion (Fig. 13.10).[24] The results are summarized in Figures 13.11-13.13. Hearts treated with PICSO had significantly less tissue acidosis during the periods of cardioplegic arrest and reperfusion (Fig. 13.11), significantly higher wall motion scores (Fig. 13.12) and a significantly lower area of necrosis ($27 \pm 4\%$ vs $73 \pm 4\%$; $p<.02$; Fig. 13.13). These results strongly suggested that retroperfusion with PICSO significantly reduces ischemic damage during urgent surgical revascularization. It also suggested that PICSO should be started as soon as possible in an attempt to limit the degree of ischemic damage during the period prior to cardioplegic arrest. Despite these favorable results, nearly 27% of the myocardium at risk had infarcted using PICSO alone. PICSO was successful because it redirected blood flow to the jeopardized myocardium and enhanced the washout of acidic metabolites. Our previous studies had shown that substrate enhancement with amino acids such as L-glutamate resulted in enhanced recovery of regional and global ventricular function in hearts subjected to ischemic injury.[25,26] We, therefore, undertook an additional series of

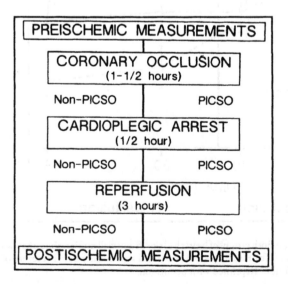

Fig. 13.10. Experimental Protocol. Reprinted with permission.

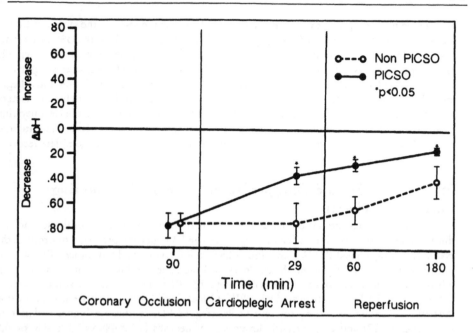

Fig. 13.11. Myocardial pH. Values are expressed as the change in pH from control (Δ pH) NOTE: PICSO treated hearts had significantly less tissue acidosis during the periods of cardioplegic arrest and reperfusion. Reprinted with permission.

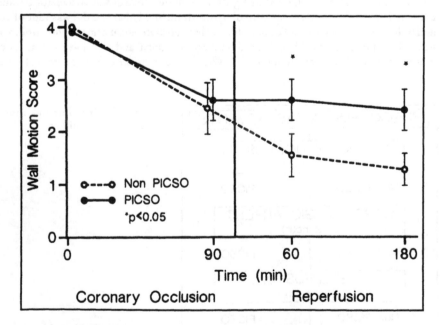

Fig. 13.12. Regional Wall Motion. Note: (a) Both groups of hearts had significant wall motion abnormalities following the period of coronary occlusion. (b) PICSO treated hearts had significantly better recovery of wall motion following 3 hours of reperfusion. Reprinted with permission.

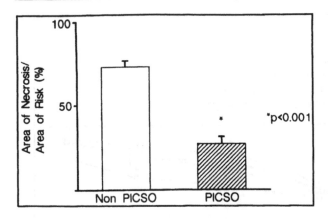

Fig. 13.13. Area Necrosis/Area Risk. PICSO treated hearts had a significantly lower area of necrosis. Reprinted with permission.

experiments to determine whether substrate enhancement with glutamate enriched blood in combination with PICSO would decrease the area of necrosis in acutely ischmic myocardium.[27]

Substrate Enhanced Coronary Venous Retroperfusion

Experimental studies in animals with totally occluded LAD vessels have shown that the retroinfusion of various pharmacological agents such as streptokinase, procainamide, and oxygen free radical scavengers result in substantially higher drug concentrations in the ischemic area of jeopardized myocardium than can be achieved with systemic intravenous administration.[28-31] This has resulted in decreased infarct size and improved ventricular function. The mechanism of retrograde perfusion to the ischemic myocardium was elucidated by Meesman and his coworkers who injected Monastral blue dye through a catheter in the coronary sinus in dogs with and without LAD occlusion.[32] They found that in the absence of an LAD occlusion with normal mean arterial pressure, there was no significant retroperfusion of myocardial tissue. However, in the presence of an LAD occlusion, the myocardium distal to the LAD occlusion was selectively perfused. Furthermore, during systemic hypotension (systolic blood pressure <50 mm Hg), retroperfusion occurred in both the myocardium beyond the LAD occlusion and in unobstructed myocardial tissue. This was associated with a reversal of the normal arteriovenous gradient such that the venous pressure now exceeded arterial pressure. Hence, they concluded that retrograde flow is primarily directed to areas of the myocardium with low antegrade perfusion pressure. Since there is less antegrade flow to the ischemic myocardium, there is less washout of tissues and hence the retrograde-delivered drug has a better chance to accumulate at the microvascular level.

Using these principles, we returned to our model of 90 minutes of diagonal occlusion, 30 minutes of cardioplegic arrest and 3 hours of reperfusion and added two additional groups. In 10 animals, in addition to the standard PICSO technique, blood obtained from a donor animal was passed through a membrane oxygenation (Sarns Membrane Oxygenator, Sarns, Inc., Ann Arbor, MI) and delivered through one of the lumens of the PICSO catheter at a rate of 7 ml/min. In another 10 animals, PICSO was combined with blood to which L-glutamate (13 mM) was added and also administered at a rate of 7 ml/min during the 1.5 hour period of coronary occlusion. The results are summarized in Figs. 13.13-13.16. All PICSO groups showed less tissue acidosis (Fig. 13.14) and better recovery of wall motion (Fig. 13.15). The least amount of necrosis was seen in the hearts treated with PICSO + L-glutamate (Fig. 13.16). Hence, these studies proved that retroperfusion combined with substrate enhancement resulted in the least amount of myocardial necrosis.

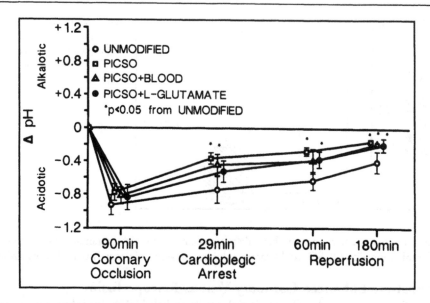

Fig. 13.14. Myocardial pH and Substrate Enhancement. All three PICSO groups had significantly fewer changes in pH from preischemic values during the period of cardioplegic arrest and reperfusion. Reprinted with permission from Lazar HL et al. Circ 1992; 86:II:352-257.

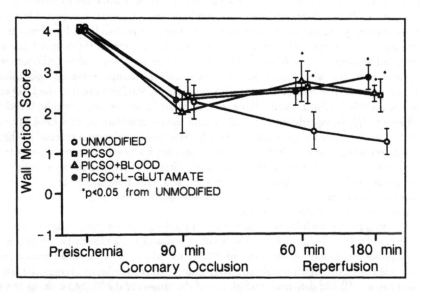

Fig. 13.15. Recovery of Wall Motion. Wall motion scores continued to deteriorate after reperfusion in the unmodified group and are significantly lower than the PICSO, PICSO plus blood, and PICSO plus L-Glutamate groups. Reprinted with permission from Lazar HL et al. Circ 1992; 86:II:352-257.

Retroperfusion and Intraaortic Balloon Pump (IABP) Support

Our experimental studies had clearly demonstrated that PICSO effectively decreases myocardial necrosis, results in better washout of metabolic acid end-products and provides better access for cardioplegic solutions and substrates. However, it has no effect on preload or afterload and cannot independently support the circulation should severe mechanical failure occur. Its major benefits result from its ability to increase myocardial oxygen supply. In contrast, the IABP effectively lowers afterload and provides some mechanical support to the failing myocardium. However, it does not directly increase coronary blood flow, is limited in the presence of severe peripheral vascular disease, and is ineffective in the presence of malignant atrial and ventricular arrhythmias. Both the IABP and PICSO used individually have been shown to reduce infarct size following the reperfusion of an acute coronary occlusion.[2,3,5,15,24,27,33] We therefore undertook an experimental study to determine whether combining coronary venous retroperfusion using PICSO with the principle of ventricular unloading using the IABP would result in superior salvage of ischemic myocardium following acute coronary occlusion.[34]

We used our standard protocol of 90 minutes of acute coronary occlusion followed by 30 minutes of cardioplegic arrest and 3 hours of reperfusion (Fig. 13.17). During the 90 minute period of coronary occlusion, hearts were treated with one of four different interventions:

Unmodified Group: Ten animals received no IABP support or PICSO.

IABP Group: in 10 animals a 9 F IABP (Kontron Laboratories, Everett, MA) was positioned in the descending aorta just below the left subclavian artery via a cutdown in the right femoral artery. Balloon pumping was instituted at a 1:1 cycle with inflation at the beginning of diastole and deflation at the beginning of systole as timed from the surface electrocardiogram.

PICSO Group: Ten animals received PICSO with an inflation:deflation cycle of 8:4 seconds.

IABP-PICSO Group: Ten animals received both the IABP and PICSO.

The results are summarized in Figures 13.17–13.20. The combination of IABP + PICSO did not significantly improve regional wall motion nor did it decrease tissue acidosis compared to the IABP and PICSO groups alone (Figs. 13.18, 13.19). However, the combination of IABP + PICSO did significantly decrease the area of necrosis compared to the other groups (Fig. 13.20). As in our previous studies, we suspect that the inability to improve wall motion was related to myocardial stunning. The decrease in myocardial necrosis supports the concept of using the IABP with retroperfusion techniques to obtain a more favorable alteration of the supply-demand imbalance.

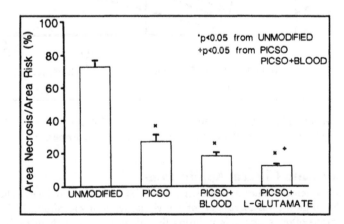

Fig. 13.16. Area Necrosis/Area Risk With Substrate Enhancement. Note: (a) All three PICSO groups had significantly less necrosis than the unmodified group. (b) The least amount of necrosis was seen in hearts treated with PICSO plus L-Glutamate. Reprinted with permission from Lazar HL et al. Circ 1992; 86:II:352-257.

Fig. 13.17. Experimental Protocol.
PICSO & IABP. Reprinted with permission.

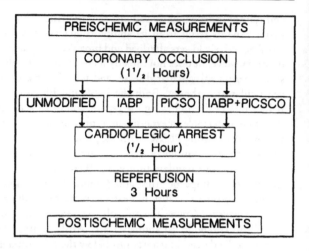

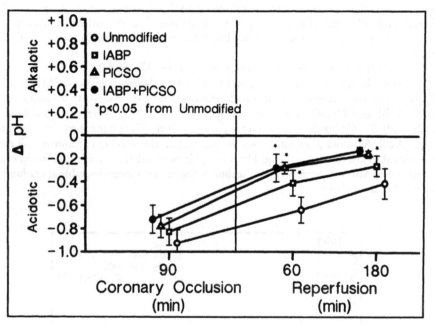

Fig. 13.18. Myocardial pH—PICSO & IABP. Hearts treated with PICSO, IABP, and PICSO and IABP
had significantly less tissue acidosis during reperfusion. Reprinted with permission.

Conclusions and Clinical Applications

Our experimental studies have shown that PICSO effectively reduces ischemic damage
following the surgical revascularization of acutely ischemic myocardium. PICSO is helpful
during all aspects of revascularization; during the initial period of ischemia following a coronary occlusion where it can be used to deliver substrate to areas of jeopardized myocardium;
during the period of cardioplegic arrest when it results in better distribution of cardioplegic
solutions; and during the period of reperfusion where it results in better washout of acid
metabolites. We feel that there will be numerous clinical applications for PICSO for both

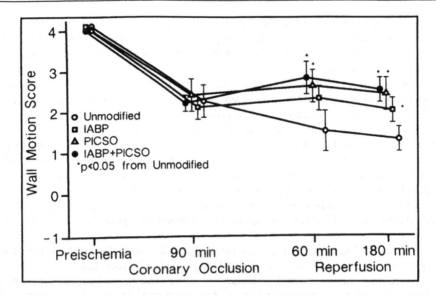

Fig. 13.19. Wall Motion Scores - PICSO and IABP. Wall motion scores in the PICSO, IABP, and PICSO and IABP groups are significantly better during reperfusion than the unmodified group. Reprinted with permission.

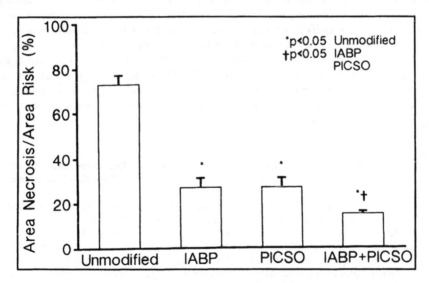

Fig. 13.20. Area Necrosis/Area Risk—PICSO and IABP. The least amount of necrosis occurred in hearts treated with the IABP and PICSO. Reprinted with permission.

cardiologists and cardiac surgeons during acute coronary ischemia syndromes. PICSO may help to minimize ischemic damage during high risk PTCA procedures. This would be particularly helpful for patients with ongoing ischemia with a large area of myocardium at risk. PICSO may also be of benefit to patients with an acute myocardial infarction. In these patients, PICSO can be initiated at local community hospitals that have access to fluoroscopy but do not have a catheterization laboratory. Inotropic, antiarrhythmic, lytic, substrate, and free radical scavenger agents can then be delivered as the patient is being transported to a tertiary care center for diagnostic catheterization. This helps to expand the time window so that cardiac catheterization can be performed to determine what type of revascularization procedure (PTCA vs CABG) will be required.

We feel that PICSO will be especially helpful for patients with a failed PTCA who require urgent surgical revascularization. As noted earlier, most patients who develop perioperative infarctions following emergent CABG for a failed PTCA develop EKG changes in the catheterization laboratory.[22,23] The initiation of PICSO in the catheterization laboratory may help to limit infarct size during the time the patient is being transported to the operating room and prior to the completion of all bypass grafts. This is especially true in those situations where a bailout or autoperfusion catheter cannot be used to restore flow across the occluded vessel. The PICSO catheter can also be used to deliver retrograde cardioplegia in the operating room thus assuring that there will be more uniform cooling and distribution of cardioplegia to the area at risk. Furthermore, PICSO can be used during the reperfusion period and left in place in the ICU.

Finally, PICSO appears to enhance such support devices as the IABP and percutaneous bypass by increasing myocardial blood supply to jeopardized myocardium.

As noted earlier, the research laboratory provides a more optimal setting to determine the efficacy of new techniques since biochemical, functional, and histological recovery can be more closely defined. In order to determine the role of PICSO and other retroperfusion techniques in clinical practice, carefully matched randomized studies in patients with evolving myocardial infarctions and unstable angina will be necessary to further define their roles in clinical practice. More sophisticated diagnostic techniques such as PET scanning and echocardiography may be needed to quantify infarct size and the recovery of wall motion. Finally, newer catheter designs will have to be tested and introduced which will withstand the rigors of clinical practice and be approved by government regulatory agencies. Nevertheless, our experimental studies have shown that coronary sinus interventions such as PICSO have the potential to play a major role in limiting infarct size and decreasing morbidity and mortality in patients requiring urgent revascularization. The challenge will be for clinicians to begin to implement this new technology into their clinical practices.

References

1. Mohl W. The development and rationale of pressure controlled intermittent coronary sinus occlusion: A new approach to protect ischemic myocardium. Wien Klin Wochenschr 1984; 96:205-9.
2. Mohl W, Glogar DH, Mary H et al. Reduction of infarct size induced by pressure-controlled intermittent coronary sinus occlusion. Am J Cardiol 1984; 53:923-8.
3. Mohl W, Punzengruber C, Moser et al. Effects of pressure-controlled intermittent coronary sinus occlusion on regional ischemic myocardial function. J Am Coll Cardiol 1985; 5:939-947.
4. Mohl W, Glogar D, Kenner T et al. Enhancement of washout induced by PICSO in the canine and human heart. In: Mohl W, Wolner E, Glogar D, eds. The Coronary Sinus. New York: Spring-Verlag, 1984:537-48.
5. Lazar HL, Rajaii A, Roberts AJ. Reversal of reperfusion injury after ischemic arrest with pressure-controlled intermittent coronary sinus occlusion. J Thorac Cardiovasc Surg 1988; 95:637-42.
6. Lange R, Kloner RA, Zierler M et al. Time course of ischemic alternations during normothermic and hypothermic arrest and its reflection by on-line monitoring of tissue pH. J Thorac Cardiovasc Surg 1984; 86:418-22.
7. Khuri SF, Josa M, Martson J et al. First report of intramyocardial pH in man. Assessment of adequacy of myocardial preservation. J Thorac Cardiovasc Surg 1983; 86:667-672.

8. Lazar HL, Haasler GB, Spotnitz WD et al. Compliance, mass, and shape of the canine left ventricle after global ischemia analyzed with two-dimensional echocardiography. J Surg Res 1985; 39:199-208.
9. Nachlas MM, Shnitka TK. Macroscopic identification of early myocardial infarcts by alterations in dehydrogenase activity. Am J Pathol 1963; 42:379-84.
10. Schaper J, Schaper TK. Reperfusion of ischemic myocardium: Ultrastructural and histochemical aspects. J Am Coll Cardiol 1983; 4:1037-41.
11. Lazar HL, Rivers S. Importance of topical hypothermia in reducing ischemic damage during heterogenous cardioplegic arrest. J Thorac Cardiovasc Surg 1989; 98:251-57.
12. Heineman FW, MacGregor DC, Wilson GJ, Ninomiya J. Regional and transmural myocardial temperature distribution in cold chemical cardioplegia: Significance of critical coronary artery stenosis. J Thorac Cardovasc Surg 1981; 81:851-55.
13. Grondin CM, Helias J, Vouche PR, Pierre R. Influence of a critical coronary artery stenosis on myocardial protection through cold potassium cardioplegia. J Thorac Cardiovasc Surg 1981; 82:608-12.
14. Dorsey LM, Colgan TK, Silverstein JI et al. Alterations in regional myocardial function after heterogenous cardioplegia. J Thorac Cardiovasc Surg 1983; 86:70-5.
15. Lazar HL, Khoury T, Rivers S. Improved distribution of cardioplegia with pressure-controlled intermittent coronary sinus occlusion. Ann Thorac Surg 1988; 46:202-7.
16. Gundry SR, Kirsh MM. A comparison of retrograde versus antegrade cardioplegia in the presence of coronary artery obstruction. Ann Thorac Surg 1984; 38:124-7.
17. Partington MT, Acar C, Buckberg GD, Julia PL. Studies of retrograde cardioplegia: II Advantages of antegrade/retrograde cardioplegia to optimize distribution in jeopardized myocardiu. J Thorac Cardiovasc Surg 1989; 97:613-22.
18. Bhayana JN, Kalmbach T, Booth F, Mentzer RM, Schimert G. Combined antegrade/retrograde cardioplegia for myocardial protection: A clinical trial. J Thorac Cardiovasc Surg 1989; 98:956-60.
19. Fiore AC, Naunheim KS, Kaiser GC et al. Coronary sinus versus aortic root perfusion wit blood cardioplegia in elective myocardial revascularization. Ann Thorac Surg 1989; 47:684-8.
20. Haan C, Lazar HL, Bernard S, Rivers S, Zallnick J, Shemin RJ. Superiority of retrograde cardioplegia after acute coronary occlusion. Ann Thorac Surg 1991; 51:408-12.
21. Kloner RA, Ellis SG, Carlson NV, Braunwald E. Coronary reperfusion for the treatment of acute myocardial infarction/postischemic ventricular dysfunction. Am J Cardiol 1983; 70:233-46.
22. Lazar HL, Haan CK. Determinants of myocardial infarction following emergency coronary artery bypass for failed percutaneous coronary angioplasty. Ann Thorac Surg 1987; 44:646-50.
23. Lazar HL, Faxon DP, Paone G et al. Changing profiles of failed coronary angioplasty patients: Impact on surgical results. Ann Thorac Surg 1992; 53:269-73.
24. Lazar HL, Haan C, Bernard S, Rivers S, Shemin RJ. Reduction of infarct size following revascularization of an acute coronary sinus occlusion (PICSO). J Mol Cell Cardiol 1990; 22:515.
25. Lazar HL, Buckberg GD, Manganero AJ, Becker H, Maloney JF. Reversal of ischemic damage with amino acid substrate enhancement during reperfusion. Surgery 1980; 88:702-10.
26. Lazar HL, Buckberg GD, Manganaro AM, Becker H. Myocardial energy replenishment and reversal of ischemic damage by substrate enhancement of secondary blood cardioplegia with amino acids during reperfusion. J Thorac Cardiovasc Surg 1980; 80:350-9.
27. Lazar HL, Haan CK, Yang X, Rivers S, Bernard S, Shemin RJ. Reduction of infarct size with coronary venous retroperfusion. Circ 1992; 86 II:352-7.
28. Meerbaum S, Lang TW, Pouzhitkov M. Retrograde lysis of coronary artery thrombus by coronary venous streptokinase adminsitration. J Am Col Cardiol 1983; 1:1262-7.
29. Karagueozian HS, Ohta M, Drury JK. Coronary venous retroinfusion of procainamide: A new approach for the management of spontaneous and inducible sustained ventricular tachycardia during myocardial infartction. J Am Coll Cardiol 1986; 7:551-63.

30. Hatori N, Miyasaki A, Todokoro H. Beneficial effects of coronary venous retroinfusion of superoxide dismutase and catalase on reperfusion arrhythmias, myocardial function and infarct size in dogs. J Cardiovasc Pharmacol 1989; 14:396-404.
31. Kobayashi S, Tadokoro H, Wakida Y et al. Coronary venous retroinfusion of deferoxamine reduces infarct size in pigs. J Am Coll Cardiol 1991; 18:621-7.
32. Meesman M, Karagueozian HS, Takashi I et al. Selective perfuison of ischemic myocardium during coronary venous retroinjection: A study of the causative role of venoarterial and venoventricular pressure gradients. J Am Coll Cardiol 1987; 10:887-97.
33. Lazar HL, Yang XM, Rivers S, Treanor P, Shemin RJ. Role of percutaneous bypass in reducing infarct size after revascularization for acute coronary insufficiency. Circ 1991; 84:II:416-21.
34. Lazar HL, Yang XM, Rivers S, Treanor P, Bernard S, Shemin RJ. Retroperfusion and balloon support to improve coronary revascularization. J Cardiovasc Surg 1992; 33:538-44.

CHAPTER 14

Coronary Venous Retroinfusion During Interventional Cardiology

Peter Boekstegers

Introduction

D uring the past decade, several percutaneous support devices for coronary angioplasty have been developed with the aim of improving myocardial tolerance to ischemia, thereby increasing the safety of coronary angioplasty and allowing the expansion of its indications. Thus, supported coronary angioplasty has been applied in patients with high risk conditions such as multivessel disease, unstable angina, impaired left ventricular function and myocardial infarction complicated by cardiogenic shock.[1-5] In the event of abrupt vessel closure during coronary angioplasty, mechanical support devices may provide a bridge until reperfusion is established[1,4] either by repeated coronary angioplasty or by emergency bypass surgery. The broader application of percutaneous support devices for high risk coronary angioplasty, however, is still limited by their inadequate efficacy or by complications associated with their use.[1,5-7]

Three main approaches have been chosen for mechanical support of acutely ischemic myocardium during coronary angioplasty: antegrade methods, whole heart support and retroinfusion of coronary veins (Fig. 14.1).

Antegrade methods provide regional support of the ischemic myocardium through the balloon catheter, i.e. autoperfusion[8] or pumping of either autologous blood[9,10] or synthetic oxygen carriers.[11-14] Regional myocardial protection, however, is not ensured until the stenotic lesion has been passed. Thus, antegrade methods may be difficult to apply in patients with unstable hemodynamic conditions, in patients with tortuous, small or diffusely disease vessels as well as in patients with sequential stenoses.[1]

Support of the whole heart independent of the stenotic lesion is possible using cardiopulmonary bypass,[2,15] intraaortic balloon counterpulsation[1] as well as left ventricular assist devices.[5] Though hemodynamic stability may be preserved using these techniques,[2,5,15] regional myocardial ischemia persists during coronary angioplasty. Furthermore, significant complications increasing morbidity and mortality of high risk coronary angioplasty have been observed using cardiopulmonary bypass.[7]

The third approach is through the backdoor of the heart by retroinfusion of coronary veins. Retrograde techniques combine both 1) regional support of ischemic myocardium and 2) their application being independent of the passage of the stenotic lesion. Thus, prophylactic installation or treatment is possible as well as its application in the event of abrupt vessel closure.[4] Furthermore, retroinfusion methods have the advantage of being less invasive than most other support devices and no major complications have been described in their clinical use.[3,4,16]

Coronary Sinus Interventions in Cardiac Surgery, Second Edition edited by Werner Mohl.
©2000 Eurekah.com.

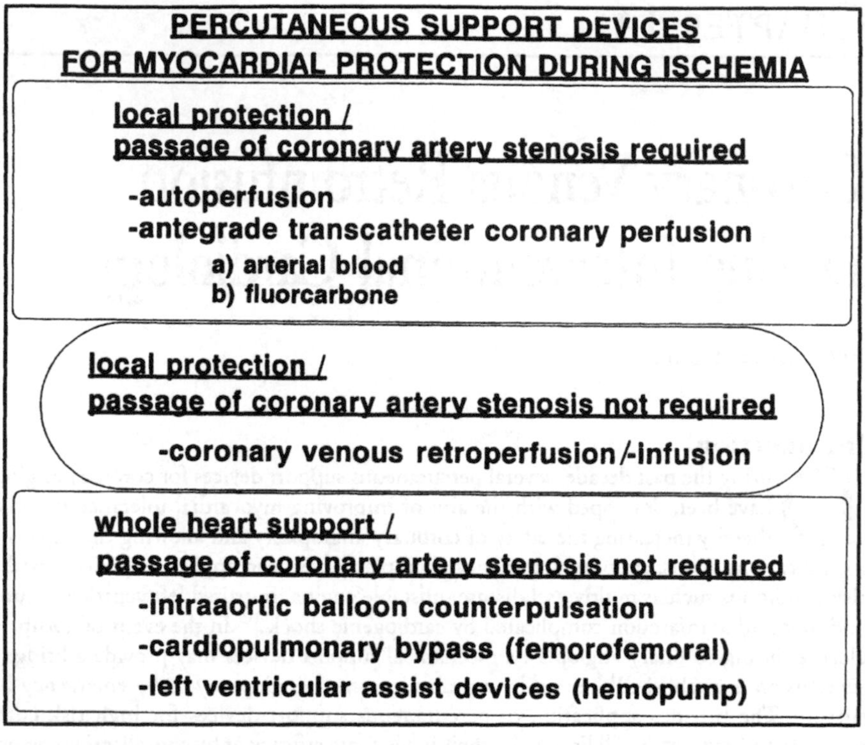

```
┌─────────────────────────────────────────────────────────────┐
│              PERCUTANEOUS SUPPORT DEVICES                     │
│       FOR MYOCARDIAL PROTECTION DURING ISCHEMIA               │
│   ┌───────────────────────────────────────────────────────┐  │
│   │  local protection /                                    │  │
│   │  passage of coronary artery stenosis required          │  │
│   │                                                        │  │
│   │   -autoperfusion                                       │  │
│   │   -antegrade transcatheter coronary perfusion          │  │
│   │       a) arterial blood                                │  │
│   │       b) fluorcarbone                                  │  │
│   └───────────────────────────────────────────────────────┘  │
│   ╭───────────────────────────────────────────────────────╮  │
│   │  local protection /                                    │  │
│   │  passage of coronary artery stenosis not required      │  │
│   │      -coronary venous retroperfusion/-infusion         │  │
│   ╰───────────────────────────────────────────────────────╯  │
│   ┌───────────────────────────────────────────────────────┐  │
│   │  whole heart support /                                 │  │
│   │  passage of coronary artery stenosis not required      │  │
│   │   -intraaortic balloon counterpulsation                │  │
│   │   -cardiopulmonary bypass (femorofemoral)              │  │
│   │   -left ventricular assist devices (hemopump)          │  │
│   └───────────────────────────────────────────────────────┘  │
└─────────────────────────────────────────────────────────────┘
```

Fig. 14.1. Different concepts of percutaneous support devices for myocardial protection during ischemia.

The efficacy of retroinfusion support, however, is the crucial limitation so far. Therefore, our review first discusses the efficacy of three different techniques of coronary venous retroinfusion in the light of recent experimental data. Secondly, the results of clinical pilot studies obtained with synchronized coronary venous retroperfusion (SRP) are compared to antegrade methods. Thirdly, potential clinical applications and future perspectives for retroinfusion support in interventional cardiology are discussed.

Different Concepts of Coronary Venous Retroinfusion

Today, three retroinfusion techniques are available with different underlying concepts (Fig. 14.2). These concepts substantially influence selectivity and efficacy of retrograde support and, thus, their potential clinical application.

Synchronized coronary venous retroperfusion (SRP) was developed in 1976 with the idea of providing augmented diastolic retroperfusion of arterial blood and to facilitate coronary venous drainage during systole.[17] Since then, the retroperfusion system and catheters were improved with respect to the autoinflatable balloon and to the possibility of higher pump flows.[4,18] The basic concept, however, was not changed. Using diastolic arterial retroperfusion, venous drainage is achieved by systolic squeezing around the deflated balloon at the catheter tip (Fig. 14.2). This form of venous drainage with SRP implies that, in order to avoid obstruction, catheterization is restricted to veins of sufficient size. Therefore, selective retroinfusion of the veins draining the ischemic myocardium is not possible, and, hence, nonischemic myocardium is also retroinfused using SRP. In animal models with occlusion of the left anterior

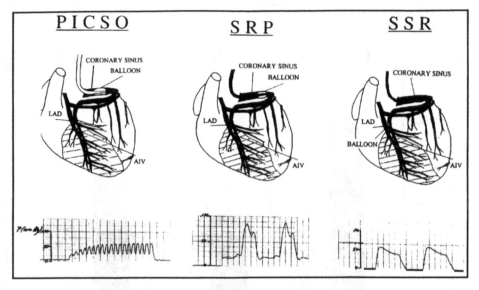

Fig. 14.2. Comparative schemes of the three concepts of coronary venous retroinfusion with particular regard to the site of regional support (position of the catheter balloon). Typical recordings of coronary venous pressure (P) from each system during treatment in pigs are shown. PICSO = pressure controlled intermittent coronary sinus occlusion, SRP = synchronized coronary venous retroperfusion, SSR = selective ecg-synchronized suction and retroinfusion of coronary veins. LAD = left anterior descending artery. AIV = anterior interventricular vein.

descending artery, the tip of the retroperfusion catheter was usually placed in the coronary sinus or great cardiac vein (Fig. 14.2). Using these catheter positions it was demonstrated that SRP resulted in nutritive blood flow to the ischemic myocardium.[19] Though sensitive methods for determination of metabolism were used, the amount and distribution of oxygen delivery as well as of nutrient exchange induced by SRP has not yet been defined.

Pressure controlled intermittent coronary sinus occlusion (PICSO) was developed in 1984[20] based on the concept that increasing coronary venous pressure by intermittent occlusion of the coronary sinus (Fig. 14.2) results in venous retroperfusion predominantly of the ischemic myocardium. Indeed, there is evidence that PICSO results in alternating venous blood flow over the ischemic region[21] and enhances washout of metabolites accumulating during ischemia.[22] PICSO, similar to SRP, is a nonselective approach of retroinfusion.

In contrast to SRP and PICSO, the concept of selective synchronized suction and retroinfusion of coronary veins (SSR)[23] is, first, to approach as near as possible to the ischemic myocardium in order to selectively retroinfuse only the veins draining the ischemic region. Second, an ECG-synchronized suction device reduces coronary venous pressure and residual blood volume in the veins draining the ischemic region before each retrograde pumping stroke (Fig. 14.2). The suction device guarantees adequate venous drainage despite permanent occlusion of the vein by the retroinfusion catheter balloon during SSR. Furthermore, the concept was based on the assumption that pumping into empty veins using a catheter position close to the ischemic myocardium increases effective blood exchange. Using SSR, the venous blood or the desaturated arterial blood is not pumped retrogradely first in contrast to SRP. Thus, the probability of reaching nutritive capillaries with each retrograde pumping cycle increases. Effective retrograde oxygen delivery with the use of SSR has been demonstrated by direct measurements of myocardial tissue oxygenation.[23,24]

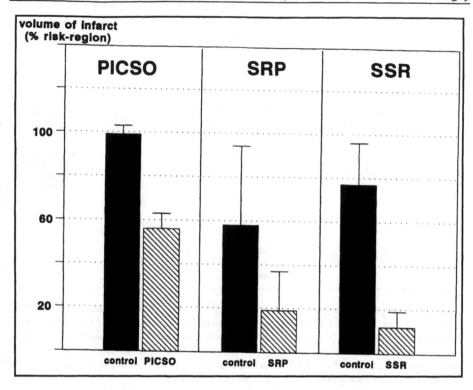

Fig. 14.3. Comparison of the efficacy of the three concepts of coronary venous retroinfusion to reduce myocardial infarction in dogs (results according to 18, 20, 23). PICSO = pressure controlled intermittent coronary sinus occlusion; SRP = synchronized coronary venous retroperfusion; SSR = selective ECG-synchronized suction and retroinfusion of coronary veins.

Comparison of the Efficacy of PICSO, SRP and SSR in Experimental Models

The efficacy of each retroinfusion support has been determined in experimental models of myocardial infarction with several hours of ischemia and, more recently, in models with transient brief occlusion of the coronary artery to simulated ischemia occurring during coronary angioplasty. In models of myocardial infarction the primary goal was to prevent cell necrosis in contrast to preservation of regional myocardial function in settings with brief ischemia. Apparently, retrograde oxygen delivery and nutrient exchange have to provide only basal requirements to maintain viability of myocardial cells. Preservation of myocardial function, however, needs nutrient exchange equivalent to at least 30–50% of normal antegrade blood flow.[25] This difference between preservation of basal metabolism and metabolic requirements for myocardial function has to be kept in mind when considering the potential clinical indications of each retroinfusion technique.

For each retroinfusion technique significant protection against myocardial infarction was demonstrated in dog models with several hours of ischemia (Fig. 14.3). Direct comparison of PICSO and SRP in the same experimental setting showed that reduction of myocardial necrosis was similar.[26] SSR using oxygenated Ringer's lactate solution instead of arterial blood resulted in 84% reduction of infarct size (Fig. 14.3) which seems to be favorable compared to SRP and PICSO. The efficacy of SSR in reduction of infarct size, however, was not directly compared to PICSO or SRP.[23] In all studies with the use of SRP or SSR, infarct size was determined 5–6 hours after coronary artery occlusion without reperfusion. Therefore, it cannot be decided definitively whether myocardial necrosis was prevented or just delayed by SRP and SSR. Only in the case of PICSO during ischemia, was infarct size determined 10 days after reperfusion, and, thus, ultimate reduction in the amount of myocardial cell necrosis was demonstrated.[27] Nevertheless, taking into account all experimental data available so far, it might be assumed that at least similar protection against myocardial infarction is possible using SRP or SSR compared to PICSO. On the other hand, the superiority of SRP or SSR to reduce infarct size has also not been demonstrated. Hence, if the aim is to preserve basal metabolism and to prevent myocardial infarction, PICSO might be sufficient and is the least invasive technique of coronary venous retroinfusion.

The efficacy of preserving myocardial function, however, is substantially different between PICSO, SRP and SSR. In dog as well as in pig models, PICSO did not prevent complete loss of regional myocardial function.[28,29] In contrast, SRP was able to preserve 52% of baseline regional myocardial function during a two minute occlusion of the left anterior descending artery in a dog model.[30] As indicated by earlier studies,[31] arterialization of the coronary veins draining the ischemic region is necessary to achieve retrograde oxygen delivery and nutrient exchange[19] sufficient to preserve regional myocardial function. The results obtained using SRP, however, are influenced by the specific anatomy of coronary arteries and veins. In pigs with the characteristic feature of rare arterial collaterals,[32] the efficacy of SRP was too low to prevent loss of regional myocardial function during ischemia (Fig. 14.4).[33-35] Residual blood flow delivered through arterial collaterals into the ischemic region during complete coronary artery occlusion is very low (<5% of baseline value) in pigs.[32,34] In contrast, it

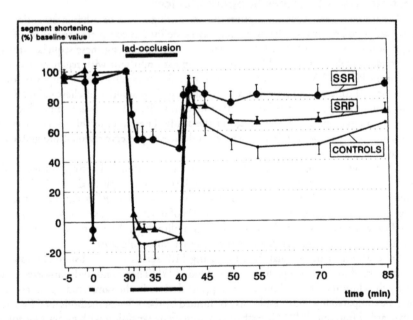

Fig. 14.4. Comparison of the efficacy of the three concepts of coronary venous retroinfusion to preserve regional myocardial function in pigs (results according to 24). Black bars indicating occlusion of the left anterior descending artery (LAD). First lad-occlusion (1 min) without treatment in all pigs. Second LAD-occlusion (10 min) a) with treatment by selective ECG-synchronized suction and retroinfusion of coronary veins (SSR, n = 10) b) with treatment by synchronized coronary venous retroperfusion (SRP, n = 10) c) without treatment (CONTROLS, n = 10).

reaches about 20–25% of baseline arterial flow in dogs.[36] Assuming a threshold for preservation of myocardial function of about 30–40% of baseline arterial flow, it is evident that similar retrograde nutrient flow induced by SRP, e.g., 20%, will result in substantial preservation of myocardial function in dogs but not in pigs.

In contrast to SRP, SSR was able to preserve 70% of baseline regional myocardial function after 1 min of ischemia and 51% after 10 min of ischemia in pigs (Fig. 14.4). Thus, direct comparison of SSR with SRP in an animal model with very low arterial collaterals showed that the efficacy of SSR was substantially higher than SRP.[24] Preservation of regional myocardial function using SSR[24] was even similar to results obtained by continuous "actual" retroperfusion of the anterior interventricular vein with simultaneous venting of left anterior descending artery to zero pressure in pigs, a technique which was not designed for clinical use.[37] This suggests that SSR resulted in a retrograde oxygen delivery and nutrient exchange comparable to actual nonsynchronous retrograde perfusion. In the same study[37] it was demonstrated that only a small amount (<30%) of retrogradely delivered blood passed through the capillary bed to reach the left anterior descending artery (determined by arterial outflow measurements). These findings imply that oxygen delivery and nutrient exchange may occur via extensive thin-walled intramyocardial venous plexus in addition to retrograde capillary filling.[37] Furthermore, the individual anatomy of the veins leading to different volume capacities and pressure/volume dependencies within the venous system seems to influence the efficacy of retroperfusion. Therefore, further studies investigating the pressure/flow relationship to preservation of myocardial function by SSR have been started.

Clinical Results Using Synchronized Retroperfusion (SRP) in Comparison to Other Support Devices

The primary goal of cardiac support devices during PTCA or other interventional procedures leading to brief myocardial ischemia may be defined as complete prevention of ischemia or significant reduction of sequelae induced by ischemia. Among these sequelae, impairment of regional or global myocardial function is the most important with regard to complication rate during PTCA.[38] Myocardial function is an efficacy variable which might be of use for comparison of different support devices. Variables such as severity of chest pain, ST-segment changes or prolongation of balloon inflation during PTCA are less comparable and may depend to a larger extent on the design of the study. Therefore, in this short review we will focus mainly on the efficacy of regional support devices to preserve regional and global myocardial function during PTCA.

Of the three retroperfusion techniques, only synchronized retroperfusion (SRP) has already been applied in patients with elective, high risk and complicated PTCA.[3,4,16] Using the human ischemic model of PTCA with and without support by SRP, a significant preservation of regional myocardial function of about 40–50% of baseline value was observed (Table 14.1). The efficacy of SRP, however, showed a large variability depending not only on the anatomy of the coronary veins but also on the extent of arterial collateralization.[4]

Preservation of myocardial function using SRP seems to be substantially lower (Table 14.1) compared to antegrade perfusion using Fluosol.[11,14] There is no study, however, comparing directly the clinical efficacy of these two support devices in the same study protocol. Furthermore, the comparability of the results may be limited by the different methods used for assessment of myocardial function.[4,11,14] Nevertheless, if antegrade perfusion with either Fluosol or atrial blood can be obtained, myocardial protection against ischemic sequelae appears to be more complete than with the use of the currently available technique of coronary venous retroperfusion (SRP) (Table 14.1).[1] This assumption is supported by the observations that using antegrade catheter perfusion techniques, extended balloon inflations up to several minutes were associated with only minor changes in ECG or chest pain compared to SRP.[3,4,6,14,40]

Global support devices such as percutaneous cardiopulmonary bypass have been developed to support systemic circulation and to prevent cardiogenic shock during PTCA. Though they may also ameliorate myocardial ischemia, preservation of regional myocardial function is not the primary goal. Hence, the efficacy of global support devices cannot be compared to regional support devices using efficacy variables such as myocardial function.[15]

Prevention of cardiogenic shock and successful support after failed angioplasty has been reported in studies using SRP,[3,4] antegrade perfusion,[8] percutaneous cardiopulmonary bypass[1,5] as well as hemopump devices.[5] These studies, however, cannot be compared retrospectively due to selection bias especially in the high risk population. Study endpoints such as prevention of cardiogenic shock or mortality rate in association with supported coronary angioplasty require comparative studies preferably in a prospective multicenter fashion.

Retrospective analysis of complications (Table 14.2) associated with the application of support devices are troublesome for similar reasons. Furthermore, complications occurring during supported PTCA may be related to the angioplasty procedure itself, e.g., acute closure of the vessel, or to the application of the support device. It was a remarkable finding, however, that in a larger study including 105 patients, percutaneous cardiopulmonary bypass increased morbidity and mortality in high-risk coronary angioplasty.[2,7] Furthermore, the combination of percutaneous cardiopulmonary support with regional support devices seemed to improve patient outcome indicating that a higher potential benefit might result from the application of regional support devices.[7]

In contrast to global support devices, regional support devices had a lower complication and mortality rate (Table 14.2). Patients selection, however, in addition to the lesser invasive procedures, might influence complication rate. Synchronized coronary venous retroperfusion appears to have a very low incidence of complications associated with the application of the support device (Table 14.2). Again, definite conclusions with respect to safety cannot be drawn from this retrospective analysis (Table 14.2) and await prospective clinical trials comparing different support devices within the same study.

Potential Clinical Applications and Future Perspectives for Retroinfusion Support in Interventional Cardiology

Species-specific anatomy of coronary arteries and veins has to be considered for interpretation and extrapolation of animal data to humans. Dog and pig models have been used most frequently to study retroinfusion support of ischemic myocardium after complete occlusion of the coronary artery. In dogs, residual blood flow delivered through arterial collaterals into the ischemic region reaches about 20–25% of baseline arterial flow[36] during complete coronary artery occlusion in contrast to pigs with very low residual blood (<5% of baseline value).[32,34] In patients with coronary artery disease, the amount of residual blood flow during coronary artery occlusion depends on the existence of collaterals and, therefore, is different from patient to patient. This implies, that, in a patient with relatively high residual blood flow, retroperfusion support by SRP might be sufficient to preserve regional myocardial function. In a patient with few collaterals, however, SRP might fail to improve regional myocardial function whereas SSR should still be able to maintain regional myocardial function even in these patients. Extrapolation of animal data to humans must be applied with caution; however, preservation of more than 50% of regional myocardial function without a reduction of cardiac output during 10 minutes of ischemia in pigs (Fig. 14.4)[24] suggests that, in patients supported by SSR, prolonged balloon inflations during PTCA or acute closure of the vessel should have only minor effects on regional and global myocardial function.

An obvious limitation of the application of selective synchronized suction and retroinfusion of coronary veins (SSR) in patients is the necessity to selectively catheterize the veins draining the ischemic zone. Catheterization of the anterior ventricular vein should be possible and sufficient to

Table 14.1. Efficacy of regional and global support devices during elective and high risk percutaneous angioplasty

Author	Method	Application	Number of patients (treated patients)	Preservation of regional myocardial function	Preservation of global myocardial function	Balloon inflation time (untreated→treated)	ST-segment (untreated→treated)	Chest pain (score/pts.)
Kar et al[4]	SRP PTCA	elective	43	37%	EF:55%	73s→81s mV	0.16→0.11	1.2→0.8
Nienaber et al[16]	SRP	elective PTCA	26	53%	nd	60s→62s	nd	1.2→1.0
Constantini et al[3]	SRP	high risk PTCA (unstable angina)	20	42%	EF:43% CI:50%	44s→145s	nd	nd
Jaffe et al[12]	antegrade perfusion/Fluosol	elective PTCA	42	nd	EF:86%	nd	nd	nd
Kent et al[14]	antegrade perfusion Fluosol	elective PTCA	245[101]	89%	nd	71s→72s	2.2→1.7mV	nd
Cleman et al[11]	antegrade perfusion/Fluosol	elective PTCA	20	94%	nd	nd	nd	nd
Banka et al[10]	antegrade hemo-perfusion	elective PTCA	43	nd	nd	nd	2.5→0.1mV	6.0→2.4

Author	Method	Application	Number of patients (treated patients)	Preservation of regional myocardial function	Preservation of global myocardial function	Balloon inflation time (untreated →treated)	ST-segment (untreated →treated)	Chest pain (score/pts.)
Di Sciascio et al[39]	antegrade hemoperfusion	elective PTCA	110	nd	nd	1.3 min→7.0 min	2.6→0.7mV	2.9→1.4
Lehmann et al[9]	antegrade hemoperfusion	elective PTCA	15	nd	nd	nd	1.9→0.5mV	6.0→4.1
Muhlestein et al[6]	auto-perfusion	elective PTCA	62	nd	nd	14 min (without control group)	na	na
Pavlides et al[15]	percutaneous cardiopulmonary bypass	elective PTCA	20	na	nd	na	na	nd
Vogel et al[2]	percutaneous cardiopulmonary bypass	high risk PTCA	105	na	na	na	na	na
Feld et al[7]	percutaneous cardiopulmonary bypass	high risk PTCA	56	na	na	na	na	na

nd = not determined; na = not applicable; nr = not reported; PTCA = percutaneous transluminal coronary ; SRP = coronary venous retroperfusion; CABG = coronary artery bypass grafting; EF = ejection fraction.

Table 14.2. Complications related to regional and global support devices during elective and high risk percutaneous angiolasty

Author	Method	Application	Number of patients (treated patients)	Feasibility	Major complication rate	Minor complication rate	Sort of complication	Mortality
Kar et al[4]	SRP	elective PTCA	43	79%	0%	23%	transient atrial fibrillation (n = 2), atrial wall contrast agent staining (n = 1), local hematoma at catheter insertion site (n=4)	0%
Nienaber et al[16]	SRP	elective PTCA	26	77%	0%	11%	transient atrial fibrillation (n = 2), atrial wall contrast agent staining (n=1)	0%
Constantini et al[3]	SRP	high risk PTCA (unstable angina)	20	75%	0%	40%	transient atrial fibrillation (n = 4), local hematoma at catheter insertion site (n = 2)	0%
Jaffe et al[12]	antegrade perfusion/Fluosol	elective PTCA	42	100%	0%	0%	nr	0%
Kent et al[14]	antegrade perfusion/Fluosol	elective PTCA	245[101]	79%	5%	2%	ventricular fibrillation (n = 2), myocardial infarction (n = 1), coronary embolism (n = 1), emergency CABG (n=1), low back pain(n=2)	1%
Cleman et al[11]	antegrade perfusion/Fluosol	elective PTCA	20	100%	0%	0%	nr	0%

Author	Method	Application	Number of patients (treated patients)	Feasibility	Major complication rate	Minor complication rate	Sort of complication	Mortality
Banka et al[10]	antegrade hemoperfusion	elective PTCA	43	nr	nr	nr	nr	nr
Di Sciascio et al[39]	antegrade hemoperfusion	elective PTCA	110	nr	6.3%	6.3%	myocardial infarction (n = 2), emergency CABG (n = 2), transient complete heart block (n = 2), entry site hematoma (n = 5)	1.8%
Lehmann et al[9]	antegrade hemoperfusion	elective PTCA	15	nr	nr	nr	nr	nr
Muhlestein et al[6]	autoperfusion	elective PTCA	62	nr	4.8%	nr	emergency CABG (n = 3)	0%
Pavlides et al[15]	percutaneous cardiopulmonary bypass	elective PTCA	20	100%	10%	nr	bleeding (n = 2)	0%
Vogel et al[2]	percutaneous cardiopulmonary bypass	high risk PTCA	105	100%	40%	nr	injury of femoral vessels (n = 30), superior mesenteric embolism (n = 2), myocardial infarction (n = 7)	7.6%
Feld et al[7]	percutaneous cardiopulmonary bypass	high risk PTCA	56	100%	7.1%	3.6%	myocardial infarction (n = 1), emergency CABG (n = 3), bleeding (n = 1), nerve injury (n = 1)	0%

nd = not determined; na = not applicable; nr = not reported; PTCA = percutaneous transluminal coronary angiopmlEty; SRP = coronary venous retroperfusion; CABG = coronary artery bypass grafting; EF = ejection fraction.

retroinfuse the ischemic zone in most patients with stenosis of the left anterior descending artery.[4] During percutaneous angioplasty of the circumflex artery, however, selective synchronized suction and retroinfusion of coronary veins (SSR) might be less effective than synchronized coronary venous retroperfusion (SRP) if more than one vein is draining the ischemic zone. This is the case in approximately 25% of humans.[41] Furthermore, long term application of selective synchronized suction and retroinfusion of coronary veins (SSR) might be more difficult than synchronized coronary venous retroperfusion (SRP) since the sucked blood must be reinfused or replaced. Reinfusion of the blood and the use of synthetic oxygen carriers for selective synchronized suction and retroinfusion of coronary veins (SSR) are currently under investigation. For the reasons mentioned above, selective synchronized suction and retroinfusion of coronary veins (SSR) and synchronized coronary venous retroperfusion (SRP) do not exclude each other. In contrast, a retroinfusion device allowing one to perform either selective synchronized suction and retroinfusion of coronary veins (SSR) or synchronized coronary venous retroperfusion (SRP) should provide the highest flexibility for retrograde support of percutaneous coronary angioplasty with normal duration and prolonged ischemia as well as in high risk and in failed angioplasty.

In addition to myocardial protection against ischemia during angioplasty or related procedures, coronary venous retroinfusion might help to detect chronic regional myocardial dysfunction (hybernating myocardium).[42] Furthermore, as has been demonstrated in animal models,[43,44] coronary venous retroinfusion may be a unique approach to deliver drugs into ischemic myocardium which cannot be reached by arterial perfusion. Particularly with regard to substances directed against reperfusion injury, coronary venous retroinfusion may offer the opportunity to deliver these substances before injury by arterial reperfusion occurs.

Summary

In this short review, three different concepts of coronary venous retroinfusion—pressure controlled intermittent cornary sinus occlusion (PICSO), coronary venous retroperfusion (SRP) and selective synchronized suction and retroinfusion of coronary veins (SSR)—are elucidated with regard to their application in interventional cardiology. The efficacy of these three systems to protect against the sequelae of ischemia are compared on the basis of recent experimental data. The potential implications for the clinical use of coronary venous retroinfusion devices are discussed. Furthermore, the results from the first clinical studies with the use of synchronized coronary venous retroperfusion (SRP) during elective and high risk PTCA are compared to results from clinical studies using antegrade transcatheter coronary perfusion or whole heart assist devices. In a retrospective analysis, the efficacy, complications and limitations of the different support devices are briefly summarized. The definitive role, however, of coronary venous retroinfusion as well as of other regional or whole heart support devices for prevention of ischemic sequelae in patients undergoing interventional procedure in cardiology still needs to be clarified and awaits comparative studies between these support devices.

References

1. Lincoff MA, Popma JJ, Ellis SG et al. Percutaneous support devices for high risk or complicated coronary angioplasty. J Am Coll Cardiol 1991; 17:770-780.
2. Vogel RA, Shawl F, Tommaso C et al. Initial report of the national registry of elective cardiopulmonary bypass supported coronary angioplasty. J Am Coll Cardiol 1990; 15:23-29.
3. Constantini C, Sampaolesi A, Serra CM et al. Coronary venous retroperfusion support during high risk angioplasty in patients with unstable angina: Preliminary experience. J Am Coll Cardiol 1991; 18:283-292.
4. Kar S, Drury JK, Hajduczki I et al. Synchronized coronary venous retroperfusion for support and salvage of ischemic myocardium during elective and failed angioplasty. J Am Coll Cardiol 1991; 18:271-282.

5. Gacioch GM, Ellis SG, Lee L et al. Cardiogenic shock complicating acute myocardial infarction: The use of coronary angioplasty and the integration of new support devices into patient mangement. J Am Coll Cardiol 1992; 19:647-653.

6. Muhlestein JB, Quigley PJ, Ohman EM et al. Prospective analysis of possible myocardial damage of prolonged autoperfusion angioplasty in humans. J Am Coll Cardiol 1992; 20:594-598.

7. Feld H, Herz I, Fried G et al. Cardiopulmonal support increases morbility and mortality in high-risk coronary angioplasty. Am J Cardiol 1991; 68:790-792.

8. Stark KS, Satler LF, Krucoff MW et al. Myocaridal salvage after failed coronary angioplasty. Am Heart J 1990; 15:78-82.

9. Lehmann KG, Atwood JE, Syder E et al. Autologous blood perfusion for myocardial protection during coronary angioplasty: A feasibility study. Circulation 1987; 76:312-232.

10. Banka VS, Trivedi A, Patel R et al. Prevention of myocardial ischemia during coronary angioplasty: A simple new method for distal antegrade arterial blood perfusion. Am Heart J 1989; 118:830-836.

11. Cleman M, Jaffee CC, Wohlgelernter D. Prevention of ischemia during percutaneous transluminal coronary by transcatheter infusion of Fluosol DA 20%. Circulation 1986; 74:555-561.

12. Jaffe CC, Wohlgelernter D, Cabin H et al. Preservation of left ventricular ejection fraction during percutaneous transluminal coronary by distal transcatheter coronary perfusion of oxygenated Fluosol DA 20%. Am Heart J 1988; 155:1156-1163.

13. Forman MB, Perry JM, Wilson BH et al. Demonstration of myocardial reperfusion injury in humans: Results of a pilot study utilizing acute coronary angioplasty with perfluorchemical in anterior myocardial infarction. J Am Coll Cardiol 1991; 18:911-918.

14. Kent KM, Cleman MW, Cowley MJ et al. Reduction of myocardial ischemia during percutaneous transluminal coronary with oxygenated Fluosol. Am J Cardiol 1990; 66:279-284.

15. Pavlides GS, Hauser AM, Stack RK et al. Effect of peripheral cardiopulmonary bypass on left ventricular size, afterload and myocardial function during elective supported coronary angioplasty. J Am Coll Cardiol 1991; 18:499-505.

16. Nienaber CA, Rehders TC, Abend M et al. Synchronisierte koronarvenöse Retroperfusion: Ischämieprotektion bei Koronarangioplastie (PTCA). Z Kardiol 1992; 81:645-655.

17. Meerbaum S, Lang TW, Osher JV et al. Diastolic retroperfusion of acutely ischemic myocardium. Am J Cardiol 1976; 37:588-598.

18. Drury JK, Yamazaki S, Fishbein MC et al. Synchronized diastolic coronary venous retroperfusion: Results of a preclinical safety and efficacy study. J Am Coll Cardiol 1985; 6:328-335.

19. O'Byrne GT, Nienaber CA, Miyazaki A et al. Positron emission tomography demonstrates that coronary sinus retroperfusion can restore regional myocaridal perfusion and preserve metabolism. J Am Coll Cardiol 1991; 18:257-270.

20. Mohl W, Glogar DH, Mayr H et al. Reduction of infarct size induced by pressure-controlled intermittent coronary sinus occlusion. Am J Cardiol 1984; 53:923-928.

21. Beyar R, Guerci AD, Halperin HR et al. Intermittent coronary sinus occlusion after coronary arterial ligation results in venous retroperfusion. Circulation Res 1989; 65:695-707.

22. Ciuffo AA, Guerci AD, Halperin H et al. Intermittent obstruction of the coronary sinus following coronary artery ligation in dogs reduces ischemic necrosis and increases myocardial perfusion. In: Mohl W, Wolner E, Glogar D, eds. The Coronary Sinus. New York: Springer 1984:454-464.

23. Boekstegers P, Diebold J, Weiss CH. Selective ecg synchronized suction and retroinfusion of coronary veins: First results of studies in acute myocardial ischaemia in dogs. Cardiovasc Res 1990; 24:456-464.

24. Boekstegers P, Peter W, v.Degenfeld G et al. Preservation of regional myocardial function and myocardial oxygen tension during actue ischemia in pigs: Comparison of selective synchronized suction and retroinfusion of coronary veins to synchronized coronary venous retroperfusion. JACC 1992; 23:459-469.

25. Guth BD, Wisneski JA, Neese RA et al. Myocardial lactate release during ischemia in swine. Circulation 1990; 81:1948-1958.

26. Jacobs AK, Simon P, Hogfeldt V. Increase in myocardial salvage by combining coronary sinus occlusion and retroperfusion. J Am Coll Cardiol 1989; 13:53A (abstr).

27. Guerci AD, Ciuffo AA, DiPaula AF et al. Intermittent coronary sinus occlusion in dogs: Reduction of infarct size 10 days after reperfusion. J Am Coll Cardiol 1987; 9:1075-1081.

28. Jacobs AK, Faxon DP, Coats WD et al. Coronary sinus occlusion: Effect on ischemic left ventricular dysfunction and reactive hyperemia. Am Heart J 1991; 121:442-449.

29. Toggart E, Nellis S, Whitesell L. Intermittent coronary sinus occlusion in swine. In: Mohl W, Wolner E, Glogar D, eds. The Coronary Sinus. New York: Springer 1984:323-327.

30. Hajduczki I, Jaffe M, Areeda J et al. Preservation of regional myocardial ultrasonic backscatter and systolic function during brief periods of ischemia by snychronized coronary venous retroperfusion. Am Heart J 1991; 122:1300-1307.

31. Zalewski A, Goldberg S, Slysh S et al. Myocardial protection via coronary sinus interventions: Superior effects of arterialization compared with intermittent occlusion. Cirulation 1985, 71:1215-1223.

32. Sjöquist PO, Duker G, Almgren O. Distribution of the collateral blood flow at the lateral border of ischmic myocardium after aucte coronary occlusion in the pig and the dog. Basic Res Cardiol 1984; 79:164-175.

33. Carlson C, Ratajczyk-Pakalska E, Cogan JJ et al. Effect of venous retroperfusion on experimental myocardial ischemia in the open chest pig. J Surg Res 1985, 38:105-12.

34. Verdouw, PD, Beatt K, Berk L et al. Does effective diastolic coronary venous retroperfusion depend on arterial-like blood pressure in the coronary sinus? Am J Cardiol 1988; 61:1148-1149.

35. Berk L, Schmeets OL, Sassen MA et al. On the time course of systolic myocardial wall thickening during coronary artery occlusion and reperfusion in the absence and presence of synchronized diastolic coronary venous retroperfusion in anesthetized pigs. In: Mohl W et al. eds. Clinics of CSI. Steinkopff, Darmstadt, 1986:277-280.

36. Jugdutt BJ, Hutchins GM, Bulkley BH et al. Myocardial infarction in the conscious dog: Three dimensional mapping of infarct, collateral flow and region at risk. Circulation 1979; 60:1141-1150.

37. Oh BH, Volpini M, Kambayashi M et al. Myocardial function and transmural blood flow during coronary venous retroperfusion in pigs. Circulation 1992; 86:1265-1279.

38. Ellis SG. Elective coronary angioplasty: Technique and complications. In: Topol EJ, ed. Textbook of Interventional Cardiology. WB Saunders Company, 1990:199-222.

39. Di Sciascio G, Angelini P, Vandormael MG et al. Reduction of ischemia with a new flow-adjustable hemoperfusion pump during coronary angioplasty. JACC, 1992; 19: 657-62.

40. V. Lüdinghausen M, Schott C. Microanatomy of the human coronary sinus and its major tributaries. In: Meerbaum S, ed. Myocardial Perfusion, Reperfusion, Coronary Venous Retroperfusion. New York: Steinkopf Darmstadt: Springer 1990: 93-122.

41. Hajduczki I, Kar S, Areeda J et al. Reversal of chronic regional myocardial dysfunction (hybernation myocardium) by synchronized diastolic coronary venous retroperfusion during coronary angioplasty. J Am Cardiol, 1990; 15:238-242.

42. Miyazaki A, Tadokoro H, Drury K et al. Retrograde coronary venous administration of recombinant tissue-type plasminogen activator: A unique and effective approach to coronary artery thrombolysis. J Am Coll Cardiol 1991; 18:613-620.

43. Kobayashi S, Tadokoro H, Wakida Y et al. Coronary venous retroinfusion of deferoxamine reduces infarct size in pigs. J Am Coll Cardiol 1991; 189:621-627.
44. Hatori H, Tadokoro H, Satomura K et al. Beneficial effects of coronary venous retroinfusion but not left atrial administration of superoxide dismutase on myocardial necrosis in pigs. European Heart J 1991; 12:442-450.

Addendum

New Developments in Coronary Venous Retroinfusion Support During Interventional Cardiology

Peter Boekstegers

Introduction

Several percutaneous support devices for coronary angioplasty have been developed with the aim to improve myocardial tolerance to ischemia, thereby increasing the safety of coronary angioplasty and allowing to expand its indications. Thus, supported coronary angioplasty has been applied in patients with high risk conditions such as main stem and main stem equivalent stenosis, severely impaired left ventricular function and myocardial infarction complicated by cardiogenic shock.[1-5] Although stent implantation has certainly reduced the incidence of unmanageable "bail-out" situations and increased the safety of high risk coronary interventions,[6-10] there are still a number of advantages which might be offered by an efficient support device in high risk patients and "bail out" situations. Preventing myocardial ischemia and hemodynamic alterations in high risk patients may help to correctly place and extend a stent without the otherwise imminent risk of the patient rapidly developing cardiogenic shock during coronary occlusion. The same benefit should be offered by the support device in case of "bail out" situations with interruption of blood flow where it is difficult or even not possible to place a stent. Finally, if the "bail out" situation cannot be resolved, a continued regional support against myocardial ischemia using retroinfusion should be able to at least prevent the development of myocardial infarction.[1,11]

Three main approaches have been chosen for support of acutely ischemic myocardium during coronary angioplasty: antegrade perfusion, whole heart support devices and retroinfusion of coronary veins. Antegrade techniques may provide regional support of the ischemic myocardium through the balloon catheter, i.e., autoperfusion[12] or pumping of either autologous blood[13,14] or oxygen carriers.[15-18] Regional myocardial protection, however, is not ensured until the stenotic lesion has been passed. Thus, antegrade techniques are difficult to apply in patients with tortuous vessels and in patients with unstable hemodynamic conditions. Furthermore, during all procedures of stent implantation, the perfusion catheter has to be removed at least temporarily thereby interrupting regional protection against ischemia in the most critical situation. Hence, in the era of stent implantation perfusion balloons have been omitted for two reasons:

1. longer balloon inflations in case of large dissections are not necessary if a stent can be placed correctly;
2. perfusion catheters may hamper and delay stent implantation.

Support of the whole heart independent from the stenotic lesion is possible using cardiopulmonary bypass,[2,19] intraaortic balloon counterpulsation[1] and left ventricular assist devices.[5] Though hemodynamics may be preserved using these techniques,[2,5,19] regional myocardial ischemia persists during coronary angioplasty and particularly in the case of an unmanageable "bail out" situation. A major drawback of cardiopulmonary bypass in high risk interventions is the high incidence of vascular complications increasing morbidity and mortality in these patients.[20]

The third approach for myocardial protection is through the "backdoor" of the heart by retroinfusion of coronary veins. Retrograde techniques combine regional support of ischemic myocardium with an application being independent of the passage of the stenotic lesion. Thus, prophylactic installation of the retroinfusion support device as well as a continuous support during stent implantation and in case of unmanageable "bail out" situation is possible. Furthermore, retroinfusion techniques have the advantage of being less invasive than whole heart support devices. The efficacy and feasibility of previous retroinfusion devices, however, may have limited their clinical application.

Therefore, this review first discusses experimental data providing a pathophysiological basis for the development of a more selective and efficacious retroinfusion device. Secondly, recent clinical studies using selective suction and pressure-regulated retroinfusion are compared to previous retroinfusion devices in terms of efficacy and feasibility.

The Concept of Selective Suction and Pressure-Regulated Retroinfusion

The potential of retroinfusion of coronary veins to protect acutely ischemic myocardium is dependent on the individual venous anatomy, in particular with regard to the venous capacity, arteriovenous and venovenous shunts or Thebesian veins.[21,22] Moreover, the heterogeneity of the venous systems implies that efficient nutritive blood flow by retroinfusion may occur at different flow rates and venous pressures. Using high retroinfusion flow rates and pressures may be potentially harmful[23,24] and may hamper myocardial function,[25] whereas insufficient retroinfusion flow rates will reduce the efficacy of myocardial protection.[25] In studies using nonpulsatile retrograde blood flow of the anterior interventricular vein with simultaneous venting of the left anterior descending artery, a system, which is not applicable clinically, efficacy of retroperfusion increased with increasing flow but reached a plateau at different flow rates depending on the coronary venous system.[25] However, retrograde flow rates at least twice as high as normal arterial flow were necessary to obtain the highest efficacy and were associated with the formation of myocardial edema.[25] Moreover, pressure-flow relationships were not uniform and resulted in different degrees of retroperfusion efficacy in each animal at different venous pressures. These findings suggest that adaptation of retroinfusion flow to the individual coronary venous system should improve both safety and efficacy.

The first technique of retroinfusion which in part took into account the individual venous anatomy and coronary venous filling capacity was pressure-controlled intermittent coronary sinus occlusion (PICSO) (Fig. A14.1).[26] PICSO was based on the concept that increasing coronary venous pressure by intermittent occlusion of the coronary sinus results in venous retroinfusion predominantly of the ischemic myocardium. Indeed there is experimental and clinical evidence that PICSO provides alternating venous blood flow in the ischemic region[27] and enhances washout of metabolites accumulating during ischemia.[28] Early in 1984 Mohl et al realized that the systolic coronary venous occlusion pressure (SCVOP) is an indicator of venous filling capacity. Therefore, by using certain algorithms for PICSO the blocking balloon in the coronary sinus was deflated if the plateau of SCVOP was reached in order to optimize retrograde venous flow into the ischemic region and at the same time to avoid impairment of arterial blood flow in nonischemic regions. Though PICSO was able to reduce infarct size,[26] its efficacy was not high enough to preserve regional myocardial function in case of acute ischemia.

The idea of providing retrograde arterial blood flow and, thus, to improve efficacy was realized already in 1976 by synchronized coronary venous retroperfusion (SRP) with diastolic retroperfusion and systolic drainage of the venous system.[29] Although the retrograde delivery of arterial blood improved efficacy to a certain degree, major limitations of the SRP system were given by the necessity of venous drainage around the deflated catheter balloon lying in the coronary sinus (Fig. A14.1). Thus, catheterization was restricted to cardiac veins of sufficient size such as the coronary sinus or the beginning of the great cardiac vein. In addition to the nonselective approach of SRP, neither the experimental nor the clinical studies using SRP took into consideration the individual venous anatomy and pressure/flow relationships.

In order to overcome the above mentioned drawbacks of previous retroinfusion systems, selective suction and retroinfusion (SSR) was developed in 1990.[11] The basic concept was

1. to approach as near as possible to the ischemic myocardium by selective catheterization of the vein draining the ischemic region (i.e., the anterior ventricular vein in case of an LAD stenosis)
2. to reduce coronary venous pressure and residual filling of the veins by an ECG-synchronized suction device combining adequate venous drainage—despite a constantly inflated balloon at the tip of the retroinfusion catheter—with retroinfusion into an empty venous system thereby increasing the probability to reach the microcirculation.

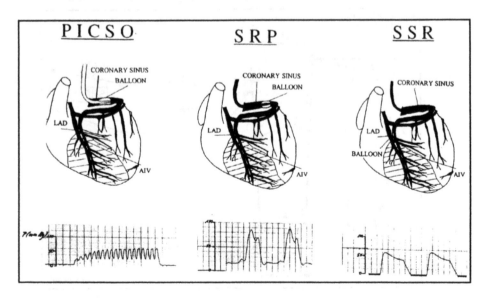

Fig. A14.1. Comparative schemes of the three concepts of coronary venous retroinfusion with particular regard to the site of regional support (position of the catheter balloon). Typical recordings of coronary venous pressure (P) from each system during treatment in pigs are shown. PICSO = pressure controlled intermittent coronary sinus occlusion, SRP = synchronized coronary venous retroperfusion, SSR = selective ECG-synchronized suction and retroinfusion of coronary veins.

Indeed, selective suction and retroinfusion was able to substantially increase the efficacy which was demonstrated by direct comparison of SSR with SRP in a pig model.[23] In contrast to SRP, SSR preserved 70% of regional myocardial function after 1 min of ischemia and 51% after 10 min of ischemia (Fig. A14.2).

The next important step in the development of the SSR system was its adaptation to the individual venous system by introducing pressure regulation of retroinfusion (Fig. A14.3). Previous devices for retroinfusion including SSR[3,4,11,23] did not allow control of retroinfusion flow during each pumping period with the consequence of unpredictable peak pressures and pressure kinetics. However, if retroinfusion flow can be adjusted to a certain venous pressure during treatment of acute ischemia, the optimal retroinfusion pressure should be determined before treatment for efficacy and safety reasons. During normal antegrade blood flow, coronary venous occlusion pressure reflects differences in capacity and anatomy of individual coronary venous systems.[31,32] At the systolic and diastolic plateau of venous occlusion, additional blood entering the occluded venous system is shunted to the systemic circulation.[31] We therefore hypothesized, that the individually different venous occlusion pressure obtained before ischemia may indicate the coronary venous pressure, at which blood is shunted to the systemic circulation also during retroinfusion of a balloon occluded vein. Hence, increasing retroinfusion flow and venous pressure above the previously determined venous occlusion pressure should not result in a higher nutritive blood flow but only a higher proportion of retrograde blood flow shunted to the systemic circulation. In order to test this hypothesis, in a pig model coronary venous occlusion pressure determined before ischemia was compared to the retroinfusion pressure with the highest efficacy during ischemia using a newly developed pressure-regulated SSR system ("Myoprotect", Pro-Med, Austria).

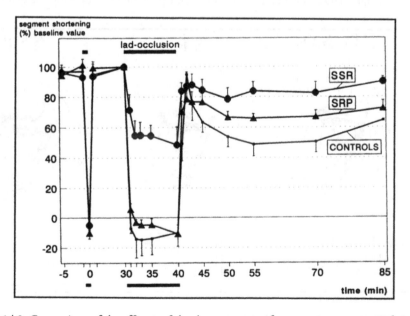

Fig. A14.2. Comparison of the efficacy of the three concepts of coronary venous retroinfusion to preserve regional myocardial function in pigs (results according to 24). Black bars indicating occlusion of the left anterior descending artery (LAD). First LAD-occlusion (1 min) without treatment in all pigs. Second LAD-occlusion (10 min) a) with treatment by selective ECG-synchronized suction and retroinfusion of coronary veins (SSR, n = 10) c) without treatment (CONTROLS, n = 10).

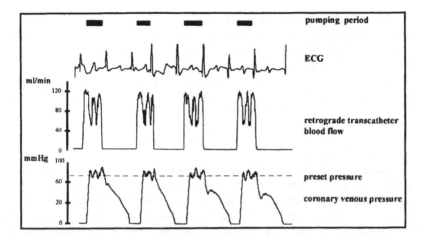

Fig. A14.3. Development of the SSR system. Adaptation to the individual venous system by introducing pressure regulation of retroinfusion.

In this experimental study it was demonstrated that preservation of regional myocardial function during ischemia supported by selective suction and pressure-regulated retroinfusion stepwise increased with retroinfusion pressure unless the individual systolic coronary venous occlusion pressure determined before ischemia was exceeded by more than 20 mm Hg. The individual systolic venous occlusion pressure was related linearly (r=0.89) to the maximal preservation of regional myocardial function. As a consequence the individual systolic coronary venous occlusion pressure (SCVOP) determined before ischemia can be used as an estimate for the optimal retroinfusion pressure and for the efficacy of selective suction and pressure-regulated retroinfusion during ischemia. Furthermore, it was shown that pressure-regulation of the SSR-system was able to deliver arterial blood at a preset retroinfusion pressure with an acceptable accuracy.

Finally, the concept of selective suction and pressure-regulated retroinfusion was supported further by an experimental study showing selectivity of drug delivery.[33] Targeting of dobutamine by SSR in low concentrations to the ischemic myocardium (LAD region) thereby increasing regional myocardial function was possible without affecting the nonischemic myocardium (circumflex region) and without systemic effects.

Clinical Efficacy and Feasibility of Selective Suction and Pressure-Regulated Retroinfusion

In a clinical pilot study in 52 patients, selective suction and pressure-regulated retroinfusion was analyzed in terms of safety, feasibility and efficacy.[34]

Considering feasibility, an overall high success rate of 95% was observed for correct placement of the retroinfusion catheter in the anterior interventricular vein at the corresponding side of the proximal stenosis of the left anterior descending artery. In contrast to previous studies,[3,4,35,36] the femoral approach[37] was used for the catheterization of the coronary sinus and final placement of the retroinfusion catheter in the anterior interventricular vein. No complications related to the application of selective suction and pressure-regulated retroinfusion occurred and the system was safe at least during short term treatment (10 min). Though in the present study peak and mean coronary venous pressures were higher than reported in previous retroperfusion studies,[3,4] there was no evidence for coronary venous damage. Thus, selective suction and pressure-regulated retroinfusion aiming to achieve systolic coronary venous occlusion pressures determined before ischemia (mean 51 mm Hg) do not appear to be associated with a higher risk of inducing damage to the coronary venous system or ischemic myocardium.[24]

Though the preset coronary venous pressures during retroinfusion were not reached in all patients due to the limited retrograde transcatheter blood flow of the initial device, regional myocardial function was preserved at approximately 75% of baseline value during supported ischemia (Fig. A14.4). Thus, selective suction and pressure-regulated retroinfusion (SSR) substantially increased efficacy if compared to previous retroinfusion devices such as SRP in similar clinical studies.[3,4]

The reduction of ischemia leading to preservation of regional myocardial function during retroinfusion supported balloon inflations was consistent with the reduction of ST segment changes as well as semiquantitative angina score. A linear relationship (r=0.73, p=0.002) between individual systolic plateau of coronary venous occlusion pressure determined before ischemia and the preservation of regional myocardial function (% of baseline, centerline method) during ischemia supported by retroinfusion was observed, which is in agreement with experimental data.[38]

From all parameters used for assessment of regional myocardial protection during retroinfusion, we infer that ischemia was not completely prevented in all patients with the limited retrograde flow rates of the retroinfusion catheters used in this study. It was an important finding, however, that similar efficacy to preserve regional myocardial function was obtained in high risk patients and that during prolonged balloon inflations of up to 10 min this effect of retroinfusion was maintained (Fig. A14.4).

The observed effects of selective suction and pressure-regulated retroinfusion on regional myocardial function were associated with a stabilization of hemodynamics during ischemia although a slight decrease of mean arterial blood pressure was not completely prevented in normal and in high risk patients. It was a consistent finding in the small group patients supported by retroinfusion and selective application of low dose dobutamine, however, that mean arterial blood pressure remained unchanged even if ischemia was prolonged to 120 sec. Since we did

Fig. A14.4. Regional myocardial function with and without SSR in 31 patients [results according to ref. 34].

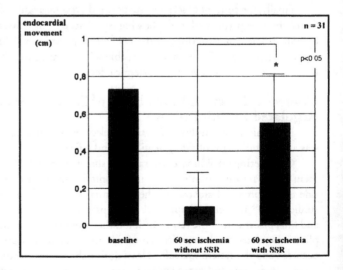

not observe any undesired systemic effects (e.g., heart rate did not change) or regional effects using selective dobutamine administration in combination with arterial retroinfusion, it seems to be a promising approach particularly in high risk patients.

The concept of preventing severe ischemia and hemodynamic alterations by selective suction and pressure-regulated retroinfusion in patients with high risk coronary interventions in combination with stent placement was associated with a high primary success rate and an excellent clinical outcome in this first clinical study. These preliminary data, however, from a small group of selected high risk patients do not indicate whether the high success rate was due to the application of retroinfusion or due to stent placement.

A major limitation of retroinfusion support during myocardial ischemia is its limited efficacy in case of circulatory standstill. Although the system of selective suction and pressure-regulated retroinfusion may operate in an untriggered mode and might prevent myocardial infarction hemodynamic support is not provided during circulatory standstill. Hence, selective suction and pressure-regulated retroinfusion might prevent regional ischemia and the development of cardiogenic shock in high risk patients. However, other support devices such as the cardiopulmonary bypass or the hemopump[5] have to be considered in the rare but difficult situation of circulatory standstill without immediate successful resuscitation.

The application of selective suction and pressure-regulated retroinfusion during high risk coronary interventions is now being studied in a recently initiated randomized multicenter trial in patients with main stem and main stem equivalent stenosis and high risk for bypass surgery.

References

1. Mohl W, Wolner E, Glogar D, eds. The Coronary Sinus. Darmstadt: Steinkopff Verlag, 1984.
2. Meerbaum S. Coronary venous retroperfusion delivery of treatment to ischemic myocardium. Herz 1986; 11:41-54.
3. Corday E, Meerbaum S, Drury JK. The coronary sinus: An alternate channel for administration of arterial blood and pharmacologic agents for protection and treatment of acute cardiac ischemia. J Am Col Cardiol 1986; 7:711-714.
4. Mohl W, Faxon DP, Wolner E, eds. Clinics of CSI. Darmstadt: Steinkopff Verlag, 1986.
5. Faxon DP, Jacobs AK. Coronary sinus retroperfusion and intermittent occlusion. In: Topol EJ, ed. Acute Coronary Intervention. New York: Alan Liss 1988:255-269.
6. Colombo A, Goldberg SL, Almagor Y et al. A novel strategy for stent deployment in the treatment of acute or threatened closure complicating balloon coronary angioplasty. J Am Coll Cardiol 1993; 22:1887-1891.
7. Schömig A, Kastrati A, Mudra H et al. Four-year experience with Palmaz-Schatz Stenting in coronary angioplasty complicated by dissection with threatened or present vessel closure. Circulation 1994; 90:2716-2724.
8. George BS, Voorhess III WD, Roubin GS et al. Multicenter investigation of coronary stenting to treat acute or threatened closure after percutaneous transluminal angioplasty: Clinical and angiographic outcomes. J Am Coll Cardiol 1993; 22:135-143.
9. Serruys PW, Keane D. The bailout stent: Is a friend in need always a friend indeed? Circulation 1993; 88:2455-2457.
10. Ruygrok PN, Serruys PW. Intracoronary stenting. From concept to custom. Circulation 1996; 94:882-890.
11. Boekstegers P, Diebold J, Weiss C. Selective ECG synchronized suction and retroinfusion of coronary veins: First results of studies in acute myocardial ischaemia in dogs. Cardiovasc Res 1990; 24:456-464.
12. Haendchen RV, Corday E. Coronary sinus interventions for reduction of myocardial ischemia. In: Kulick DL, Rahmintoola SH, eds. Techniques and Applications in Interventional Cardiology. New York: Mosby Year Book, 1991.

13. Corday E, Haendchen R. Introduction. In: Seminar on Coronary Venous Delivery Systems for Support and Salvage of Jeopardized Ischemic Myocardium. J Am Coll Cardio 1991; 18 (No. 1):253-256.
14. Beck CS. Revascularization of the heart. Surgery 1949; 26:82-88.
15. Gensini GG, DiGiorgi S, Murad-Nettor S. Coronary venous occluded pressure. Arch Surg 1963; 86:72-80.
16. Gensini GG, DiGiorgi S, Murad S et al. Percutaneous retrograde venous perfusion of the myocardium (Abstract #22). 1962; 6th Scientific Session of the American College of Cardiology.
17. Meerbaum S, Lang TW, Osher J et al. Coronary venous retroperfusion treatment of jeopardized myocardium. (Abstract P1.67).
18. Meerbaum S, Lang TW, Osher JV et al. Diastolic retroperfusion of acutely ischemic myocardium. Am J Cardiol 1976; 37:588-598.
19. Markov AK, Lehan PH, Hellems HK. Reversal of acute myocardial ischemia in closed chest animals by retrograde perfusion of the coronary sinus with arterial blood. Acta Cardiol 1976; 31:185-190.
20. Jacobs AK, Faxon DP. Retroperfusion and PTCA. In: Topol EJ, ed. Textbook of Interventional Cardiology. New York: WB Saunders Co, 1990:477-495.
21. von Lüdinghausen M, Schott C. Microanatomy of the human coronary sinus and its major tributaries. In Meerbaum S (ed): Myocardial perfusion, reperfusion, coronary venous retroperfusion. Steinkopff, Darmstadt, Springer, New York, 1990; 93-122.
22. Verdouw PD, Wolffenbuttel BH, van der Giessen WJ. Domestic pigs in the study of myocardial ischemia. Eur Heart J 1983; 4 Suppl C:61-67.
23. Boekstegers P, Peter W, von Degenfeld G et al. Preservation of regional myocardial function and myocardial oxygen tension during acute ischemia in pigs: Comparison of selective synchronized suction and retroinfusion of coronary veins to synchronized coronary venous retroperfusion. J Am Coll Cardiol 1994; 23:459-469.
24. Boekstegers P, Peter W, Werdan K et al. Letter to the editor. J Am Coll Cardiol 1994; 24:578-581.
25. Oh BH, Volpini M, Kambayashi M et al. Myocardial function and transmural blood flow during coronary venous retroperfusion in pigs. Circulation 1992; 86:1265-1279.
26. Gundry SR. Modification of myocardial ischemia in normal and hypertrophied hearts, utilizing diastolic retroperfusion of the coronary vein. J Thor Cardiovasc Surg 1982; 83:659.
27. Hatori N, Utiuda Y, Isozima K et al. Short term treatment with synchronized coronary venous retroperfusion before full reperfusion significantly reduces myocardial infarct size. Am Heart J 1992; 123:1166-1174.
28. Yamazaki S, Drury JK Meerbaum S et al. Synchronized coronary venous retroperfusion: Prompt improvement of left ventricular function in experimental myocardial ischemia. J Am Coll Cardiol 1985; 5:655-663/
29. Berdeaux A, Farcot JC, Boudarias JP et al. Effects of diastolic synchronized retroperfusion on regional coronary blood flow in experimental myocardial ischemia. Am J Cardiol 1981; 417:L033-L040.
30. Meerbaum S. Coronary venous retroperfusion delivery of treatment to ischemic myocardium. Herz 1986; 11:41-54.
31. Meesmann M, Karagueuzian HS, Ino T et al. Selective perfusion of ischemic myocardium during coronary venous retroinjection: A study of the causative role of venoarterial and venoventricular pressure gradients. J Am Coll Cardiol 1987; 10:887-897.
32. Mohl W, Punzengruber C, Moser M et al. Effects of pressure-controlled intermittent coronary sinus occlusion on regional ischemic myocardial function. J Am Coll Cardiol 1985; 5:939-947.
33. von Degenfeld G, Giehrl W, Boekstegers P. Targeting of dobutamine to ischemic myocardium without systemic effects by selective suction and pressure-regulated retroinfusion. Cardiovasc Res 1997; 35:233-240.

34. Boekstegers P, von Degenfeld G, Giehrl W et al. Selective Suction and Pressure-regulated Retroinfusion: an Effective and Safe Approach to Retrograde Protection against Myocardial Ischemia in Patients undergoing Normal and High Risk Percutaneous Transluminal Coronary Angioplasty. JACC 1998 (in press).

35. Freedman RJ, Lasorda DM, O'Neill WW. Combined intraaortic balloon counterpulsation with synchronized coronary venous retroperfusion: the united states experience. J Cathet Cardiovasc Diag 1994; 33:362-367.

36. Barnett JC, Freedman RJ, Touchon RC et al. Coronary venous retroperfusion of autologous arterial blood for the treatment of acute myocardial ischemia in the community hospital. J Cathet Cardiovasc Diag 1993; 28:206-213.

37. Nitsch J. Femoral vein approach to the coronary sinus during electrophysiology studies. Am J Cardiol 1995; 75:651.

38. Giehrl W, von Degenfeld G, Boekstegers P. Die druckgesteuerte selektive Retroinfusion von Koronarvenen (SSR) erlaubt die Anpassung des Retroinfusionsdruckes an das individuelle Koronarvenensystem zur Optimierung der Myokardprotektion während koronarer Ischämie. Z Kardiol 1996; 85:169.

Index

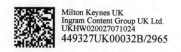

9 780367 447342